SECOND EDITION

POLICY AND POLITICS

for Nurses
and Other Health Professionals

ADVOCACY AND ACTION

Donna M. Nickitas, PhD, RN, NEA-BC, CNE, FNAP, FAAN
Professor
Hunter College
Hunter-Bellevue School of Nursing
The City University of New York
Executive Officer, Doctor of Philosophy in Nursing Program
Graduate Center, The City University of New York
New York, New York
Editor
Nursing Economic$, The Journal for Health Care Leaders
Pitman, New Jersey

Donna J. Middaugh, PhD, RN
Associate Dean for Academic Programs
College of Nursing
University of Arkansas for Medical Sciences
Little Rock, Arkansas

Nancy Aries, PhD
Professor of Social Policy
School of Public Affairs
Director of Baruch Honors Program
The City University of New York
Baruch College
New York, New York

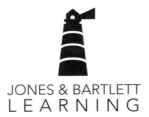

JONES & BARTLETT
LEARNING

World Headquarters
Jones & Bartlett Learning
5 Wall Street
Burlington, MA 01803
978-443-5000
info@jblearning.com
www.jblearning.com

Jones & Bartlett Learning books and products are available through most bookstores and online booksellers. To contact Jones & Bartlett Learning directly, call 800-832-0034, fax 978-443-8000, or visit our website, www.jblearning.com.

Substantial discounts on bulk quantities of Jones & Bartlett Learning publications are available to corporations, professional associations, and other qualified organizations. For details and specific discount information, contact the special sales department at Jones & Bartlett Learning via the above contact information or send an email to specialsales@jblearning.com.

03248-2

Production Credits
VP, Executive Publisher: David Cella
Executive Editor: Amanda Martin
Associate Acquisitions Editor: Rebecca Myrick
Production Editor: Amanda Clerkin
Senior Marketing Manager: Jennifer Stiles
Art Development Editor: Joanna Lundeen
Art Development Assistant: Shannon Sheehan
VP, Manufacturing and Inventory Control: Therese Connell

Composition: Cenveo Publisher Services
Cover Design: Kristin E. Parker
Manager of Photo Research, Rights & Permissions: Lauren Miller
Cover Image: © PinnacleAnimates/ShutterStock, Inc.
Printing and Binding: Edwards Brothers Malloy
Cover Printing: Edwards Brothers Malloy

Library of Congress Cataloging-in-Publication Data
Policy and politics for nurses and other health professionals : advocacy and action / edited by Donna M. Nickitas, Donna J. Middaugh, and Nancy Aries. — Second edition.
    p. ; cm.
Includes bibliographical references and index.
ISBN 978-1-284-05329-6
I. Nickitas, Donna M., editor. II. Middaugh, Donna J., editor. III. Aries, Nancy, editor.
[DNLM: 1. Health Policy—United States. 2. Health Care Costs—United States. 3. Lobbying—United States. 4. Policy Making—United States. WA 540 AA1]
RA395.A3
362.10973—dc23
                                                                                                                    2014019231
6048

Printed in the United States of America
18 17 16 15   10 9 8 7 6 5 4 3 2

Dedication

Donna Nickitas

To my husband, Michael and my children Nick, Kate, and Jon-Philip, who allowed me to model the importance of self –advocacy, so that I could teach and model the way for others. Your love and encouragement has made all the difference and for that I am grateful. Also, I dedicate this book, in the memory of my sister, Grace M. Shanahan, a librarian, who taught me the importance of reading, and that readers are leaders!

Nancy Aries

To the memory of my father, Leon J. Aries, a surgeon, who taught me that caring for one's patients was the fundamental job of all health professionals, and my mother, Marie L. Aries, whose organizational and political insights suggested how this might be done.

Donna J. Middaugh

To my husband Robert and our son Robert Guy, who have awakened my soul and are my inspiration in everything I do. They have taught me to love unconditionally, enjoy life, live with purpose, and to strive for excellence. Robert Guy: you will be such a compassionate, dedicated nurse! I could not be more proud! Also, to the memory of my mother, Alpha Duff, a teacher, who taught me to never stop learning.

Contents

Chapter 6
Physicians: From Solo Practitioners to Team Leaders... 113
Nancy Aries and Barbara Caress

Chapter 7
Healthcare Quality.. 137
Donna Middaugh

Section 4
Healthcare Providers: Understanding How Power, Markets, and Government Impact Organization and Delivery of Care

Chapter 13
Private Health Insurance Market 261
Joyce A. Hahn and Brenda Helen Sheingold

Chapter 14
Medicare: From Protector to Innovator 279
Lucas Pauls

Chapter 15
Medicaid and the Financing of Care for Vulnerable Populations:
A Story of Misconceptions..299
Barbara Caress and Nancy Aries

Preface

Numerous texts describe the healthcare delivery system in the United States or explain how politics and policy making influence the organization of healthcare delivery. Why are we committed to a second edition of our text when other texts purport to address many of the same questions? Our answer is both simple and complex.

Simply put, we believe that many of these texts fail to address the reality of health care as experienced by nurses and other healthcare practitioners. Often, the students and practitioners with whom we work are totally absorbed in the day-to-day demands of their jobs and fail to recognize how policy shapes and influences their clinical practice. They work hard just to keep up with the needs of patients and their families, physicians, and administrators. Many describe themselves as running up a down escalator that speeds up every time they think they might make some forward progress. One consequence of this consuming daily struggle is that there is no time to step back and reflect on the larger institutional, social, political, and economic forces that impact their profession and the healthcare industry at large. This text is intended to provide an understanding of health policy, public policy, and social policy so our students can be conversant with the politics and economics that generate the rules of the game under which they work with such skill and dedication.

The more complex answer is that our students often recognize that the healthcare settings that employ them (hospitals, nursing homes, community-based agencies, ambulatory clinics, and schools) are under severe regulatory and financial pressure and that they, as frontline workers, often bear the brunt of complying with the demands of internal and external forces. When their units or organizations are understaffed and the demand for productivity is increased, nurses and other health professionals must be better equipped at identifying, acknowledging, and managing the larger institutional, social, political, and economic forces that impact their profession and productivity. Our commitment in writing this text is further based on our belief that healthcare professionals can no longer be prepared solely for clinical practice. They must ready themselves to be engaged in the economic, political, and policy debates in the field. They must stand ready to inform, educate, and advocate to leaders at their own institutions and other stakeholders—including the federal, state, and local government, insurance companies, health suppliers (such as the pharmaceutical industry)—about health policy, planning, and management.

To be engaged they need to know exactly how health policy and public policy are connected to the care and treatment of patients. In this text we put the opportunities and constraints that confront our profession in a larger perspective. Policy making is an interactive process. In some instances, government dictates the response of providers. In other cases, providers dictate the response of government. Then there is the business sector—insurance companies, public health organizations, professional associations, and advocacy groups. Each one is trying to be heard and push the system to be more responsive to its needs and the needs of its constituents. In this text we recognize that practitioners can play a similar role in this process.

By developing a more nuanced understanding of the ways policy shapes how the healthcare system is organized, we hope to provide those working in healthcare delivery with the tools they need to influence these decisions. For nurses in particular, obtaining a seat at the table has not always been easy. They have had less influence on the organization and delivery of health care than some of the other constituencies previously mentioned. We believe that nurses must have increased influence and equity compared to other important decision makers or revenue generators on national issues relating to influencing healthcare

reform. However, the lessons from this text are addressed to all healthcare professionals because together with nurses they have insights that are not otherwise represented. Given their role as caregivers, nurses bring a unique perspective to policy making concerns. Our hope is that in the not-so-distant future nurses and other healthcare professionals will assume their rightful place at the table and speak with equal voice and influence.

The ideas presented in this text offer our combined thoughts about the ways nursing and other healthcare professionals who are interested in improving healthcare systems and services in local, regional, national, and global communities can be involved in healthcare advocacy and action. This text offers an interdisciplinary approach to understanding health care, health finance, health professionals, and health policy. We have sought contributions from a group of diverse experts who recognize the internal and external forces influencing health care in America. Our rationale for seeking a transdisciplinary approach is the understanding that no one individual or discipline has a comprehensive understanding of the challenges and complexities confronting the healthcare system and the potential for healthcare reform. These challenges include, but are not limited to, increasing access to care and improving quality by such actions as reducing medical errors, promoting health and wellness, and improving efficiency and reducing costs.

As the nation explores ways to reform the healthcare system, health professionals recognize that our healthcare system is broken and needs a complete, comprehensive reform to assure that future generations may enjoy a delivery system that will ensure their health and well-being. As this text goes to press, the first major reform since the passage of Medicare and Medicaid will take effect. Starting in January 2014 uninsured people have access to statewide health insurance exchanges that have increased access to health care by making health insurance more widely available. The Affordable Care Act strives for increased quality through wellness and preventive care initiatives and holds promise of reduced costs through payment reform.

This is just a beginning. Every day, healthcare professionals will need to exercise their clinical judgment, political acumen, and leadership skills to make important and much-needed changes that further increase access to and improve the quality and affordability of health care. This text offers future healthcare practitioners and others who are committed to improving health disparities and health care equality, keen insight, and understanding that clinical practice is derived from regulations, laws, and policies that are initiated from public policy and politics. This text demonstrates that we are in a position to advocate for our professions and for the patients that we serve by making sure healthcare reform meets its intended goals. Our collective voices must and should be heard. The combination of describing the healthcare system and explaining how complex policy processes shape it and the ways nurses and other healthcare professionals can be instrumental in that process is what distinguishes this text. By more fully understanding the healthcare system and the levers for change, it becomes possible to influence the direction the system takes through advocacy and action.

Donna M. Nickitas

Donna J. Middaugh

Nancy Aries

Contributors

Danette Alexander, DNP
Nurse Director
Emergency Medical Services and Lifestar
Hartford Hospital
Hartford, Connecticut

Terri Ameri, DNP, CNE, CPN, FNP-BC
Regional Medical Director
Presbyterian Medical Services
New Mexico Health
Farmington, New Mexico

Nancy Aries, PhD
Professor of Social Policy
School of Public Affairs
Director of Baruch Honors Programs
Baruch College
The City University of New York
New York, New York

Steven Baumann, PhD, APRN-BC, RN
Professor
Hunter College
Hunter-Bellevue School of Nursing
New York, New York

Elyse Berkman, MPA
Project Manager
Private Industry
New York, New York

Claudia J. Beverley, PhD, RN, FAAN
Professor (Secondary), Department of
    Health Policy and Management
Professor
College of Nursing
Professor (Secondary)
College of Medicine
Director, Arkansas Aging Initiative, Donald
    W. Reynolds Institute on Aging

Barbara Caress
Senior Consultant
Service Employees International Union
New York, New York

Ellen Chesler
Senior Fellow
Roosevelt Institute
New York, New York

Jonathan Engel, PhD
Professor of Public Affairs
School of Public Affairs
Baruch College
New York, New York

Jeanne Gargiulo, DNP
Nurse Practitioner
Huntington Hospital
Huntington, New York

Joyce Hahn, PhD, APRN-CNS, NEA-BC, FNAP
Association Professor
School of Nursing
George Washington University
Washington, D.C.

Juliet Harris-Brown, NP, DNP

Eileen Levy, RN, PhP
Nurse Practitioner at NSLIJ
Huntington Hospital
Huntington, New York

Sandra B. Lewenson, EdD, RN, FAAN
Professor
College of Health Professions
Lienhard School of Nursing
Pleasantville, New York

Donna J. Middaugh, PhD, RN
Associate Dean
College of Nursing
University of Arkansas for Medical Sciences
Little Rock, Arkansas

Donna M. Nickitas, PhD, RN
Professor
Hunter College
Hunter-Bellevue School of Nursing
The City University of New York
Executive Officer, Doctor of Nursing
    Science Program
Graduate Center, The City University of
    New York
New York, New York
Editor
*Nursing Economic$, The Journal for Health
    Care Leaders*
Pitman, New Jersey

Kathleen Nokes, PhD, RN, APHN-BC, FAAN
Professor Emeritus
Hunter College
The CUNY Graduate Center
New York, New York

Lucas Pauls, MPT, MPA
Director of Health Fund Research and
    Planning
Building Services 32BJ Health Fund
New York, New York

Janice Phillips, MS, PhD, RN, FAAN
Director of Government and Regulatory
    Affairs
CGFNS International, Inc.
Philadelphia, Pennsylvania

Roby Robertson, PhD
Professor of Public Administration
Institute of Government
University of Arkansas at Little Rock
Little Rock, Arkansas

Franklin A. Shaffer, EdD, RN, FAAN
Chief Executive Officer
CGFNS International, Inc.
Washington, D.C.

Brenda Helen Sheingold, PhD, MBA, BSN
Assistant Professor
Director
Health Care Quality Graduate Programs
George Washington University
Washington, D.C.

Stephanie Stephens, DNP

Marie Truglio-Londrigan, PhD, RN
College of Health Professions
Lienhard School of Nursing
Pace University
Pleasantville, New York

Carol A. Tuttas, PhD, RN
CGFNS International, Inc.
Philadelphia, Pennsylvania

Ralph Vogel, PhD, RN
Clinical Assistant Professor
College of Nursing
University of Arkansas for Medical Sciences
Little Rock, Arkansas

Helen Werner, PhD, RN
Assistant Professor
Program Coordinator, Upper Division
Monroe College School of Nursing
Monroe, New York

Introduction

CHAPTER 1

Nursing's History of Advocacy and Action

Sandra B. Lewenson and Donna M. Nickitas

Overview

The American Nurses Association (ANA) reminds nurses of the social contract between nurses and the public that "reflects the profession's long-standing core values and ethics, which provide grounding for health care in society" (American Nurses Association [ANA], 2010, p. 10). The ANA *Social Policy Statement* has articulated nursing's social obligation since it was first published in 1980. Nurses turn to this document to understand how nursing fulfills this obligation by providing ethical and culturally competent care to individuals, families, communities, and populations. It also helps nurses explain their role to the larger society, to new members of the profession, and to nurses already working in the field.

This chapter explores political advocacy in light of nursing's role and responsibility to advocate for and act on behalf of those for whom nurses have contracted to provide care. The first section of the chapter explains why nurses need to know history to be effective advocates and why knowing history matters to advocacy. It provides historical exemplars to highlight how history informs the profession as it continues to invoke the social contract that nursing maintains with society. The second part of the chapter examines a more contemporary look at nursing's political advocacy efforts and what it means for nurses, the profession, and the health of the public at large.

Objectives

- Discuss why nursing history is relevant to health policy and nursing advocacy and action.
- Explore historical exemplars that provide evidence of nursing's ability to advocate for individuals, families, communities, and populations.
- Analyze nursing's role in how political advocacy impacts nurses, the profession, and the health of the public at large.

Nurses as Advocates

Although society reportedly trusts nurses to work toward accomplishing the goals set forth for them by the profession (ANA, 2010), nurses may not be grounded in how they reached these "long-standing core values" that the nursing profession developed over time. As nurses advocate for their patients—whether seen as individuals, families, communities, or populations—an understanding of nursing's enduring and longstanding values that are rooted in its history provide depth and breadth to their efforts. To this end, it is important to know nursing's historical role in ensuring access to care; it is important to know nursing's contributions toward patient quality and safety measures; it is important to know how nursing interventions changed over time in response to the context in which nurses practiced; and it is important to know how nurses and the profession adapted to shifts in the social, political, economic, and cultural environment (D'Antonio & Lewenson, 2011).

Why Study Nursing History?

Historian and nurse educator Ellen Baer and colleagues respond to the question of why nursing history should be studied:

> Just as a nurse can make little progress caring for or curing a patient's presenting problem without knowing the patient's physiological, psychological, and cultural history so is it for a nurse trying to make sense out of the persistent problems and possibilities in nursing and health care. To make good decisions in planning nursing's future in the context of our complex health-care system, nurses must know the history of the actions

being considered, the identities and points of view of the major players, and all the states that are at risk. These are the lessons of history. (Baer, D'Antonio, Rinker, & Lynaugh, 2001, p. 7)

Some lessons from the past that support the understanding of political advocacy and action can be learned by examining how Florence Nightingale influenced the development of nursing education programs that started in 1873 and led to what became known as the Modern Nursing Movement. It began with the first three Nightingale training schools: the Bellevue Training School for Nurses in New York City; the Boston Training School for Nurses at Massachusetts General in Boston; and the Connecticut Training School in New Haven, Connecticut. Following the opening of these three schools, hospitals around the country recognized the value that student nurses bring to the hospital because care could be provided at relatively low cost and the hospital would have no obligation to hire the nurses when they graduated. Nurses, after their training was complete, would need to find work elsewhere, typically in private duty or in the emerging field of public health nursing.

Twenty years after the opening of these schools of nursing, early nursing leaders recognized the need to organize nurses to control the quality of practice and training as a way to protect the public. Between 1893 and 1912, four professional nursing organizations formed to do just that: the National League for Nurses, formed in 1893 (originally called the American Society of Superintendents of Training Schools for Nurses); the American Nurses Association, started in 1896 (originally named the Nurses' Associated Alumnae of the United States and Canada); the National Association of Colored Graduate Nurses, which formed to address racial bias in nursing and health care and was in existence between 1908 and 1952; and finally, in 1912, the National Organization of Public Health Nursing, formed to control practice and educational standards during the rising movement of public health and public health nursing in the United States. This organization ended in 1952, when the National League for Nursing assumed its role (Lewenson, 1993).

Even before women in the United States gained the vote in 1920, nurses sought legislation that would define nursing practice, and they advocated for the protection of the public by prohibiting anyone who was not professionally trained from calling him- or herself a nurse. This required convincing lawmakers, at that time only men, to support nursing legislation; the nurses knew they could not vote into law the early nurse practice acts. While nurses struggled for statewide nursing registration, they had to "fight battles against long hours of work and opposition to nursing education" (Lewenson, 1993, p. 171). To accomplish their goals, some nurses, either individually or through the early nursing organizations, began to support the work of the suffragist movement and aligned themselves with the larger women's movement of the early 1900s. Individual nursing leaders, like public health pioneer Lillian Wald and nursing suffragist Lavinia Dock, advocated for healthcare reforms in the community and in the legislative arena. The professional organizations that formed during this period did so to protect the public from uneducated nurses and to develop standards for nursing education and practice.

Although an in-depth history of this time period is beyond the scope of this chapter, it is important for nurses to understand that

political advocacy was part of the profession's early identity. Political advocacy and action in nursing is not new or innovative. Nurses have always been political advocates for those in their care (Lewenson, 2012). As a result, the early efforts made by nurses and their professional organizations provide a narrative for and insight into today's advocacy efforts where protection of the public means ensuring a level of education for all nurses, the development of quality and safety standards, and the ability of nurses to practice to the fullest extent of their education, as recommended by an Institute of Medicine report (2010).

History Counts

Fairman and D'Antonio (2013) wrote, "history counts in health policy debates" (p. 346). Bringing a historical perspective to discussions about health care deepens our understanding of the issues by recognizing the evolution of ideas across time. In the debate about control of the "newly" minted medical homes of today, understanding the roles of early public health nurses in providing primary healthcare services to individuals, families, communities, and populations in both urban and rural settings can trigger some useful ideas or solutions about what to call the new entity, who should finance it, and who should lead it (Keeling & Lewenson, 2013).

The current debate centered on medical homes provides such an example. The term was first coined in the 1960s and defined a medical model of care for chronically ill pediatric patients that looked at control issues, inter- and intradisciplinary issues of providing care, and the financial aspects of care. Physicians led the earlier medical home movement that has evolved to mean "a model of primary care that is accessible, continuous, comprehensive, family-centered, coordinated, compassionate and culturally effective" (American Academy of Pediatrics, 2002, as cited in Keeling & Lewenson, 2013, p. 360). Nurses use the words that define the medical home of today to describe nursing's work of providing accessible, continuous, comprehensive, family-centered, coordinated, compassionate, and culturally effective care. Knowing the history of nursing serves to highlight the profession's strong contribution to health care in the United States.

Advocacy and Public Health Nursing

Exploring some of the public health initiatives that Wald established—the Henry Street Settlement and the American Red Cross Town & Country—offer excellent examples of how nursing, history, and political advocacy and action intersect. By studying the work of those nurses and nursing leaders within these settings, we not only learn about the role nurses played in primary health care (as described by Keeling & Lewenson, 2013), but we can also learn about the healthcare advocacy that public health nurses sought for those individuals, families, and communities. The next section uses these two early-20th-century public health initiatives as examples of political advocacy by public health nurses.

Advocacy at Henry Street

Lillian Wald graduated from nurses' training in 1891 from the 2-year diploma-based program at New York Hospital in New York City. Within 2 years of graduating, she and her school friend Mary Brewster recognized the overwhelming healthcare needs of immigrant families living in the overcrowded and unclean conditions of the tenement houses on the Lower East Side of New York City. Filled with a sense of social obligation to improve the health of society, Wald and Brewster began the Henry Street Settlement and found support for the venture from philanthropists and other nursing leaders. Wald's work expanded from just nine public health nurses working in one settlement house that was established in 1893 to more than 250 nurses working throughout the New York City area in at least seven different locations (Buhler-Wilkerson, 2001; Keeling, 2007; Lewenson, 1993).

While caring for the families, Wald clearly saw a close relationship between the health of the public and civil responsibility. In a speech she delivered in 1900 at the sixth annual meeting of the American Society of Superintendents of Training Schools for Nurses, Wald said that "among the many opportunities for civic and altruistic work pressing on all sides nurses having superior advantages in their practical training should not rest content with being only nurses, but should use their talents wherever possible in reform and civic movements" (Wald, 1900, as cited in Birnbach & Lewenson, 1991, p. 318). In keeping with her beliefs, Wald and her colleagues at Henry Street introduced several legislative initiatives that would improve the health of children, such as the introduction of nurses in public schools (Wald, 1915). Wald (1915) described how she advocated for hiring nurses in the local public schools to decrease truancy rates, given that children were sent home due to illness and lack of treatment. As of 1897, physicians had only recently been hired by the New York City Department of Health to assess children in school. Doctors sent children home from school when any contagious illnesses were found. However, this did not address some of the pressing health issues because the physicians did not provide treatment for conditions such as trachoma, a contagious eye infection that plagued school-age children at the time. Wald (1915) wrote about her experience convincing legislators of the value of assigning public health nurses in the schools in her book *The House on Henry Street*.

In 1902, when a reform administration came into power, the medical staff was reduced and the physicians' salary was increased to $100 per month, and they were expected to work only 3 hours per day. The health commissioner ordered an examination of all public school pupils and was horrified to learn of the prevalence of trachoma. Thousands of children were sent away from school because of this infection. Where medical inspections were the most thorough, the classrooms were empty. It was ironic that Wald watched the children who had been turned away from school playing with the children they had been sent home to protect. Few children received treatment, and it followed that truancy was encouraged:

> The time had come when it seemed right to urge the addition of the nurse's service to that of the doctor. My colleagues and I offered to show that with her assistance few children would lose their valuable school time and that it would be possible to bring under treatment those who needed it . . . I exacted a promise from several of the city officials that if the experiment were successful they would use their influence to have the nurse, like the doctor, paid from public funds. Four schools from which there had been the greatest number of exclusions for medical causes were selected, and an experienced nurse, who possessed tact and initiative, was chosen

from the settlement staff to make the demonstration . . . Many of the children needed only disinfectant treatment of the eyes, collodion applied to ringworm, or instruction as to cleanliness, and such were returned at once to the class with a minimum loss of precious school time. Where more serious conditions existed the nurse called at the home. (Wald, 1915, pp. 51–52)

Within 1 month, the experiment was deemed successful and an "enlightened Board of Estimate and Apportionment voted $30,000 for the employment of trained nurses, the first municipalized school nurses in the world" (Wald, 1915, p. 53).

Advocacy in the Town & Country

Wald's advocacy extended to families living in rural settings. One of the most compelling examples is the establishment of the American Red Cross Rural Nursing Service (later known as the Town & Country). As Keeling and Lewenson wrote (2013), this organization "served as the point of contact for families in rural communities where remoteness, isolation, and fewer physicians and nurses created barriers to care" (p. 362). Wald believed that the American Red Cross—already organized to provide nursing services during wartime and natural or manmade disasters—was the right vehicle in which to organize public health nursing services throughout the country during peacetime (Dock, Pickett, Clement, Fox, & Van Meter, 1922; Keeling & Lewenson, 2013). Through Wald's influence, philanthropists supported the implementation of this new rural public health nursing service. During the first year, criteria were established for nurses who would collaborate with community leaders, physicians, and families to provide both curative and preventive health care in rural settings. The requirements to become a rural public health nurse were far reaching and included pragmatic skills. Nurses were expected to ride a bicycle or a horse, or drive a car, so they could access their patients.

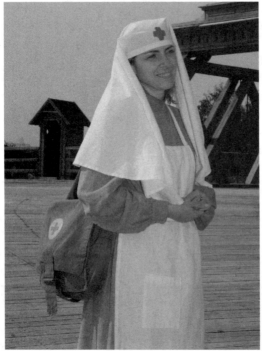

© fotorobs/ShutterStock, Inc.

More important, and often difficult to find, were nurses who had an education that prepared them to negotiate and collaborate with others in the community. Typical nurses' training programs did not provide these skills. It was determined that a minimum of a 4-month education was needed to prepare nurses to work independently in communities across America (American Red Cross Rural Nursing Service, 1912–1914). Educational programs were established, like the one at Teachers College in New

York, in conjunction with the Henry Street Settlement and the rural District Nursing Service of Northern Westchester, soon after the American Red Cross Rural Nursing Service formed. By 1914 the new public health nurse curriculum offered courses in sociology, municipal and rural sanitation, and experiences in rural and urban public health settings. These courses were valuable for nurses who practiced in rural settings because they did not have the same support systems as urban areas.

Wald's advocacy extended to the use of media to show the public what a rural public health nurse could do and to garner support for the initiative. While she was at the third meeting of the American Red Cross Committee on Rural Nursing—the committee established by the American Red Cross in 1912 to develop the criteria for the Town & Country—Wald suggested that the committee "get in touch with the Publication Syndicate, and Rural Nursing written up possible [*sic*] in story form for the Ladies' Home Journal and other popular magazines" ("Minutes of the Third Meeting," 1913, p. 2). At the same meeting, it was noted that Wald and others supported establishing a relationship with the Metropolitan Life Insurance Company and the Steel Corporation whereby the Rural Nursing Service would "undertake nursing for these large concerns" ("Minutes of the Third Meeting," 1913, p. 4). Many of the communities in question were rural mining communities that required public health nursing services. The committee believed this relationship would be beneficial in many ways, including possibly raising the standards of other nursing associations and economically supporting the cost of nursing supervision in these locations.

Advocacy took many forms, which ranged from sitting on national committees to seeing that care was provided at local levels. The work of the public health nurse was framed by the needs of the community, the kinds of public healthcare organizations that were organized, and the geographical location. Each Red Cross rural nurse chapter—whether in the mountains of New Hampshire, in Kentucky, or in the West—directed the kinds of work that public health nurses would do, including bedside care for frostbite, well-baby clinics, school nursing, industrial nursing, classes in home hygiene and care of the sick, advocacy on town boards, and educational and publicity efforts about their work (Fox, 1921). Sometimes there was only one public health nurse in an area. At other times, public health nurses shared a district. Sometimes a nurse faced barriers by communities that were uncomfortable with outsiders offering care. Yet the success of these American Red Cross Town & Country nurses relied on the ability to recruit and retain those who could handle the challenges of rural settings. This concern remained a constant and enduring problem throughout the life span of the American Red Cross Town & Country.

History and Political Advocacy

Political advocacy requires the depth and breadth of an evolving historical narrative to inform contemporary debates in health care, to reflect the variety of perspectives that history can bring to the debate, and to offer a "way to think about the future" (Fairman & D'Antonio, 2013, p. 346). The work of the nurses at Henry Street Settlement and the American Red Cross Town & Country are two examples that can stimulate discussions about healthcare reform today. Readers are encouraged to explore the many historical studies being completed and the early writings of

nurses that can be found in nursing journals, such as the *American Journal of Nursing*. This journal has digitalized its entire collection from 1900 to the present, allowing readers to easily access articles online and explore nursing advocacy over time. The American Association for the History of Nursing (AAHN) (www.aahn.org) also provides information and resources for where one can go to find nursing archives, learn more about historical methods, and attend the association's annual meeting where the latest in historical research is presented. The AAHN also publishes a well-respected journal, *Nursing History Review*, where readers can find outstanding historical research by leading historians. There are also many archival centers around the country, such as the Barbara Bates Center for the Study of Nursing History at the University of Pennsylvania and the Eleanor Crowder Bjoring Center for Nursing Historical Inquiry at the University of Virginia. Centers such as these provide a wealth of archival data and support for those interested in historical research. The websites for these centers and other resources are available on the AAHN website.

Nursing's Political Advocacy and Action

The next part of this chapter moves from the historical to the contemporary and further explores the meaning of advocacy and action, as well as what that means for nurses, the profession, and the health of the public. Today nurses must be politically active in professional nursing practice and health policy issues like the nurse reformers and activists before them. Nursing's historical roots in meaningful advocacy and action have shaped the profession's political astuteness and action to keep pace with professional regulatory, statutory, and legal changes in education, practice, and research. The profession must remain nimble and responsive to policy changes by promoting and protecting the well-being of the population and nurses themselves. To effectively manage the emerging needs of populations and the profession, every nurse must be engaged in the advocacy process. The American Nurses Association suggests that high-quality nursing practice include advocacy as an essential aspect of patient care (ANA, n.d.). Advocacy is considered both a philosophical principle of the profession and a part of ethical nursing practice that ensures that the rights and safety of the patient are protected and safeguarded. Advocacy is the one professional construct that demonstrates a complex interaction among nurses, patients, professional colleagues, and the public (Selanders & Crane, 2012).

To become engaged in advocacy, nurses must be informed about policy and how to influence nursing, health, and public policy at local, regional, national, and global levels. This engagement requires sound evidence and a political strategy that allows for increased understanding of the potential impact of linking the nursing workforce with the globalization of health care, the implementation of the Patient Protection and Affordable Care Act (PPACA), and the ongoing disparities in health care and health outcomes. The demands for increased access and better healthcare outcomes will require nursing to widen its influence in policy areas that address the health and healthcare needs of underserved and minority populations (Villarruel, Bigelow, & Alvarez, 2014).

As political advocates, nurses are uniquely positioned to lead system change to improve care for patients and families, influence the implementation of the PPACA, and conduct a political environmental scan. As leaders, administrators, educators, and researchers, nurses have demonstrated the ability to manage complex processes and related data analytics around disparities, health outcomes, quality, and costs. The next section of this chapter discusses how nurses will continue to amplify their voices and advocate to meet the changing landscape of health care.

Nursing Strong

Professional nursing care is essential to the healthcare system. Of the more than 3.1 million registered nurses (RNs), approximately 84.7% are employed in nursing (62.2% in hospitals), making registered nursing the largest healthcare profession (ANA, n.d.). As such, nurses must advocate by bringing problems to the government and seek decisions in the form of programs, laws, regulations, or other official responses that create new innovations and care models to transform delivery and advance the nation's health.

To begin, nursing must advocate for changes within the profession. To successfully advance health care, the nursing profession must make significant strides to change the composition of the future workforce. This will require greater efforts toward the successful recruitment of underrepresented minority groups into nursing. Phillips & Malone (2014) report that nurses from minority backgrounds represent 16.8% of the RN workforce. The 2008 National Sample Survey of Registered Nurses showed that the RN workforce is composed of 5.4% African American, 3.6% Hispanic, 5.8% Asian/Native Hawaiian, 0.3% American Indian/Native Alaskan, and 1.7% multiracial individuals (U.S. Department of Health and Human Services, 2010). The workforce is involved in the policy process and gives nurses ample opportunity to create a culturally and linguistically diverse care environment.

A diverse healthcare workforce increases both minority participation in the health professions and the cultural competency of all patients. A U.S. Department of Health and Human Services report (2006) shows that increased diversity among healthcare professionals leads to improved patient satisfaction, improved patient–nurse communication, and improved access to care for racial and ethnic minority patients who are best served by providers who are knowledgeable about their backgrounds and cultures. The intersecting goals of increasing workforce diversity, ensuring fair and equal access to quality health care and healthcare resources, eliminating health disparities, and achieving health equity is where nursing's political advocacy and action will have its greatest impact.

Achieving health equity for all requires a collective effort across all disciplines and all sectors, including those outside nursing. Therefore, nurses must align themselves with other healthcare professionals to address health disparities and health equity, specifically within the context of the social determinants of health. As an interprofessional healthcare team, all professionals must "draw upon their moral responsibility to respond to human suffering and become acknowledged participants in the nation's efforts to correct health disparity" (Harrison & Falco, 2005, p. 261).

To promote the health of the public, nurses must work to eliminate the overuse, underuse, and misuse of services and resources (Orszag, 2008). Reducing healthcare spending is seen as one of the greatest challenges in health care. In 2011, U.S. healthcare spending grew 3.9% to reach $2.7 trillion, marking the third consecutive year of relatively slow growth. Growth in national healthcare spending closely tracked growth in nominal gross domestic product (GDP) in 2010 and 2011, and health spending as a share of GDP remained stable from 2009 through 2011 at 17.9% (Hartman, Martin, Benson, & Catlin, 2013). To address care gaps and avoid service duplication, the PPACA has invoked care coordination to improve the public's health.

With the provisions of the PPACA focused on improving the quality of patient-centered care and controlling costs within and across settings, nurses need to understand and interpret this legislation and health policy. By being able to interpret healthcare reform from a nursing perspective, nurses can determine how to best distribute resources to individuals, families, and populations. The law stimulates payment and delivery reforms that are highly relevant to nurses, particularly those working in primary care and ambulatory settings.

Nurses play a vital role in creating opportunities for better health, better health care, and lower costs through improvement. For example, chronic conditions such as diabetes, arthritis, hypertension, and kidney disease account for 7 of 10 deaths among Americans each year, and they account for 75% of the nation's healthcare spending (Conway, Goodrich, Macklin, Sasse, & Cohen, 2011). The obesity epidemic and growing levels of preventable diseases and chronic conditions greatly contribute to the high costs of health care. Additionally, an aging population has increased the demand to address end-of-life care in a cost-effective manner (Rice & Betcher, 2010). By understanding the burdens of caring for individuals with chronic conditions and the economic realities of controlling costs while achieving value in health care, nurses are using care coordination models as an integrative service. These models use case managers, health information technology, and other strategies to manage care delivery and support services for patients. Care coordination has been reported to have significant outcomes in high-risk populations and in patients with chronic conditions to reduce treatment costs and repeated hospitalizations.

Discussion Questions

1. How does history inform nursing's efforts to provide primary health care?
2. What is the relevance of nursing's history to political advocacy today?
3. Describe the role of advocacy within the history of nursing's development in the United States.

References

American Nurses Association. (2010). *Nursing's social policy statement: The essence of the profession (2010 edition)*. Silver Spring, MD: Author.

American Nurses Association. (n.d.). *Advocacy*. Retrieved from www.nursingworld.org/Main-MenuCategories/The Practiceof Professional-NursingPatientSafetyQuality/Advocacy.aspx

American Red Cross Rural Nursing Service. (1912–1914). Circular for application. Rockefeller Sanitary Commission microfilm (Reel 1, Folder 8, Rockefeller Archives). Pocantico, NY: American Red Cross Town & Country Nursing Service.

Baer, E. D., D'Antonio, P., Rinker, S., Lynaugh, & J. E. (2001). *Enduring issues in American history*. New York, NY: Springer.

Birnbach, N., & Lewenson, S. (Eds.). (1991). *Work of women in municipal affairs. First words: Selected addresses from the National League for Nursing 1894–1933*. New York, NY: National League for Nursing.

Buhler-Wilkerson, K. (2001). *No place like home: A history of nursing and home care in the United States*. Baltimore, MD: Johns Hopkins University Press.

Conway, P. H., Goodrich, K., Macklin, S., Sasse, B., & Cohen, J. (2011). Patient-centered care categorization of U.S. health care expenditures. *Health Services Research*, *46*(2), 479–490.

D'Antonio, P., & Lewenson, S. B. (Eds.). (2011). *Nursing interventions over time: History as evidence*. New York, NY: Springer.

Dock, L. L., Pickett, S. E., Clement, F., Fox, E. G., & Van Meter, A. R. (1922). *History of American Red Cross nursing*. New York, NY: Macmillan.

Fairman, J., & D'Antonio, P. (2013). History counts: How history can shape our understanding of health policy. *Nursing Outlook*, *61*(5), 346–352.

Fox, E. (1921). Red Cross public health nursing, out to sea. *Public Health Nurse*, *13*, 105–108.

Harrison, E., & Falco, S. M. (2005). Health disparity and the nurse advocate: Reaching out to alleviate suffering. *Advances in Nursing Science*, *28*(3), 252–264.

Hartman, M., Martin, A. B., Benson, J., & Catlin, A. (2013). National health spending in 2011: Overall growth remains low, but some payers and services show signs of acceleration. *Health Affairs*, *32*(1), 87–99. doi:10.1377/hlthaff.2012.1206

Institute of Medicine. (2010). *The future of nursing: Leading change, advancing health*. Washington, DC: National Academies Press.

Keeling, A. (2007). *Nursing and the privilege of prescription*, 1893–2000. Columbus: Ohio State University Press.

Keeling, A., & Lewenson, S. B. (2013). A nursing historical perspective on the medical home: Impact on health care policy. *Nursing Outlook*,

61(5), 360–366. http://dx.doi.org/10.1016/j. outlook.2013.07.003.

Lewenson, S. B. (1993). *Taking charge: Nursing, suffrage, and feminism in America, 1873–1920.* New York, NY: Garland.

Lewenson, S. B. (2012). A historical perspective on policy, politics, and nursing. In D. J. Mason, J. K. Leavitt, & M. W. Chafee (Eds.), *Policy and politics in nursing and health care* (6th ed., pp. 12–18). St. Louis, MO: Elsevier Saunders.

Making medical homes work: Moving from concept to practice. (2008, December). *Policy Perspective: Insights into Health Policy Issues.* Retrieved from http://www.hschange.org/CONTENT/1030/1030.pdf

Minutes of the third meeting of the Committee on Rural Nursing. (1913). Rockefeller Sanitary Commission microfilm (Reel 1, Folder 8, Rockefeller Archives). Pocantico, NY: American Red Cross Town & Country Nursing Service.

Orszag, P. R. (2008). *The overuse, underuse, and misuse of health care.* Testimony before the U.S. Senate Committee on Finance. Retrieved from http://www.cbo.gov/sites/default/files /cbofiles/ftpdocs/95xx/doc9567/07-17-health-care_testimony.pdf

Phillips, J., & Malone, B. (2014). Increasing racial /ethnic diversity in nursing to reduce health disparities and achieve health equity. *Public Health Reports, 2*(129), 45–50.

Rice, E., & Betcher, D. (2010). Palliative care in an acute care hospital: From pilot to consultation service. *MEDSURG Nursing, 19*(2), 107–112.

Selanders, L. C., & Crane, P. C. (2012). The voice of Florence Nightingale on advocacy. *Online Journal of Issues in Nursing, 17*(1).

U.S. Department of Health and Human Services. (2006). *The rationale for diversity in the health professions: A review of the evidence.* Retrieved from http://bhpr .hrsa.gov/healthworkforce /reports/diversityreviewevidence.pdf

U.S. Department of Health and Human Services. (2010). *The registered nurse population: Findings from the 2008 National Sample Survey of Registered Nurses.* Rockville, MD: Author.

Villarruel, A., Bigelow, A., & Alvarez, C. (2014). Integrating the 3Ds: A nursing perspective. *Public Health Reports, 2*(129), 37–44.

Wald, L. (1915). *The House on Henry Street.* New York, NY: Henry Holt & Company.

CHAPTER 2

Policy and Politics Explained

Nancy Aries

Overview

Nurses and other healthcare professionals must understand how the government, providers, consumers, and insurers interact in the health policy process. This chapter provides an overview of the essential cornerstones that drive and shape health policy in America. By understanding the framework within which policy is made, and the politics of policy making and program implementation, all healthcare professionals, regardless of where they perform their duties, will be better prepared to advocate for a healthcare system that best meets the needs of the population.

Objectives

- Define policy (generally) and health policy (specifically).
- Explain the role of the market and the government in framing policy.
- Describe the policy-making process, including the following:
  - Competing concepts of federalism that create the structure within which policy is determined
  - The policy-making process
  - The role of competing interests and their influence on policy outcomes
  - The implementation of policy and its ramification for future action
- Identify different ways that healthcare advocates can impact policy and programmatic outcomes.

Introduction

Early in President Obama's first term, when healthcare reform was being proposed, he reported receiving a letter from a woman who did not know the difference between a government and a private health insurance plan. She said, "I don't want government-run health care. I don't want socialized medicine. And don't touch my Medicare" (Cesca, 2009). Since President Obama received that letter, healthcare reform legislation has become a reality. The Affordable Care Act (ACA), also known as "Obamacare," was signed into law in 2010. Starting January 1, 2014, millions of Americans—many of whom had been uninsured—have bought affordable health insurance. But confusion still characterizes the discussion. Some persons who think of themselves as informed do not know that the ACA and Obamacare are the same thing (Jimmy Kimmel Live, 2013). While both stories reference a small number of people, they suggest a collective failure to understand how the organization and delivery of health care are shaped by government policies and programs.

This chapter explains the role of government in the policy and policy-making process as a first step to providing the necessary tools to those who want to shape the organization and delivery of care. The first section defines policy and considers the ways policy shapes our experience of the healthcare system. Policy refers broadly to actions that advance the well-being of society. Most often policy is formed and carried out by government, which is empowered to act on behalf of the whole. When health care works, it is often because of policies that enable it to succeed. When there is failure, it is often because policies have created an environment in which it is difficult to operate.

The second section of this chapter highlights the different ways government policy and programs intervene in the organization and delivery of health services to ensure greater social equity in the access to affordable and high-quality health care. The choice of tools is determined by the balance established between the market and the government in overseeing the organization of healthcare delivery.*

Although the United States operates under a mixed system, the market and the government each present a different set of opportunities and constraints for policy makers.

The third section examines the framework within which policy is constructed. This includes the competing concepts of federalism and the ways it impacts the development of government programs and the actual programmatic tools the government uses to achieve its goals. In the fourth section, the policy-making process is explained. To understand policy is to understand the groups that have a stake in the development of government programs and how their interests are expressed in the political process. The fifth section considers the politics of decision making. This chapter does not explain legislative procedures; that is better left to a civics text. Rather, this chapter explains how interest groups influence the decision-making process to achieve what they perceive to be a more favorable outcome. Policy making, however, does not stop with the passage of legislation. Implementation, which is equally

---

*The terms *market* and *government* are shorthand expressions that describe the two ways in which society conducts its business. *Market* means reliance on generally voluntary exchanges between private parties. Sometimes these exchanges are mandated and regulated by government, as is the case with mandatory liability insurance to own a motor vehicle. *Government* means reliance on the direct provision of a service by government employees, as is the case with Veterans Affairs hospitals. It is not uncommon to use a combination of markets and government, as is the case with Medicare and Medicaid, where government makes payments to private providers to care for individuals who are being served by the government.

important, although sometimes overlooked, is also an opportunity to influence how policy is realized on a day-to-day basis. The final section of this chapter brings the discussion back to the nurses and other healthcare professionals for whom this text is written. A better understanding of policy not only impacts the experiences of those seeking and providing health care; it also provides a framework for understanding how healthcare professionals can be more effective players within the system and have greater influence as a result.

Policy Defined

Policy in the broadest sense is the manifestation of ideology or belief systems concerning public purpose (Weissert & Weissert, 2012). Public purpose refers to those actions that benefit the population as a whole. In the United States, ethnic and religious communities were historically the primary providers of social and economic support for persons in need of assistance. This responsibility shifted to the state during the Great Depression with the passage of the Social Security Act in 1935, which included the Social Security Program, Aid to Dependent Children, and Maternal and Child Health Services, among others. It was further advanced by President Johnson's War on Poverty, whose healthcare initiatives included Medicare, Medicaid, and funding for community health centers. The pendulum is currently moving back in the opposite direction. Rather than looking to government to secure social welfare, there is a desire for the government to retreat from the role of social provider and move to social advocacy. The call for smaller government is grounded in the belief that the market is capable of meeting the needs of individuals.

The concept of public purpose is not easily defined. One writer has labeled it paradoxical (Stone, 2012), and others say it is ambiguous (Weissert & Weissert, 2012). It is paradoxical in that the same words can convey multiple meanings. This can lead to agreement at the highest possible expression of policy, but it can break down when more detail is required. Take, for example, the concept of social equity. Does the argument pertaining to social equity refer to the process by which goods or services are provided, or the resulting outcomes? In education, for example, access is no longer considered an adequate measure of success given the achievement gap among black, Hispanic, white, and Asian students. It is ambiguous because there is no certainty that our actions will result in predictable ends. Given the diversity of thought about how best to achieve a stated goal, there is often no telling whether the outcome will be the one that was intended. Take another example: the government's response to the fiscal crisis in 2008. Whether there should have been a government bailout and the size of the bailout was fervently debated. The government settled on a bailout that was smaller in scale than some had proposed. The consequence was that the situation stabilized, but the economy did not recover as quickly as some—both those who called for no government intervention and those who called for greater government intervention—had suggested.

Markets versus Government

How best to define public interest poses a challenge, in terms of balancing individual versus group interests and the role of the market versus the role of government (Stone, 2012). Most goods and services, including health care, are acquired through the market. In the market, the assumption is made that the aggregate of individual interests results in the community's interest. In other words, the outcome that best serves the individual is enhancing the collective good. Our decisions and choices are influenced by signals from sellers in terms of the prices at which they offer products. An obvious example is the way the cost of gasoline is shifting consumer preferences away from large fuel-guzzling automobiles toward smaller fuel-efficient cars. Less obvious, perhaps but more important, are the ways in which the market responds to broader shifts in society. Consider the housing market's response to an aging population. The number of persons looking for housing alternatives that offer services not readily available in single-family or multi-unit dwellings is growing. Companies such as Marriott are entering the senior housing market in response to this demand. In these cases, consumers influence producers. There are also cases in which business tries to influence consumer behavior. The direct marketing of pharmaceuticals through television and print advertising is intended to influence consumer perceptions about possible remedies for their health conditions.

A fundamental problem of the market is its inability to respond to individual and social needs or preferences that cannot be expressed in terms of price. In a market, one has a right to purchase only the goods and services that one can afford. Those who cannot afford their desired goods and services are not entitled to them. What if, however, the service is essential to an individual's welfare or the welfare of a society? In these cases, the market is an inadequate distributive mechanism because competition puts those with fewer resources at a disadvantage in terms of accessing services such as health care. Most Americans younger than age 65 rely on health insurance as the means by which they can afford and therefore access health services. However, 5 million persons lost their health insurance during the recession that began in 2007 (Holahan, 2011). The market is limited in its ability to ensure distributive justice for those persons as the market assumes an exchange among equals. Such an exchange is not possible in a society with an unequal distribution of income (Arrow, 1963).

The government intervenes in these situations (Stone, 2012). The government's role derives from this fundamental tension between the economic organization of the production and the distribution of goods and services. The market may pull in the direction of economic inequality, but political beliefs demand a counterbalance in terms of the distribution of rights and opportunities. The government becomes the counterbalance for persons who cannot provide for themselves through the exchange of goods and services in the market (Arrow, 1974). Through its policies and programs, government mediates the interests of the market and interests that have no expression in the market. This is the mechanism by which a society seeks to achieve greater equality. Its policies and programs are redistributive, which means that actions that benefit the larger group may result in losses for some individuals.

Framework for Governmental Action

Public policy, the term used to describe government action, is typically divided into three areas: foreign policy, economic policy, and social policy (Lowi & Ginsberg, 1998). The objective of foreign policy is to defend national sovereignty. Economic policy is designed to promote and regulate markets. Although foreign and economic policy seek to promote the political and economic well-being of American society, policies in these areas typically do not have equal impact on all sectors of society. Some groups may benefit, whereas others might suffer undue consequences. The North American Free Trade Agreement benefited the overall economy, but many persons who held manufacturing jobs found themselves unemployed as production moved from the United States to countries with lower production costs. Social policy often becomes the means by which the unintended consequences of policies that seek to better the overall condition of American society are addressed. Government actions are the ways in which the provision of the basic necessities—food, shelter, health care, and education—is ensured (Midgley & Livermore, 2008). Social policy is redistributive by its very nature. Its goal is to achieve greater social equity.

Health policy exists within this larger realm of social policy. Because policy generally is rooted in social values and ideologies, the discussion of health policy begins with the recognition of the values and ideology that shape the organization of the healthcare system. The historic course of American health policy is best described in terms of shifting beliefs about access to care. Sometimes we have stridently pursued health care as a right for all. Sometimes we have treated it as a privilege (Knowles, 1977). These competing values (i.e., a right versus a privilege) are simultaneously and continually at work.

This duality can be observed in the public provision of health care. Medicare covers practically all Americans older than age 65. Medicare is a universal entitlement, which means a defined population is eligible for care

regardless of ability to pay. One argument underscoring the creation of Medicare was that the older population had worked for the benefit of society and should not risk poverty in old age due to high healthcare costs. For those older than age 65, health care was deemed a right. Such programs tend to be more expensive because of their all-inclusive nature, but they also tend to have broad political support because all persons can expect to receive the program's benefits (Brown & Sparer, 2003). Despite Medicare being understood as a right, the rising cost of Medicare has led to proposals that seek to balance the market and government as providers of this important benefit (Steuerle & Bovbjerg, 2008). Market-based alternatives that shift costs to the beneficiaries include means testing Medicare Part A, raising the age of eligibility, or making Medicare a premium support program. The ACA maintains the right to health care for persons over age 65 and seeks alternatives to cost shifting, such as cutting physician payments and creating greater care coordination (Eibner, Goldman, Sullivan, & Garber, 2013).

The opposite holds true for the working-age population and their dependents. No universal health insurance program is available to Americans younger than age 65. They can either obtain health insurance as a benefit of employment, or they can purchase health insurance out of pocket. Health insurance, however, is costly. The average annual premium in 2013 was $5,884 for an individual health insurance policy. For those who cannot afford to purchase insurance, there is an array of safety-net programs that are challenged to meet the needs of the uninsured, even with the implementation of the ACA in 2014 (Andrulis & Siddiqui, 2011). Medicaid, a selective program with need-based eligibility criteria, is one example of a safety-net program for some of the most vulnerable populations who cannot afford to access health services through the market (Brown & Sparer, 2003). Programs like Medicaid are less expensive because they serve a subset of the population. They also tend to have less political support because they typically serve needy populations whose claim for services is considered questionable and because they often provide a level of service that is greater than persons who are slightly above the cutoff can access. Despite Medicaid being a selective program, the ACA called for expanding program eligibility to persons at 138% of the poverty level. Nineteen states have chosen not to participate in the Medicaid expansion. As a result, a large number of people will have no access to Medicaid or subsidized private health insurance (Commonwealth Fund, 2014).

Federalism

To understand how this situation came to pass, it is important to understand the nature of the federalist system within which policy is made (Bovbjerg, Wiener, & Housman, 2003). American federalism is a system of governance in which the exercise of sovereign power is split among the 50 states and the national government. Hence, the federal government is limited in its actions in several important ways. First, there is the dual system of state and federal governance. When the nation was founded, the states ceded certain responsibilities to the federal government but retained others for themselves. In addition, within the federal government, there is a separation of powers among the legislative, executive, and judicial branches. This further constrains the power of the national government by dividing the government against itself. Finally, the Constitution limits both the federal and state governments

by protecting individual rights that cannot be denied except through extraordinary procedures.

According to the framers of the Constitution, the central government has express powers to levy taxes, declare war, and oversee interstate commerce. All power not expressly delegated to the federal government falls under the jurisdiction of the states. This system of dual federalism provides the context in which the patchwork pattern of health policy exists. Although there is a strong national government, the states were initially more important than the federal government in virtually all policies governing the lives of Americans, such as economic regulation, public health, and education. When President Pierce vetoed a law setting aside millions of acres of federal land to benefit the mentally ill, he argued that mental health was a state, not a federal, responsibility (Rothman, 1971).

Despite the fact that social policy relating to individual welfare is a state responsibility, there has been a constant expansion of federal power in this area since the Civil War. By the 1930s, scholars saw such a radical departure in the conduct of federalism that the New Deal was characterized as a shift from a system of dual federalism to a system of cooperative federalism (Kernell & Jacobson, 2006). This shift was brought on by the severe hardship of the Great Depression. At that time, the ability of states to protect the well-being of their citizens was diminished because states had limited ability to raise funds through taxation or deficit financing. Therefore, the states turned to the federal government, which initiated and funded many social programs. Using grant-in-aid programs, Congress appropriated money to state and local governments with the condition that the money be spent for particular purposes as defined by Congress. The Maternal and Child Health Services, which was created under Title V of the Social Security Act in 1935, is an example of such a grant-in-aid program. This program sought to improve the health of low-income mothers and children. From a policy perspective, cooperative federalism is important because Congress began to set national goals and influence state activity in the realm of social policy.

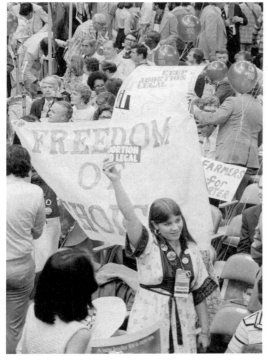

Courtesy of the Library of Congress, Prints & Photographs Division, preproduction number ppmsca 09733

Federal power increased through the 1960s as opposition grew to the various ways in which states implemented social programs. The federal government assumed a larger role in terms of shaping and funding social welfare programs by imposing national standards on the states through regulations (Conlan, 2006).

States needed to comply with the regulations or risk a penalty, such as the withholding of grant money. Typically, the costs of regulatory compliance were not funded by the federal government. Hence, these were labeled as unfunded mandates. Federal regulatory authority was further advanced by the social movements of the 1960s. Civil rights advocates demanded the expansion of federal programs in their efforts to achieve racial and social equality. One response of the federal government was to create categorical programs that made funding directly available to community-based providers (Davis & Schoen, 1978). This meant federal funding bypassed the sovereign power of the state governments. The community health centers that were funded by the Office of Economic Opportunity are an example of a categorically funded program. In this instance, the federal government contracted directly with healthcare providers for specified services.

In the late 20th century, there was one more shift in the relationship between the federal government and the states. Starting with President Nixon, and affirmed during Reagan's presidency, there has been a push to return authority to the states. Initially called *new federalism*, it involves devolution of authority to the states to define social welfare programs that are funded by the federal government (Anton, 1997). The expressed intent is to permit states to better accommodate their diversity. This is not possible when the federal government is perceived to impose a one-size-fits-all approach to social programs. The use of block grants is the mechanism by which greater discretion has been given to the states to shape programs. The block grants essentially combine funding from several grant-in-aid programs and allow states to determine how the money will be spent to achieve program goals.

The very nature of federalism is that it results in a fragmented system of governance (Steinmo & Watts, 1995). Nowhere is this clearer than in the arenas of social policy and health policy. Laws addressing similar needs are being passed at the federal, state, and local levels. One of the consequences is the fragmentation and duplication of services caused by the different programs that address a particular need. Examples of gaps in services and duplication of services due to the nonalignment of program requirements are easily recognized by those who serve older persons. An individual seeking long-term care is confronted with myriad programs, including Medicare and Medicaid, as well as social service block grants developed under both the Social Security Act and the Older Americans Act. Individuals must navigate this maze of programs to determine their eligibility for services, while providers must to integrate the various funding streams to provide coordinated and comprehensive services.

Fragmentation also impacts the ability to create a program of national health insurance, as evidenced by the problem of insurance regulation, a seemingly obscure problem. States have regulatory authority over insurance, including health insurance, but the Employee Retirement Income Security Act of 1975 supersedes state laws relating to benefit plans. This means businesses that self-insure for employee health as part of their benefits program are exempt from state insurance regulations. The significance of this dual regulatory system is that neither the states nor the federal government can easily mandate employers to offer health benefits because neither governing body has regulatory authority over all businesses in a particular area (Mariner, 1996). Unable to create an employer mandate, the ACA mandated individuals to purchase health insurance

instead. The Supreme Court upheld the constitutionality of the mandate in June 2012 as well as the penalty under the federal government's power to collect taxes (Jost, 2012).

Governmental Intervention

The government has several tools at its disposal to intervene when the market cannot adequately address a problem (Stone, 2012). Among these are taxation, service provision, and regulation. Taxation is often considered the means by which government raises money to support its spending. Medicare Part A is financed by payroll taxes that are paid by employers and employees. Taxation, however, can also be used as a way to influence behavior. Many states place a high tax on the sale of cigarettes to influence personal choices about cigarette use (DeCicca, Kenkel, Mathios, Shin, & Lim, 2008). Higher cigarette taxes have resulted in lower rates of consumption. Likewise, the penalty for not having health insurance under the ACA can be understood as a tax designed to influence behavior. The revenues raised in this way can either be targeted for programs to support the desired behavioral change or contribute to the state's general revenues.

Another tool is the use of government revenues to support service provision. In some cases, the government is the actual provider of services. Public hospitals are locally financed institutions that were organized to serve persons who cannot afford care. The Veterans Health Administration is a comprehensive healthcare system provided by the federal government to men and women who have medical problems resulting from service-related injuries after discharge from the service. Both are socialized medicine in that the programs are managed and provided by government agencies. Alternatively, the government can purchase services from the private sector. Medicaid is an example of such a program. Medicaid enrollees seek services from providers who have contracted with the state government to provide services. These providers bill the government for their services and are reimbursed for the medical care they provide. Such spending is designed to increase access to the market for persons with limited resources. The government can also be a producer and a purchaser of services. This is the case with biomedical research. The National Institutes of Health has a large biomedical research complex that supports numerous researchers. In addition, the National Institutes of Health funds independent researchers at universities and research laboratories across the country.

The purchase of services may also take an indirect form whereby the government subsidizes specific sellers to encourage their participation in markets that might not be competitive based on price. For example, medical education is an extremely costly endeavor (Koenig et al., 2003). Hospitals that train physicians cannot compete on price with nonteaching hospitals given the additional costs incurred for resident and faculty salaries and the additional resources used for each patient seen by a resident. As a result, Medicare assists with physician training by funding the salaries of residents and subsidizing the hospitals where residents are trained. Another example is the orphan drug program (Grabowski, 2005). The government subsidizes pharmaceutical companies to research drugs that are used by a very small number of persons and are therefore not profitable to develop and produce. Through these types of programs, the government offsets what might be the high cost of services or encourages program expansion in specific areas.

A third programmatic tool is government regulation of the market. Regulations are legal restrictions aimed to produce outcomes that otherwise might not occur. Examples of regulation include the licensure of physicians and other healthcare professionals (Grumbach, 2002). These regulations were adopted in the early 20th century as a way to protect the public from practitioners who were not qualified to provide care. Through a series of educational and practice requirements and an examination, states regulate who can and cannot provide medical and healthcare services. Another example of government regulation is state-mandated nursing-to-patient ratios for hospital-based care (Conway, TamaraKonetzka, Zhu, Volpp, & Sochal, 2008). These regulations are designed to protect patients by maintaining a minimum number of nurses in a department at all times.

The Policy-Making Process

Federalism creates the structure within which social policy is made. Federalism, however, does not explain the content of a particular program and how programs are changed over time. The substance is determined by individuals and groups that have an interest in the field, and change occurs as the environment within which health care operates, as well as the power of these groups to shape policy alternatives and influence policy outcomes, rises and falls (M. Smith, 1993). The healthcare field is composed of many players both inside and outside government. There are physicians, nurses, hospital administrators, insurance companies, and on and on. They represent multiple interests, and each one is trying to influence the direction of government policy. The challenge for someone interested in the policy-making process is to understand how these interests are organized and which ones have the most influence in shaping what policy is adopted. In the following section, the major stakeholders or interest groups in the health-care arena are described. This is followed by a more complete discussion of the ways problems are identified and how policy options are articulated based on the problem definition.

Interest Groups

Because health and health care are fundamental to our well-being, it is a sphere of activity that garners everyone's interest. It is possible to speak generally about the public's interest in health care, but the term typically refers to people and organizations that have a stake in an issue and the determination of the solution (Stone, 2012). These groups are generally known and identifiable. They shape the content of health policy making. Figure 2-1 provides a schema for understanding which groups are part of the healthcare delivery system and how their interests can be understood in relationship to one another and the field as a whole. Healthcare providers are most central to the discussion of health policy. They are surrounded by persons who use the healthcare system and by three groups that support the operation of the system: payers, the medical supply industry, and knowledge producers. Although there are stronger and weaker ties among these groups, the impact of each group's actions reverberate throughout the field.

Healthcare providers can broadly be categorized in two groups: clinicians and the organizations where they work. On the clinical side, one can speak about physicians, nurses, and other clinicians and technicians. On the institutional side, there are hospitals and nursing homes, and community-based providers such

as community health centers and physicians' offices. Although it is possible to identify broad categories of interest, none of these groups speaks with a single voice. Physicians as a group are represented by the American Medical Association (AMA); however, the AMA may avoid specific policies because the interests of specialists are at odds with those of primary care physicians. As a result, there are many physician organizations representing unique sets of interests. For example, the American Board of Internal Medicine represents internists. The American College of Surgeons represents practitioners within this medical specialty, and the list goes on. Such divisions can be found within other groups of clinicians. The nursing profession has several lead organizations that often work jointly when addressing issues surrounding health, health care, and nursing practice, but they take independent positions on specific issues such as unionization. These associations include the American Nurses Association, the American Association of Colleges of Nursing, the National League for Nursing, and the American Academy of Nursing. The same holds true for institutional providers. The American Hospital Association is the primary advocacy group for the hospital industry, but public hospitals, academic health centers, and for-profit hospitals each have their own associations: the National Association of Public Hospitals, the Association of American Medical Colleges, and the Federation of American Hospitals, respectively (Fox, 1986).

Healthcare providers are just one set of voices. There are also healthcare consumers. Again, they do not speak in a single voice. There are organizations that advocate for single diseases, such as the American Cancer Society, the American Lung Association, and the National Mental Health Association.

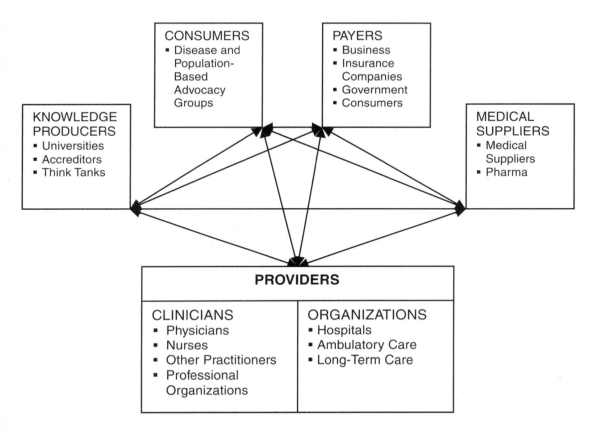

FIGURE 2-1 The health Delivery System policy field

This list also includes other diseases, such as Parkinson's disease, lupus, arthritis, and autism. In some cases, the organizations' concerns are specific to advancing the treatment of a specific illness, and in other cases, their agendas more broadly relate to better financing of a discrete set of services. In addition to disease-specific groups, there are population-based groups that speak on behalf of their membership's need for health services. The largest groups represent women, older persons, the poor, and racial and ethnic minorities: for example, the National Organization for

Women, the American Association of Retired Persons, the National Association for the Advancement of Colored People, the Urban League, and La Raza. Health care is not their primary charge, but it is an important part of each organization's agenda.

Providers depend on revenue to survive. Critical to the system are organizations that pay for the provision of health services. The business community is the prime purchaser of health care through employer-based insurance. A plethora of organizations represent business interests related to health care, including the

U.S. Chamber of Commerce. The business sector typically works in conjunction with insurance companies. The insurance companies are represented by the Health Insurance Association of America. The federal and state governments are also major purchasers of services. The federal government is represented by the Centers for Medicare and Medicaid Services. Organizations such as the National Governors Association represent the interests of state governments. Each of these groups has a concern for the well-being of the population, but each one also has a stake in how health services are financed and reimbursed to reflect its particular set of concerns.

Closely aligned to clinical providers are knowledge producers who are concerned with advancing the science that underpins medical care and establishing and maintaining standards for medical practice. The most obvious are universities and biomedical research organizations. One of the most central organizations is the American Association of Medical Colleges. Beyond the university, there are think tanks that are concerned with the production and dissemination of healthcare research, and associations such as the Institute of Medicine, the Pew Commission, the Kaiser Family Foundation, and the Commonwealth Fund. Such organizations seek to inform the public about the state of health care in this country. Last, there are organizations like The Joint Commission that are concerned with maintaining the standards of medical practice through accreditation, examinations, and licensing.

The last group to consider is the medical supply industry. This sector is assuming a larger role in health policy decisions as technology plays a greater role in the provision of health care. The fastest growing part of this sector is the pharmaceutical industry, which is represented by the Pharmaceutical Research and Manufacturers of America (PhRMA). One must also take into account the growing set of suppliers of medical devices, such as stents and medical equipment like imaging machines. The American healthcare system is known for its technological know-how. The interests of these companies must be taken into account when decisions are made that impact the use of medical devices.

Policy Framework

The term *policy framework* refers to the definition of the problem, the attribution of its causes, and the formulation of policy alternatives by varied interests. This is a more complex task than can be imagined. While there is often agreement as to the problem—for example, the rising number of uninsured individuals in the United States, the rising cost of health care, or the uneven quality of care—agreement as to the causes is far more complex and difficult to achieve.

First, it is hard to ascertain whether problems are the result of intended or unintended actions. Take a natural disaster like Hurricane Sandy in October 2012. It caused tremendous devastation to communities on the East Coast, from Connecticut all the way to southern New Jersey. On the one hand, the region has rarely experienced a hurricane of this magnitude, so Sandy can be described as a natural disaster. On the other hand, environmentalists predicted the increasing occurrence of such storms due to climate change, and policy analysts can point to numerous policies and programs that failed to take into account how extensive the damage might be when such a storm occurred and what steps could be taken to mitigate the negative outcomes.

The second problem with attributing causation is political in nature. Causal models not only explain problems but, more important, justify action. As a number of organizations and individuals interact around a policy issue, causal theories will be used to challenge or protect existing sets of rules. By attributing causation, which is a more positive way of saying assigning blame, it becomes possible to identify who should be responsible for fixing a problem, which may result in redistributing power and resources. Causal theories "have a political life independent of the evidence for them . . . The different sides in an issue act as if they are trying to find the 'true' cause, but they are always struggling to influence which causal story becomes the main guide to policy" (Stone, 2012, p. 207).

Given the difficulty of reaching agreement as to the causes of any problem, it is evident that finding solutions to which all interests can agree can be just as complex. When the causes of a problem can be explained with certainty, there tends to be greater agreement about a solution to turn the situation around. However, that is rarely the case. When multiple alternatives are being proposed, cost–benefit analysis is frequently used to determine which alternative moves the situation closest to the stated policy goals. This alternative should then be identified as the policy solution. Cost–benefit analysis, however, is not always effective at identifying policy solutions. First, it is difficult to account for every factor that impacts complex social phenomena. Second, multiple goals typically underlie any policy alternative. Different policy solutions favor different goals. In the case of healthcare policy, there are trade-offs between controlling costs and ensuring quality. Last is the need to identify policy alternatives that are also politically viable. A policy must have support from interests that play a critical role in the policy process. In the

debates leading up to passage of the ACA, the single-payer option was dropped as a policy alternative because it was not considered politically feasible. Its advocates argued that single payer was the best method to expand access and control costs (Halpin & Harbage, 2010).

The Politics of Decision Making: Interest Group Power and Influence

There are many competing policy alternatives given the number of groups that have interests in the healthcare arena, but choices must be made between them. Because the power of these groups is not equal, some ideas have a greater chance to succeed than others (Bachrach & Baratz, 1962; Smith, 2002). Some groups find themselves struggling to be heard, whereas others have greater access to policy makers, so their proposals have greater credibility. The policies and programs that are most reflective of the strongest interests in the healthcare field have the greatest chance of being taken under consideration (Schnattschneider, 1960). These are the groups that hold the most power within society generally, and the healthcare field specifically. These groups' strength is reflected in their ability to organize, the cohesion of their members, their funding, their expertise on the issue, and their legal status (Howlett & Ramesh, 2003).

The healthcare field has been characterized as being composed of five broad groups of actors. Within each broad group, some players are more powerful than others. Historically, physicians were the dominant group that shaped health policy (Morone, 1995). The power of the AMA was legendary, particularly when discussing the possibility of national health insurance. Power was ceded to the medical profession at the turn of the last century (Freidson, 1970; Starr, 1982). Physicians had a claim to technical expertise that justified their control over the organization and delivery of medical services. Second, their professional authority was extended to state-supported control over the healthcare field. Physicians determined the regulation of medicine through state licensing procedures. Physicians actively advocated against programs, such as national health insurance, that were perceived to undermine their authority by increasing the role of the state to regulate the provision of health services. Later they began to advocate for programs that enhanced their authority, such as the Peer Review Organizations (Starr, 1982).

In addition to physicians, the other centers of power until the 1980s were hospitals and academic medical centers (Tierney, 1987). The advancement of both groups augmented the work of physicians. Their growing strength can be seen post–World War II, when increased pressure was put on the federal government to provide support for health care. The federal government could not intervene directly and support the provision of health services because such proposals were aggressively opposed by physicians as being precursors to socialized medicine. Physicians acceded to government funding of hospital construction and biomedical research spending, which enhanced their ability to practice medicine (Stevens, 1971). The Hill-Burton Act of 1946 made money available to rebuild and expand the deteriorating hospital infrastructure. The federal government also dramatically increased its support for the National Institutes of Health, which became the vehicle for funding biomedical research at the universities where doctors trained (Daniels, 1971).

The balance of power among these groups is not constant. A shift began to occur in the 1980s due to a convergence of several factors. Most important was the increasing cost of health care. Healthcare expenditures rose from 5.1% of the gross domestic product (GDP) in 1960 to 9.1% by 1980 (Centers for Medicare and Medicaid Services, 2008). With the country in an economic downturn, the rising healthcare costs put pressure on payer groups to find solutions to the problem of rising costs. Second, the government was fast becoming one of the largest payers of health services, with the growth of the Medicare and Medicaid programs. A third trend was the growing corporatization of the healthcare field (Relman, 1980; Starr, 1982). The growth of for-profit facilities and multifacility corporations shifted institutional goals away from public benefit toward more narrow concerns for financial profitability. Finally, technology and demographic trends pointed to ever-increasing costs caused by the rate of medical innovation and the aging of the population that required increased services (Bodenheimer, 2005).

The growing complexity of the healthcare system led to its transformation from a physician-dominated system to a finance-driven system (Starr, 1982). When the issue was recast as one of constraining costs, professional expertise was no longer the critical skill needed to resolve the problem. Doctors' ability to influence and direct the organization and delivery of care began to give way to the administrators of the system, including third-party payers. These groups were in a better position to control the cost of care by creating financial incentives to influence physician practice patterns. By the 1990s, authority over health policy had shifted toward the payers of health services (Weissert & Weissert, 2012). These include big business, the insurance companies that are represented by the Health Insurance Association of America, and, increasingly, the federal and state governments.

The challenge to physician dominance is not limited to the financial sector of the industry. Patients are also advocating for greater autonomy and sovereignty over the decisions that affect their health (Schneider, 1998). They want to demystify the role of physicians and become active participants in their own care. Patients' loss of trust in the medical profession is manifest in many ways (Mechanic, 1996). Among these are the courts that offer recourse to care that is found negligent. The number of malpractice suits began rising in the 1980s, which led to a crisis of sorts related to the cost and availability of malpractice insurance (Studdert, Mello, & Brenna, 2004). As early as 2003, several physician groups responded with a joint statement on medical professionalism that reaffirmed the importance of the patient–physician relationship being defined by integrity, respect, and compassion (American Board of Internal Medicine, 2002).

Recently, nurses and other health professionals have found themselves with greater authority and are leading several policy-related discussions. The healthcare labor force is described as a pyramid, with physicians at the apex directing all related medical practice. As a result, nurses and other health professionals take instruction from doctors for matters related to direct patient care (Gordon, 2005). As the provision of care becomes increasingly complex, alternative practitioners have begun to seek professional status and the right to independent practice. Research demonstrates that they provided care comparable to, or of higher quality than, their physician counterparts (R. P. Newhouse et al., 2011). These practitioners are capable of providing quality care

at a lower cost. They offer a cost-effective alternative to physicians. Professional associations of groups, such as physical therapists and nurse practitioners, are lobbying on a state-by-state basis to change licensing laws so these clinicians can practice independently and receive direct reimbursement for their services. Such laws create an alternative center of authority.

Agenda Setting

The objective conditions, or what might be called the actual problem, are the necessary foundation for a social policy idea to succeed but are not a sufficient one. The first step is for an idea to become part of the public agenda. National health insurance is an interesting case study because it has moved on and off the public agenda since the early 20th century (Cairl & Imershein, 1977; Oberlander, 2010; Skocpol, 1995; Steinmo & Watts, 1995). It was not until President Obama's administration that Congress finally acted and passed the ACA in 2010.

Explaining the passage of the ACA provides insight into how advocates can advance their own causes. Several explanations can be offered as to why Congress finally passed a program to reform the healthcare system. On the one hand, problems with the healthcare system related to rising costs and the growing number of uninsured people were slowly threatening the stability of the healthcare system. As it was organized, the system could not be sustained. Changes were required to the financing and the organization of care. As a result, health reform required the support of powerful interest groups, such as the insurance industry, small businesses, and the hospital sector. Their support was obtained by making concessions to their varied interests (Oberlander, 2010). For example, the ACA relies on the private insurance market for coordinating the financing of care.

On the other hand, the problems that were threatening the stability of a system have been part of the national dialogue. This makes it important to explain why they became elevated at a particular point in time (Peterson, 1993). In some instances, there are triggering events, such as Hurricane Katrina. Many public health issues that had been ignored before the hurricane, such as emergency preparedness, were suddenly perceived as needing immediate action (Fee & Brown, 2002). Interest groups have many tools to advance their policy agenda. They can lobby and advocate for their interests by meeting with legislators and corporate executives or organizing conferences to inform policy makers and the public about a particular issue. Political action is another means to build consensus about the need for action. Whether on the National Mall or at a corporate headquarters, demonstrations are intended to be a show of support for a set of issues and thus pressure legislatures to act. Interest groups can also use the courts to advance their cause. The series of lawsuits brought against tobacco companies in the 1990s led them to seek a compromise with the government that would provide liability protection in exchange for greater regulation (Pertschuk, 2001). Persons in political power can also put issues on the public agenda. Legislators are known to advance particular interests. Harrison Wofford's special run in 1991 for U.S. senator from Pennsylvania was framed by a single issue: national health insurance. This put the issue back on the agenda after a hiatus of almost 20 years. The president also sets the agenda each year at the State of the Union address. This was the case for President Obama, who chose to make healthcare reform one of the central issues of his first term.

An even more nuanced explanation for why the ACA was passed in 2010 might be found in the convergence of three particular factors (Kingdon, 1995). The problems by this time were well defined. This was followed by the development of policy alternatives that had broad-based agreement from powerful healthcare interests. The third factor was the politics of the time. The president's campaign had been framed by the ideas of hope and change. Given the crash of the financial markets, people were looking for some assurances about the well-being of the country. There was a Democratic majority in the House and the Senate that could ensure passage of the legislation with or without partisan support. Despite opposition, President Obama moved ahead in a relatively expeditious way.

Policy Adoption

Policy is enacted through the legislative process. Elected officials decide the broad outlines of policy when they enact laws. Legislators do not act in isolation. There are many centers of power both inside and outside government that try to influence their decision-making process. Interest groups typically work on their own behalf when issues are quite specific. They form coalitions when the issues are more general. Multiple positions are typically advocated at the same time (Weissert & Weissert, 2012). As a result, legislators usually seek a middle ground that is responsive to these competing interests (D. G. Smith, 2002). When looking for this middle ground, two of the most important considerations are a proposal's technical feasibility and its acceptability among different political constituencies (Kingdon, 1995; Tierney, 1987). Legislators are often looking for programs that are small and limited in scope because implementation is not as difficult to achieve and the programs are more likely to succeed. As proposed programs become more complex and impact more groups, developing legislation that is acceptable to all the involved parties becomes more difficult (Morone, 1995). In these cases, legislators look for proposals around which they can build public support. Such proposals have often been termed *safe*. This means legislators are seeking to adjust existing programs rather than proposing fundamental change to the status quo (Bachrach & Baratz, 1962).

There are exceptional moments when programs disrupt existing social relations that define the organization and delivery of services. The passage of Medicare and Medicaid in 1965 and the Affordable Care Act in 2010 are the most notable examples in the healthcare field. These programs sought to redistribute control over access to healthcare resources. Even such major pieces of legislation are rooted in past programs and were shaped in response to existing political interests, which makes the distinction difficult to determine (Weissert & Weissert, 2012). Medicare succeeded in making health insurance available to persons older than age 65, but the legislation must also be understood as an extension of the existing healthcare system. The hospitals supported Part A because charges would be determined retrospectively based on actual costs, and they would receive reimbursement for persons who previously had trouble paying for hospital care. Physicians and the AMA, as well as the Republicans, supported Part B because it was voluntary and did not create a broader precedent for the government provision of care. The insurance companies supported Medicare because they would be responsible for claims administration. For Democrats, Medicare was a social insurance program that set a precedent for government-provided universal coverage (Marmor, 1973).

Likewise, the ACA can be understood as being both disruptive to and an extension of existing policies and programs. On one hand, it is not a program of national health insurance. The ACA extends access to private health insurance and government-funded health programs to a greater number of people. Initial estimates were that 30–33 million people who were previously uninsured would have health insurance (Congressional Budget Office, 2012). But the percentage of uninsured people will remain as high as 31% given the Supreme Court's ruling that the Medicaid expansion is a state option. This undermined the section of the law that guaranteed insurance to all persons up to 138% of the poverty level (Nardin, Zallman, McCormick, Woolhandler, & Himmelstein, 2013). The ACA also has disruptive elements. Structural changes, such as the expansion of Accountable Care Organizations under the Medicare provisions and revised payment methodologies, have the potential, over time, to transform how care is structured in the United States and, as a result, its cost and quality (Marmor, 2012).

Implementation

Policy implementation is a continuation of the politics of policy creation in the administrative arena and cannot be divorced from the policy-making process. Legislation provides the broadest possible outline of a program. The specificity of the law determines the flexibility that the administration has in its implementation (Lowi, 1979). Congress can attempt to be specific in its formulation of programs to control the actions of a possibly hostile administration, or Congress can choose to leave the details of implementation to the administering agency. There are advantages and disadvantages to both choices. A bill in which details are clearly specified may encounter difficulty in Congress because groups may oppose the particulars instead of the overarching goals. President Clinton's health insurance plan was a victim of this approach (Brady & Buckley, 1995). A consensus can be more easily built around a law with broad goals and few details (Stone, 2012). In that case, decisions about implementation are left to the administering agencies.

Program implementation is the responsibility of the federal or state executive branch and its administrative agencies. At the federal level, the Department of Health and Human Services has responsibility for the administration of programs created by Congress (Pressman & Wildavsky, 1973). Implementation can be difficult because the abstract agreements made during the legislative process often fall apart if underlying conflicts have not been resolved. This makes the administrative leadership and organizational capacity of administrative agencies even more important. How an agency chooses to implement the program can have tremendous influence on its outcome (Jacobson & Wasserman, 1999; Morone, 1995; Pressman & Wildavsky, 1973). The leadership of the agency must be in accord with the program's goals so it does not languish, and the personnel must have program expertise to implement it effectively. Implementation of the Medicaid expansion under the ACA is a case in point. States have control over whether they will participate. At the present time, 19 states have opted out, which will leave many more persons uninsured than if these states had participated (Commonwealth Fund, 2014).

Administrative agencies do not work in a vacuum. As in the case of the legislative process, organized interests that are instrumental in mobilizing and building support for policies throughout the legislative process play a comparable role during its implementation. They work with the administrative agencies to ensure that implementation meets their interests by monitoring the process (Pressman & Wildavsky, 1973). Agency staff also develop a stake in the programs they oversee (Peterson, 1993). As they become expert in a given field, they become influential in the policy-making process. It is not atypical for government employees to work with advocacy groups and Congressional committees to advance their program's interests. Given their expertise in a given field, the situation exists where professionals move between these sectors—sometimes working for the government and sometimes working in the private or nonprofit sectors.

Healthcare professionals and their patients experience the impact of the implementation process on a daily basis. How patients are recruited to programs such as Medicare Part D, and now the insurance exchanges, is determined by the regulations of these programs. Which companies offer health plans, and the scope of these plans, under the newly formed exchanges is a result of program guidelines. The same is true for the nurse-to-patient ratios specified in the laws of California or the limit on the hours that medical residents can work in New York state hospitals (which came about in response to a patient's death in a city hospital). These are all examples of programs that were developed by federal or state legislatures and implemented by federal and state administering agencies. Although their work is seemingly distant, its impact is immediate in terms of access to quality health care.

At times, programs do not achieve their stated goals. There are often unintended consequences of any legislative act. The Medicare

Advantage Program, which was created in 1998, was assumed to be a way to control Medicare spending by offering beneficiaries a managed care option. As implemented, however, the program resulted in higher costs than would have occurred if patients had remained in the traditional Medicare program. This was the result of the payment methodology that reimbursed plans at average cost, while programs enrolled beneficiaries whose costs were below average. What makes this important is that the proposed solutions in one time period set up the problems that need be addressed in the next. In the case of the Medicare Advantage Program, the federal government moved to a system of risk adjustment payments (J. P. Newhouse, Price, Huang, McWilliams, & Hsu, 2012). Thus, the policy cycle is never-ending.

What Is at Stake for Nurses and Other Health Professionals?

The work of nurses and other health professionals tends to be highly individualized. By interacting with patients, they see the many problems that result from policy decisions made at a distance. They understand how physicians' orientation toward care can overrule nurses' orientation toward care (Glouberman & Mintzberg, 2001). They observe how the loss of healthcare insurance can result in patients deferring care, much to their detriment. They understand that the pursuit of quality patient care is dependent on their ability to engage and use nursing resources effectively, which will likely become more challenging as the nursing shortage persists and resources become increasingly limited (Rother & Lavizzo-Mourey, 2009).

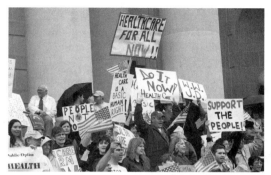

© Samuel Perry/Shutterstock, Inc.

In many cases, these professionals become the patients' advocates, but historically they have not played a major role in the initial development of the policies that have such a tremendous impact on their work and on the lives of their patients. Some have attributed this to heavy workloads. Others have discussed the educational process that socializes nurses to distance themselves from politics. Still others speak about the difficulty nurses have in asserting their professional authority when they find themselves up against dominant interests, such as physician groups, hospitals, and payers. Regardless of the cause, there is now a growing concern that nurses and other health professionals need to assert a greater voice in the policy-making process (Needleman & Hassmiller, 2009; Thomas & While, 2007; Wolf & Greenhouse, 2007).

By understanding the process and how it has shaped the organization and delivery of health care, it is possible to understand the terms of engagement. Since the 1990s, the market has been assumed to bring greater efficiency to the organization and delivery of health care. It is the failure of this approach that reinvigorates interest in its politics. We know that health costs are rising, that insurance coverage is problematic, and that quality can suffer despite the best efforts of healthcare providers. The critical challenge is determining how health care should be organized and delivered to ensure the best possible health outcomes for the population. The stresses that ordinary Americans experience are often evidenced in the healthcare arena through even greater numbers of persons, some who are seeking care and others who are delaying or forgoing care. Determining what will be the trade-offs between access, costs, and quality will impact the situation that nurses and other professionals confront every day. Nurses and other healthcare providers need to become one of the dominant voices in the policy-making and policy-implementation process if the healthcare system is to best meet the needs of the people it serves.

Discussion Questions

1. What are the limits of the market in the provision of health services?
2. Explain what is meant by the concept that policy can be paradoxical or ambiguous.
3. Why does the federalist system of government result in the fragmentation of healthcare delivery?
4. What interest groups are dominant in the current health policy debates?
5. Why are policy alternatives political in nature?
6. What makes implementation as important to the understanding of policy as the legislated programs?

References

American Board of Internal Medicine. (2002). Medical professionalism in the new millennium: A physician charter. *Annals of Internal Medicine, 136,* 243–246.

Andrulis, D. P., & Siddiqui, N. J. (2011). Health reform holds both risks and rewards for safety-net providers and racially and ethnically diverse patients. *Health Affairs, 30*(10), 1830–1836.

Anton, T. (1997). New federalism and intergovernmental fiscal relationships: The implications for health policy. *Journal of Health Politics Policy and Law, 22*(3), 691–720.

Arrow, K. J. (1963). Uncertainty and the welfare economics of medical care. *The American Economic Review, 53*(5), 941–974.

Arrow, K. J. (1974). *The limits of organization.* New York, NY: W. W. Norton.

Bachrach, P., & Baratz, M. (1962). Two faces of power. *American Political Science Review, 56,* 4632–4642.

Bodenheimer, T. (2005). High and rising health care costs. Part 2: Technologic innovation. *Annals of Internal Medicine, 142,* 932–937.

Bovbjerg, R., Wiener, J., & Housman, M. (2003). State and federal roles in health care: Rationales for allocating responsibilities. In J. Holahan, A. Weil, & J. Wiener (Eds.), *Federalism and Health Policy* (Vol. 3, pp. 25–51). Washington, DC: Urban Institute Press.

Brady, D. W., & Buckley, K. M. (1995). Health care reform in the 103d Congress: A predictable failure. *Journal of Health Politics Policy and Law, 20,* 447–454.

Brown, L. D., & Sparer, M. S. (2003). Poor program's progress: The unanticipated politics of Medicaid policy. *Health Affairs, 22*(1), 31–44.

Cairl, R., & Imershein, A. (1977). National health insurance policy in the United States: A case of non-decision-making. *International Journal of Health Services, 7*(2), 167–178.

Centers for Medicare and Medicaid Services. (2008). *National health expenditures. Aggregate and per capita amounts, annual percent change and percent distribution. Selected calendar years 1960–2012.* Retrieved from http://www.cms.hhs.gov/NationalHealthExpendData/downloads/tables.pdf

Cesca, B. (2009). *Keep your goddamn government hands off my Medicare!* Retrieved from http://www.huffingtonpost.com/bob-cesca/get-your-goddamn-governme_b_252326.html

Commonwealth Fund. (2014). *State participation in the Affordable Care Act's expansion of Medicaid eligibility.* Retrieved from http://www.commonwealthfund.org/Maps-and-Data/Medicaid-Expansion-Map.aspx

Congressional Budget Office. (2012). *Updated estimates for the insurance coverage provisions of the Affordable Care Act.* Retrieved from www.cbo.gov/sites/default/files/cbofiles/attachments/03-13-Coverage%20Estimates.pdf

Conlan, T. (2006). From cooperative to opportunistic federalism: Reflections on the half-century anniversary of the commission on intergovernmental relations. *Public Administration Review, 66,* 663–676.

Conway, P. H., TamaraKonetzka, R., Zhu, J., Volpp, K. G., & Sochal, J. (2008). Nurse staffing ratios: Trends and policy implications for hospitalists and the safety net. *Journal of Hospital Medicine, 3*(3), 193–199.

Daniels, G. H. (1971). *Science in American society: A social history.* New York, NY: Alfred Knopf.

Davis, K., & Schoen, C. (1978). *Health and the war on poverty: A ten year appraisal.* Washington, DC: Brookings Institution.

DeCicca, P., Kenkel, D., Mathios, A., Shin, Y. J., & Lim, J. Y. (2008). Youth smoking, cigarette prices, and anti-smoking sentiment. *Health Economics, 17,* 733–749.

Eibner, C., Goldman, D. P., Sullivan, J., & Garber, A. M. (2013). Three large-scale changes to the Medicare program could curb its costs but also reduce enrollment. *Health Affairs, 32*(5), 891–898.

Fee, E., & Brown, T. M. (2002). The unfulfilled promise of public health: Déjà vu all over again. *Health Affairs, 21*(6), 31–43.

Fox, D. (1986). The consequences of consensus: American health policy in the twentieth century. *The Milbank Quarterly, 64,* 176–199.

Freidson, E. (1970). *Profession of medicine: A study of the sociology of applied knowledge.* New York, NY: Dodd, Mead.

Glouberman, S., & Mintzberg, H. (2001). Managing the care of health and the cure of disease: Part I: Differentiation. *Health Care Management Review, 26*(1), 56–69.

Gordon, S. (2005). *Nursing against the odds: How health care cost cutting, media stereotypes, and medical hubris undermine nurses and patient care (the culture and politics of health care work).* Ithaca, NY: Cornell University Press.

Grabowski, H. (2005). Encouraging the development of new vaccines. *Health Affairs, 24*(3), 697–700.

Grumbach, K. (2002). Fighting hand to hand over physician workforce policy: The invisible hand of the market meets the heavy hand of government planning. *Health Affairs, 32*(5), 13–27.

Halpin, H. A., & Harbage, P. (2010). The origins and demise of the public option. *Health Affairs, 29*(6), 1117–1123.

Holahan, J. (2011). The 2007–09 recession and health insurance coverage. *Health Affairs, 30*(1), 145–152.

Howlett, M., & Ramesh, M. (2003). *Studying public policy: Policy cycles and policy subsystems.* Toronto, Canada: Oxford University Press.

Jacobson, P., & Wasserman, J. (1999). The implementation and enforcement of tobacco control laws: Policy implications for activists and the industry. *Journal of Health Politics Policy and Law, 24,* 567–598.

Jimmy Kimmel Live. (2013). *Six of one— Obamacare vs. the Affordable Care Act* [video]. Retrieved from http://www.youtube.com/watch?v=sx2scvlFGjE

Jost, T. S. (2012). The Affordable Care Act largely survives the Supreme Court's scrutiny—but barely. *Health Affairs*, *31*(8), 1659–1662.

Kernell, S., & Jacobson, G. C. (2006). *The logic of American politics* (3rd ed.). Washington, DC: CQ Press.

Kingdon, J. W. (1995). *Agendas, alternatives, and public policies*. New York, NY: Harper Collins College.

Knowles, J. H. (1977). The responsibility of the individual. In J. H. Knowles (Ed.), *Doing better and feeling worse: Health in the United States*. Cambridge, MA: American Academy of Arts and Sciences.

Koenig, L., Dobson, A., Silver, H., Jonathan, M., Siegel, J. M., Blumenthal, D., & Weissman, J. S. (2003). Estimating the mission-related costs of teaching hospitals. *Health Affairs*, *22*(6), 112–122.

Lowi, T. (1979). *The end of liberalism: Ideology, policy, and the crisis of public authority* (2nd ed.). New York, NY: Norton.

Lowi, T., & Ginsberg, B. (1998). *American government* (5th ed.). New York, NY: Norton.

Mariner, W. (1996). State regulation of managed care and the Employee Retirement Income Security Act. *New England Journal of Medicine*, *335*, 1986–1990.

Marmor, T. (1973). *The politics of Medicare*. Chicago, IL: Aldine.

Marmor, T. (2012). The rough politics of reforming health care. *Health Affairs*, *31*(5), 1121–1122.

Mechanic, D. (1996). Changing medical organization and the erosion of trust. *The Milbank Quarterly*, *74*(2), 171–189.

Midgley, J., & Livermore, M. (Eds.). (2008). *The handbook of social policy*. Los Angeles, CA: Sage.

Morone, J. (1995). Elusive community: Democracy, deliberation, and the reconstruction of health policy. In M. Landy & M. Levin (Eds.), *The new politics of public policy* (pp. 180–204). Baltimore, MD: Johns Hopkins University Press.

Nardin, R., Zallman, L., McCormick, D., Woolhandler, S., & Himmelstein, D. (2013). *The uninsured after implementation of the Affordable Care Act: A demographic and geographic analysis*. Retrieved from http://healthaffairs.org/blog/2013/06/06/the-uninsured-after-implementation-of-the-affordable-care-act-a-demographic-and-geographic-analysis/

Needleman, J., & Hassmiller, S. (2009). The role of nurses in improving hospital quality and efficiency: Real-world results. *Health Affairs*, *28*(4), w625–w633.

Newhouse, J. P., Price, M., Huang, J., McWilliams, J. M., & Hsu, J. (2012). Steps to reduce favorable risk selection in Medicare Advantage largely succeeded, boding well for health insurance exchanges. *Health Affairs*, *31*(12), 2618–2626.

Newhouse, R. P., Stanik-Hutt, J., White, K. M., Johantgen, M., Bass, E. B., Zangaro, G., . . . Weiner, J. P. (2011). Advanced practice nurse outcomes 1990–2008: A systematic review. *Nursing Economic$*, *29*(5). Retrieved from https://www.nursingeconomics.net/ce/2013/article3001021.pdf

Oberlander, J. (2010). Long time coming: Why health reform finally passed. *Health Affairs*, *29*(6), 1112–1116.

Pertschuk, M. (2001). *Smoke in their eyes: Lessons in movement leadership from the tobacco wars*. Nashville, TN: Vanderbilt University Press.

Peterson, M. A. (1993). Political influence in the 1990s: From iron triangles to policy networks. *Journal of Health Politics, Policy and Law*, *18*, 395–436.

Pressman, J. L., & Wildavsky, A. (1973). *Implementation*. Berkeley: University of California Press.

Relman, A. S. (1980). The new medical–industrial complex. *New England Journal of Medicine*, *303*, 963–970.

Rother, J., & Lavizzo-Mourey, R. (2009). Addressing the nursing workforce: A critical element for health reform. *Health Affairs*, *28*(4), w620–w624.

Rothman, D. J. (1971). *The discovery of the asylum: Social order and disorder in the New Republic*. Boston, MA: Little, Brown.

Schnattschneider, E. E. (1960). *The semisovereign people: A realist's view of democracy in America*. New York, NY: Holt, Rinehart, and Winston.

Schneider, C. E. (1998). *The practice of autonomy: Patients, doctors, and medical decisions*. New York, NY: Oxford University Press.

Skocpol, T. (1995). *Boomerang: Clinton's health security effort and the turn against government in US politics*. New York, NY: W. W. Norton.

Smith, D. G. (2002). *Entitlement politics: Medicare and Medicaid 1995–2001*. New York, NY: Aldine de Gruyter.

Smith, M. (1993). *Pressure, power, and policy: State autonomy and policy networks in Britain and the United States*. Pittsburgh, PA: University of Pittsburgh Press.

Starr, P. (1982). *The social transformation of American medicine*. New York, NY: Basic Books.

Steinmo, S., & Watts, J. (1995). It's the institutions, stupid! Why comprehensive national health insurance always fails in America. *Journal of Health Politics, Policy and Law, 20*, 329–372.

Steuerle, C. E., & Bovbjerg, R. R. (2008). Health and budget reform as handmaidens. *Health Affairs, 27*, 633–644.

Stevens, R. (1971). *American medicine in the public interest*. New Haven, CT: Yale University Press.

Stone, D. (2012). *Policy paradox: The art of political decision making* (3rd ed.). New York, NY: W. W. Norton.

Studdert, D. M., Mello, M. M., & Brenna, T. A. (2004). Medical malpractice. *New England Journal of Medicine, 350*, 283–292.

Thomas, P., & While, A. (2007). Should nurses be leaders of integrated health care? *Journal of Nursing Management, 15*, 643–648.

Tierney, J. (1987). Organized interests in health politics and policy-making. *Medical Care Review, 44*(1), 89–118.

Weissert, W. G., & Weissert, C. S. (2012). *Governing health: The politics of health policy* (4th ed.). Baltimore, MD: Johns Hopkins University Press.

Wolf, G. A., & Greenhouse, P. K. (2007). Blueprint for design: Creating models that direct change. *Journal of Nursing Administration, 37*, 9381–9387.

CHAPTER 3

A Policy Toolkit for Healthcare Providers and Activists

Roby Robertson and Donna Middaugh

Overview

What is the role of healthcare professionals in the political process? Given the range of issues, where does the political process begin and end? Healthcare policy is centered on the notion that all healthcare providers require a fundamental understanding of the healthcare system that is not limited to the knowledge required to practice their discipline. No longer can healthcare professionals be prepared solely for clinical practice. They must ready themselves to deal with the economic, political, and policy dimensions of health care because the services they provide are the outcome of these dynamics.

Objectives

- Define the role of healthcare professionals in policy advocacy and politics.
- Describe processes for becoming a policy advocate within one's own organization, profession, and community.
- Recognize the difference between expertise and internal and external advocacy in relation to stakeholders.
- Apply the concepts of health policy to case study vignettes.
- Develop one's own toolkit for becoming a health policy advocate.

Professional nurses and other allied health practitioners must have a seat at the policy table, but they must also understand the perspectives of their colleagues; therefore, we have used contributors from outside nursing, including allied health professionals, activists, politicians, economists, and policy analysts who understand the forces of health care in America. The rationale behind an interdisciplinary approach is that no one person has the right solution to the challenges confronting health care in America. These challenges include high costs, limited access, medical errors, variable quality, administrative inefficiencies, and a lack of coordination.

It is not surprising that the healthcare system is under serious stress and that a host of actors both within and beyond the system have myriad solutions to the problem. This text offers current and future healthcare practitioners who are committed to reducing health disparities and achieving healthcare equality insight into how clinical practice is derived from regulations and laws that are based on public policy and politics. This chapter suggests that politics is both necessary and critical to making changes, whether we are discussing system-level reforms (e.g., national health insurance reform) or a local hospital improving health data access (e.g., electronic medical records).

This chapter provides healthcare practitioners a toolkit, or a working model, of how to "do" policy advocacy within and beyond our organizational lines. The toolkit is based on the ability to answer these questions: What is the health professional's role in policy advocacy and politics? What are the major distinctions in affecting policy through the two primary areas addressed in this text? This chapter examines two broad components of policy change: the influence and power of stakeholders or constituencies, and the power of expertise. Although these arenas overlap, here we examine them separately to portray their specific roles more accurately.

What, then, is the healthcare practitioner's role in the political process? Where does that process take place? In this chapter, we examine the dynamics of the process. Many traditional views define the political process as external only, primarily defined at the policy-making levels of government or boards and commissions; therefore, the argument follows that professionals below senior-level decision makers are primarily reactive; that is, they respond to proposals from up the line and must calculate how to implement changes that others have imposed on them.

In public administration, this has traditionally been defined as a politics/administration dichotomy; that is, political decisions are made by higher-ups, and the administrator finds a way to carry out those decisions. That dichotomy, however, is not reflective of reality because in actual decision making and in the practicalities of day-to-day management, policy shaping and implementation within a given organization are the result of interactions at all levels of the organization. The administrators are trying to influence policy outcomes, like those in the policy arena. It is time that practitioners do the same.

There is another reason why practitioners must develop a political/policy toolkit. Politics and policy making are not a function only of the external environment of the organization. In fact, the most sophisticated and nuanced elements of such a policy/political role can also be found in the internal environment of the organization. Again, practitioners can play a role in influencing these outcomes.

Imagine the following scenario: Your senior executive pulls you aside one day and says, "Do you know that proposal you've wanted to push forward about how we reallocate the staff here in the organization? Well, why don't you put together the budget, a time line, and what we need to do to move this forward in the next budget cycle?" You have been anxious to do so for some time, and you stay in the office every evening detailing the proposal (with fancy pie charts, a time line, personnel requirements, etc.), and you turn it in to your executive.

A week goes by, and then two, then three. You are getting anxious; to start some of the time line issues, you would need to get rolling soon, but you've heard nothing. You mention it to the executive and she nods, looks solemn, and asks you back into the office. She sits on the edge of the desk (not behind the desk, not a good sign) and pulls out your proposal. You can see it has lots of red marks throughout. The executive shakes her head and says, "Well it really is a great idea; it really is the way to go in the future, but I ran it up the line, and well, you know, politics got in the way. It's just not going to fly!" She hands back your proposal. You return to your office and open the file cabinet of other projects that didn't get off the ground, and you think, politics!

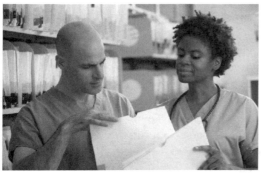

© Medioimages/Photodisc/Thinkstock

Why didn't it fly? What could have happened? Senior managers did not like the proposal? It competed with other proposed

changes that could fly. What kept yours from flying? Perhaps it was because you had not accounted for the politics of your own organization. Politics exist at the organizational level, not just at the policy-making level, and you did not take into account those considerations. Thus, our approach in this chapter suggests that the politics of the environment are both external and internal.

We suggest that the key to gaining more effective use of the policy environment, both inside and outside the organization, is to understand more effectively the power that one has to effect change. Unlike many analyses of power that are often based on the individual, our approach is to examine the organizational power that exists for the practitioner/advocate. We examine that power through two broad lenses: the power of stakeholder relationships and the power of expertise.

Figure 3-1 is a simple heuristic about power. This pyramid has been widely used in political science and policy fields for years. Power can be seen in the levels of the pyramid, with the narrowest (and thus the weakest) type of power at the top of the pyramid. It becomes broader with more effective types of power. The power to make others do things is obvious, from the actual use of force (including weapons) through the more common use of force in an organization, which is the power of the organization to enforce rules, standards, and practices. Influence is more nuanced, but its role is also obvious. Does the organization have the capacity to convince others that they should support or acquiesce to the organization's decision? There are many reasons an organization may be able to influence a decision. Possibly the organization has shown the capacity to be successful; maybe the organization has demonstrated knowledge or connections to accomplish the

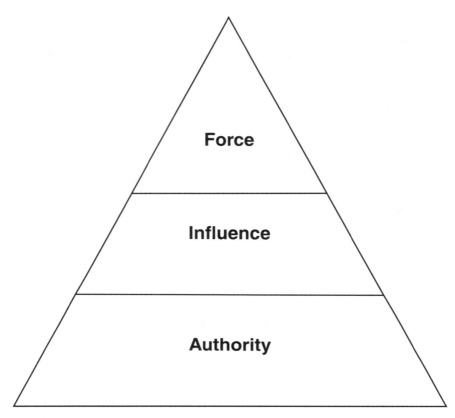

FIGURE 3-1 The power pyramid

required tasks. Nevertheless, the organization must convince others that its decisions are good. Finally, the broadest and most critical part of the pyramid is authority. At the core of a lot of political theory is authority—the acceptance of the organization to decide and the acceptance by others of its decisions without serious question. Expertise is one form of authority. It is clear that in some situations the expertise of the organization, its professionals, or the policy implementation of that expertise is simply accepted—but that is not always true!

One example of how all three elements of the power triangle work is when you are driving

your car late at night and you stop at a red light with nobody around. There you sit because a light bulb with a red cover is on. Now, that is power! Do you recognize why you stopped? Did you have to be convinced? (Maybe you think for a second that lights regulate traffic, but it is the middle of the night and there are no cars around.) You do not run the light right away because you first look around to see if there is a police car around. Now all three elements are in play. You stopped at the light in the first place because it turned red, and you stop at red lights.

Thus, how do we understand our power in organizations? There are multiple elements—from the regulatory environment, the level of federalism, the growth of the state, and so forth. Here we summarize two broad elements that undergird the organization's power: stakeholders and expertise. We are going to distinguish between internal and external power (power within the organization and beyond) (see Figure 3-2).

Stakeholder Power

For many in the healthcare arena, stakeholder power is the most obvious political tool. A simple "who do you know, who is on our side" model of developing policy change is obvious. Too often, however, our approach is to simply add up the influential players on our side and the other side. The stakeholder list becomes a roster of names rather than the nature of power relationships. If it is just a matter of numbers, any policy that is supported by a greater number of individuals or organizations should prevail. Under those conditions, we would suggest that a national health system that is effective for the poor would be the easiest to pass, but we know that organizations representing low-income groups have less influence than those representing high-income groups. It therefore cannot be just numbers!

Stakeholder analysis is tied to the network of stakeholders, and which sets of stakeholders are closer to your organization and which are more

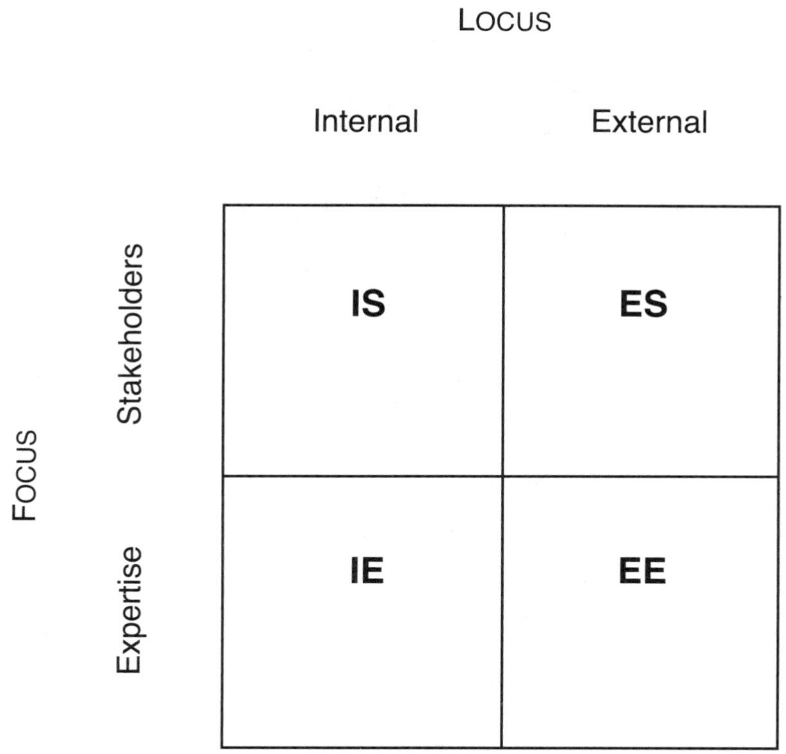

LOCUS

	Internal	External
Stakeholders	IS	ES
Expertise	IE	EE

FOCUS

FIGURE 3-2 Focus and locus of organizational power

distant. This close/distant issue is often defined in terms of natural and face-to-face relationships—ideally, which groups deal with your agency or policy arena on a routine, constant basis and which groups deal with your organization on a more limited basis. Thus, the classic stakeholder map often has concentric circles of groups and organizations that are closer and further away from the organization based on the level of interdependence and organizational closeness (Fottler, Blair, Whitehead, Laus, & Savage, 1989). If you represent a veterans' hospital,

for example, members of veterans' organizations, such as the American Legion or Veterans of Foreign Wars, are more central to your organization, but if you are working at a children's hospital, that organizational tie is irrelevant. Thus, understanding how central other stakeholders are to the organization may be the first part of a stakeholder analysis (Figure 3-3).

To understand stakeholder power for an organization, one must define it in terms of organized stakeholders. When working with various healthcare organizations, we often hear

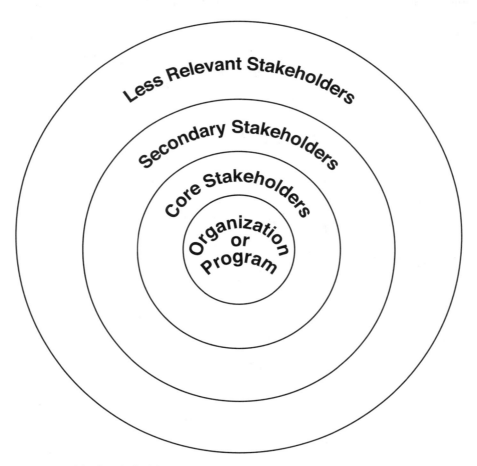

FIGURE 3-3 Simplified stakeholder map.

stakeholders described in individual terms (e.g., patients or customers), but the key is to recognize the importance of having stakeholders who are organized and have well-defined structures. For example, *veterans* is a vague definition for a set of stakeholders, but the American Legion or Veterans of Foreign Wars are two critical organized groups that represent veterans.

What if there is no organized set of stakeholders? The first question might be, why is that true? Perhaps the stakeholders in the external environment that your organization deals with are too amorphous to be defined. In James Q. Wilson's (1989) terminology, you may represent a majoritarian organization that has no discernible set of constituents or stakeholders other than the public. If that is the case, stakeholder power will be more limited for your organization. At the other end of Wilson's stakeholder organizational model are client agencies whose power is defined heavily through a strong relationship with a single client group. In those cases, the organizations must seek to avoid being captured by that single clientele group (Wilson, 1989).

However, we have found that many organizations have developed stakeholder groups over time (often for nonpolitical reasons), which generates some level of influence. One of our favorite examples comes from outside the healthcare arena—police departments. If one thinks about natural constituents or stakeholders, a police department's most obvious stakeholders are those who commit crimes—we are not sure how to build a stakeholder group there! Over time, police departments have developed a host of support organizations, including neighborhood watch groups. The reason they are created is not to influence political decisions about police departments, but strong neighborhood watch groups (organized across a city)

can become a critical secondary stakeholder group for a police department. Who organized those neighborhood watches? Generally, police departments took the lead and the neighborhood watch groups typically support what is being proposed by the police department.

The example of a children's hospital is appropriate here. One might argue that on a day-to-day basis, the constituents of such a hospital are the patients. They are children, but maybe we would include the parents. What about parent groups? Generally, they have limited interest in being stakeholders of the hospital; in fact, they want their children to get well and leave the hospital. What about children suffering from a chronic illness or a long-term disease such as cancer? Most hospitals have developed parent and children's groups that get together periodically to support each other (and to provide additional information to the hospital and to other patients and their families about coping with the illness). If the hospital's outreach department has helped organize the group so that it establishes officers and meeting dates, the group is organized! Is it the same as a veterans' organization? Clearly not, but it would be wise to include such a group in any efforts to advocate for policy changes (inside and beyond the hospital).

Finally, we suggest that most professional groups have delineated additional ways to develop clear stakeholder relationships because they have a stake in what happens within the day-to-day operations of an organization. In nursing, for example, the American Nurses Association (2013) has created an advocacy network and has detailed how to expand the relationships with both nurses and other stakeholder groups in the field. Additionally, the National League for Nursing (2013) offers a Public Policy Advocacy Toolkit to guide nurses, nursing students, and nursing faculty through the levels of governmental actions. To understand the advocacy role, one must see the importance of the professions' own expertise, to which we now turn.

Expertise

What is expert power in an organization? Some define it in terms of knowledge acquisition and professionalism. Thus, an expert organization would have a large proportion of highly educated professionals, defined by advanced education, licensure, professional norms and ethical standards, and a lifetime of continuing education. The healthcare arena has a clear advantage here. The various professions within any existing healthcare arena are often complex, and they have specialized education, training, and licensure at virtually every level of professional delivery of services. Such professionalized organizations often begin with a noticeable advantage over other organizations in which there is little or no professionalized workforce because of their expertise that lends added weight to their advocacy positions.

Thus, any definition of organizational expertise must begin with the nature of the expertise of the organization and whether it is well developed and professionalized and of the highest educational standards; however, one must be careful about defining this power simply as a set of acquired educational or professional standards. In the end, it is a bit like a traffic light—all the diplomas, certificates, and licensures do not necessarily mean the expertise is perceived as powerful. Similar to the number of stakeholders not being as important as the proximity of stakeholders to the decision makers, not all experts carry equal weight when it comes to organizational decisions.

What is the key to this expertise? It is the perception of others that the expertise is legitimate. Many healthcare professionals blunder here because they believe a variety of graduate and professional degrees automatically leads to support of their expertise. To put it in simple terms, many occupations (especially in the healthcare arena) are licensed, certified, and with advanced education, but they do not have equal expertise power. Why? Maybe because the public or the broader political and policy environment does not differentiate the various specializations, or the expertise of the profession is recognized strongly only by the profession itself. The public tends to understand expertise hierarchically. The expertise of physicians carries more weight than other professionals within the healthcare system.

The best example today is the widespread public agreement about the need for more nurses. How does that translate generally? The public does not differentiate well between LPN, RN, diploma, AD, BSN, MSN, NP, CRNA, CNS, or advanced practice nurses. But it does see the difference between a general practitioner in medicine and a specialist in oncology. What is the difference? We suggest that the public is convinced (generally through well-defined efforts by the medical establishment) that there are differences in behavior in the various medical specializations and that some of them have more expertise power because the public perceives them as more expert. Why is that not as true in nursing? We think part of the explanation is that the nursing profession has been reluctant to publicly emphasize the differences among the various areas of nursing professionalism. We suggest that this limits the political capacity of the various specializations to garner separate political support.

Buresh and Gordon (2000) proclaim that nurses are not recognized as a profession because they do not educate patients and their families, friends, and communities about nursing work. If the voice and viability of nursing were commensurate with the size and importance of nursing in health care, nurses would receive the three Rs: respect, recognition, and reward. These authors expound that if the work of nurses is unknown or misunderstood, then nurses cannot be appreciated or supported and cannot exert appropriate influence in health care. They go on to say that the general public needs to know what nurses do today and why their work is essential.

> Those in a position to influence legislation, policy making and funding must know that health care environments rich in nurses promote high levels of health whereas understaffed settings put patients at risk. They need to be aware of the incipient tragedies awaiting patients when nurses are not available to prevent falls, complications, errors in treatment and care or to rescue patients in need. (Buresh & Gordon, 2000, p. 18)

An example of how nurses fail to communicate their expertise can be found in the simple example of dress. Professionals are often recognized by their attire or uniform. The behavior and dress of nurses today tend to downplay professionalism by blurring the identity of nurses and making the place of nursing in health care more ambiguous. In healthcare settings, it is often not easy for patients or families to pick out who is a nurse and who is not. Buresh and Gordon (2000) proclaim that without a protocol to provide clarity, it is up to individual nurses to convey who they are through

their appearance, behavior, and language. It has become a common practice for nurses in hospital settings not to show their last name on name tags. Physicians would certainly not do this. When members of the largest healthcare profession (nurses) opt out of the standard professional greeting, they risk communicating that they do not regard themselves as professionals (Buresh & Gordon, 2000).

Can you imagine hospitals saying today, as they did 20–30 years ago, that they cannot afford to staff with registered or BSN-prepared nurses? What has pushed that bar? The Institute of Medicine's report on the future of nursing recommends that we "increase the proportion of nurses with a baccalaureate degree to 80 percent and double the number of nurses with a doctorate by 2020" (Institute of Medicine, 2013, p.1).

Thus, exerting expert power in an organizational setting must also include addressing some important issues, not the least of which is the belief that the expertise of the particular set of professionals has a valid place in the policy environment. When policy is being made internally, such as in a hospital, about how practices are implemented, changed, evolved, or reorganized, is the profession you represent at the table in the discussion? If not, why?

We all understand how professions develop expertise over time. They have specialized degrees, certifications, accreditations, licensures, state associations, and so forth. For the nursing profession, there is no higher recognition than a Magnet designation for a healthcare organization. The American Nurses Credentialing Center's Magnet Recognition Program recognizes healthcare organizations for quality patient care, nursing excellence, and innovations in professional nursing practice. The organization says, "Consumers rely on Magnet designation as the ultimate credential for high quality nursing" (American Nurses Credentialing Center, 2013, p. 1).

It is agreed that it is important for excellent nursing care to be recognized and rewarded, but why don't all healthcare organizations have Magnet status? Many hospitals have tried and failed, and others elect not to go for Magnet status. What does that tell us about this professional issue? It is still desirable, but not everyone is doing it; therefore, it is controversial. Many healthcare institutions cannot afford the Magnet journey. For others, they cannot meet the level of nursing education and expertise that is required due to size, location, and so forth.

Thus, as we develop the toolkit for expert power, we must ask a critical question: Who believes that this expertise of a profession is valued and should be represented in the decision-making process both within and beyond the organization?

Toolkit Case Studies

The case studies included in this toolkit chapter are designed to aid the reader in understanding the politics of organizational power. They are divided based on four categories: external stakeholder, internal stakeholder, external expertise, and internal expertise. Each of these real-life case studies illustrates how health professionals have applied the tools as highlighted within this chapter. The case study authors have included references when applicable. To guide your comprehension and application of the toolkit, the authors have included several thought-provoking questions at the end of each case study. Readers are encouraged to critically analyze the political methods and

power used in each case study, exploring the stakeholders and type of expertise involved. The questions following each case study are helpful for group discussion and individual analysis. This chapter concludes with one additional case study that has not had any political result to date, and readers are asked to analyze that case in terms of how one might build the necessary political stakeholder and expert power.

External Expert Power

The first two cases are doubtless well known to readers, but what may not be well known is the history of policy development in these areas. As you examine these two case studies, remember that their purpose is to show the role of expertise in affecting policy.

Case Study

External Stakeholder Power: Margaret Sanger as Nurse and Public Health Advocate

Ellen Chesler

"No gods, no masters," the rallying cry of the Industrial Workers of the World, was her personal and political manifesto. Emma Goldman and Bill Haywood, Mabel Dodge, and John Reed were among her earliest mentors and comrades. Allied with labor organizers and bohemians, Margaret Sanger first emerged on the American scene in those halcyon days at the turn of the 20th century, when the country seemed wide open with possibility, before world war, revolution, and repression provided a more sober reality.

She organized pickets and protests and pageants in the hope of achieving wholesale economic and social justice. What began as a callow faith in revolution quickly gave way to a more concrete agenda for reform. Working as a visiting nurse on New York's Lower East Side, she watched a young patient die from the complications of a then-common illegal abortion and vowed to abandon palliative work and devote herself to a single-minded pursuit of reproductive autonomy for women.

Sanger proudly claimed personal freedom for women. She also insisted that the price women pay for equality should not be the sacrifice of personal fulfillment. Following in the footsteps of a generation of suffragists and social welfare activists who had forgone marriage to gain professional stature and public influence, she became the standard bearer of a less ascetic breed, intent on balancing work and family obligations.

The hardest challenge in writing this history for modern audiences, for whom these claims have become routine, is to explain how absolutely destabilizing they seemed in Sanger's time. Even with so much lingering animus toward women's rights today, it is hard to remember that reproduction was once considered a woman's principal purpose, and motherhood was her primary role—women were assumed to have no need for identities or rights independent of those they enjoyed by virtue of their relationships to men. This principle was central to the long-enduring opposition women have faced in seeking rights to work, to inheritance and property, to suffrage, and especially to control of their own bodies.

Sanger needed broader arguments. By practicing birth control, women would not just serve themselves, she countered. They would also lower birthrates, alter the balance of supply and demand for labor, alleviate poverty, and thereby achieve the aspirations of workers without the social upheaval of class warfare. It would not be the dictates of Karl Marx, but the refusal of women to bear children indiscriminately, that would alter the course of history—a proposition ever resonant today as state socialism becomes an artifact of history, while family planning, although still contested, endures with palpable consequences worldwide.

In 1917, Sanger went to jail for distributing contraceptive pessaries to immigrant women from a makeshift clinic in a tenement storefront in the Brownsville section of Brooklyn. Sanger's contribution was to demand services for the poor that were available to the middle class. Her heresy, if you will, was in bringing the issue of sexual and reproductive freedom out in the open and claiming it as a woman's right. She staged her arrest deliberately to challenge New York's already anachronistic obscenity laws—the legacy of the notorious Anthony Comstock, whose evangelical fervor had captured Victorian politics in a manner eerily reminiscent of our time—and it led to the adoption, by the federal government and the states, of broad criminal sanctions on sexual speech and commerce, including all materials related to contraception and abortion.

Direct action tactics served Sanger well, but legal appeal of her conviction also established a medical exception to New York's Comstock Law. Doctors—although not nurses, as she originally intended—were granted the right to prescribe contraception for health purposes. Under that constraint, she built the modern family planning movement with independent, freestanding facilities as the model for distribution of services, a development that occurred largely in spite of leaders of the medical profession who remained shy of the subject for many years and did not formally endorse birth control until 1937, well after its scientific and social efficacy was demonstrated.

By then, Sanger and Hannah Stone, the medical director of her New York clinic, had also achieved another legal breakthrough.

They prevailed in a 1936 federal appellate court decision in New York that licensed physicians to import contraceptive materials and use the federal mail for transport. The ruling effectively realized years of failed efforts to achieve legislative reform in Congress, although it did formally override prohibitions that remained in several states until the historic ruling in *Griswold v. Connecticut,* with its claim of a constitutional doctrine of privacy, later extended so controversially to abortion in *Roe v. Wade.*

Sanger had long since jettisoned political ideology for a more reasoned confidence in the ability of education and science to shape human conduct and in the possibility of reform through bold public health initiatives.

With hard work and determination, she was able to mobilize men of influence in business, labor, academia, and the emerging professions. No less critical to her success was her decision to invest in the collective potential of women, many of whom had been oriented to activism by the suffrage movement and were eager for a new cause after finally winning the vote in 1920. She also lobbied the churches, convincing the clerical establishments of the progressive Protestant and Jewish denominations of the virtue of lifting sexuality and reproduction from the shroud of myth and mystery to which traditional faiths had long consigned them. She even won a concession from the hierarchy of the American Catholic Church, which overruled the Vatican and endorsed natural family planning, or the so-called rhythm method, as a way of countering the secular birth control movement and reasserting religious authority over values and behavior.

With an uncanny feel for the power of well-communicated ideas in a democracy, Sanger moved beyond women's rights to put forth powerful public health and social welfare claims for birth control. She proved herself a savvy public relations strategist and an adept grassroots organizer. Through the 1920s and 1930s, she wrote best-selling books, published a widely read journal, and crisscrossed the country and circled the globe to give lectures and hold conferences that attracted great interest and drove even more publicity. She built a thriving voluntary movement to conduct national- and state-level legislative lobbying and advocacy and to work in communities on the ground, sustaining affiliate organizations that organized and operated pioneering women's health clinics. Offering a range of medical and mental health services in reasonably sympathetic environments, many of these facilities became laboratories for her idealism.

Yet the birth control movement stalled during the long years of the Great Depression and World War II, stymied by the increasing cost and complexity of reaching those most in need and overwhelmed by the barrage of opposition it engendered. The issue remained mired in moral and religious controversy, even as its leadership determinedly embraced centrist politics and a sanitized message. When hard times encouraged attention to collective needs over individual rights and when the New Deal legitimized public responsibility for economic and social welfare, Sanger cannily replaced the *birth control* moniker with the more socially resonant *family planning.* She invented both terms and popularized them after consulting allies and friends. These strategies of accommodation, however, did nothing to stop officials of the National Catholic Welfare Conference and other opponents from making the most scandalous accusations that birth control was killing babies, waging war on poor families, even causing the Great Depression itself by slowing population growth and lowering consumer demand—a proposition that some economists of the day endorsed.

Having enjoyed Eleanor Roosevelt's enthusiastic support and personal friendship in New York, Sanger went to Washington in the 1930s hoping that Congress would overturn the Comstock law and legalize contraceptive practice as a first step to her long-term goal of transferring responsibility and accountability for services from small, privately funded clinics to public health programs with appropriate resources and scale; however, she failed to anticipate that the success of the Roosevelts would depend on a delicate balance of the votes of conservative urban Catholics in the north and rural fundamentalist Protestants in the south. There would be no invitations to tea at the White House and no government support, at least until Franklin Roosevelt was safely ensconced in a third term.

Like other well-intended social reformers of her day, Sanger also endorsed eugenics, the then ubiquitous and popular movement that addressed the manner in which biological factors affect human health, intelligence, and opportunity. She took away from Darwinism the essentially optimistic lesson that man's common descent in the animal kingdom makes us all capable of improvement, if only we apply the right tools. Believing that ability and talent should replace birthright and social status as the standard of mobility in a democratic society, she endorsed intelligence testing, an enduring legacy of the era, and she did not repudiate the infamous Supreme Court decision of 1929 in *Buck v. Bell* that mandated compulsory sterilization on grounds of feeblemindedness. She also supported the payment of bonuses to women who volunteered for sterilization because they wanted no more children.

These compromised views placed her squarely in the intellectual mainstream of her time and in the good company of many progressives who shared these beliefs. Still, her failure to consider the validity of standard assessments of aptitude or the fundamental rights questions inherent in these procedures has left her vulnerable, in hindsight, to attacks of insensitivity and bigotry. The family planning movement at home and abroad has long been burdened by the charges that it fostered prejudice, even as it delivered welcome services and relief from unwanted childbirth to women in need.

Embittered by these controversies and disenchanted with the country's increasing pronatalism after World War II, Sanger turned her attentions abroad. In 1952, she founded the International Planned Parenthood Federation, with headquarters in London, as an umbrella for the national family planning associations that remain today in almost every country.

By the time of her death in 1966, the cause for which she defiantly broke the law had achieved international stature. Although still a magnet for controversy, she was widely eulogized as one of the great emancipators of her time. She lived to see the U.S. Supreme Court provide constitutional protection for the use of contraceptives in *Griswold v. Connecticut*. She watched Lyndon Johnson incorporate family planning into America's social welfare and foreign policy programs, fulfilling her singular vision of how to advance opportunity and prosperity, not to speak of human happiness, at home and abroad. A team of doctors and scientists she had long encouraged marketed the oral anovulant birth control pill, and a resurgent feminist movement gave new resonance to her original claim that women have a fundamental right to control their own bodies.

In the years since, however, further controversy has surrounded the practices of what developed as often alarmist global population control efforts that adopted rigid demographic targets and imposed harsh, unwelcome, and culturally insensitive technologies on women. Population policy makers and service providers have been fairly criticized for abusing rights by ignoring or downplaying the risks of providing costly technologies where health services are inadequate to cope with potential complications and where failure rates have been high, even though these products are medically benign when properly administered.

In 1994, the United Nations International Conference on Population and Development in Cairo created a framework for state responsibility to ensure programs allowing women to make free and informed decisions about family planning, but also obligating access to comprehensive reproductive health services of high quality, including birth control. Population and development professionals, however, also committed to a doctrine that weds policies and practices to improvements in women's status—to education, economic opportunity, and basic civil rights for women subject to culturally sanctioned discrimination and violence—just as Margaret Sanger first envisioned.

Hundreds of millions of women and men around the world today freely practice some method of contraception, with increasing reliance on condoms in light of the epidemic spread of HIV/AIDS and other sexually transmitted infections. This represents a sixfold increase since rates of population growth peaked in the 1960s.

Still, half the world's population today— nearly 3 billion people—are under the age of 25 years. Problems associated with widespread poverty, food insecurity, and environmental degradation are widespread. There remains considerable unmet need for family planning, and there is tragically insufficient funding for research on new methods and for new programming to meet ever-increasing demand. Funding

for both population and development programs has slowed dramatically, as other needs compete for funds and as concern now spreads about an aging and shrinking population in many countries where birthrates have sharply declined. The cycles of history repeat themselves.

Case Study Questions

- At what points did the science of birth control precede any change in policy/practice in this area? Why do you think that was the case?

- Why was the expertise of effective birth control not widely shared, and why did it take the medical establishment so long to endorse policy change in this area? Clearly, the women's movement was part of the opening of change in this area, but how did it contribute to the creation of knowledge?

- What happened to the policy of birth control after the American Medical Association supported it in the 1930s?

- Why did it take another 30 years for birth control to be widely available to women in America?

- Have there been changes in recent years in the broader environment that are analogous to the early adoption of birth control programs (e.g., RU-486 or the so-called morning after pill)?

- Have these changes increased or limited access to birth control? Think through the acceptance of the expertise in this area and the ways in which it has contributed to (or limited) the change in policy in this environment and the ways in which it has not been taken into account.

- Can you illustrate how expertise is still about perception, both within professional fields and in the broader public?

Case Study

External Stakeholder Power: Successful Efforts to Pass Advanced Practice Nurse Legislation

Claudia J. Beverly

The Arkansas State Legislature meets every other year to conduct the business of the state. In the year preceding the legislative session, the Policy Committee of the Arkansas Nurses Association (ArNA) examines the healthcare needs of the state and designs a strategic health policy plan for nursing that will be introduced in the upcoming session. The work is always initiated with a clear understanding of the needs of the state's citizens. In this rural state, 69 of the 75 counties are medically underserved. The poverty level is one of the worst in the country. The health statistics of Arkansans are in the bottom four states, and several counties do not have a single primary care provider. Given the many healthcare challenges facing the state, nursing is in a key position to address these needs, and society expects them to do so.

In the early 1990s the ArNA, which represents all nurses in Arkansas, concluded that advanced practice nurses were best prepared to address the primary healthcare needs of Arkansans. At that time, however, there was no standardization or clear regulation for this level of nurse other than national certification and the registered nurse (RN) license that is basic for all levels of registered nurses.

The ArNA's first attempt to address the primary healthcare needs of the citizens was in 1993. Their attempt to pass legislation that would allow prescriptive authority by advanced practice nurses failed. After this failure, the ArNA, with the assistance of its lobbyist, began to develop legislation for introduction in the

1995 legislative session to provide a mechanism for advanced practice nurses to practice to the extent to which they are academically prepared. Additionally, a mechanism whereby society could be assured of safe practice by all providers needed to be in place.

The process began when a legislator from a rural area with the greatest need introduced a study bill. This bill provided an opportunity for the ArNA to educate legislators about advanced practice nursing and how this type of nurse could address the healthcare needs of Arkansans. The study bill was assigned to the Interim Public Health, Welfare, and Labor Committee of both the House of Representatives and the Senate. Several public hearings were held by the committee, and various groups and individuals both in support and in opposition were given the opportunity to voice their opinions.

During the hearings, there were opportunities to provide correct information supported by the literature. Clarification of the proposed legislation was also on the agenda. At one point, concern was raised about the use of the term *collaboration with medicine*, as some persons preferred to use *supervision* or a definition that would limit the practice to one being supervised. The task force initiated a process to define the term *collaboration*. A review of the literature showed that collaboration had already been defined in the 1970s by both medicine and nursing. Armed with that information and definitions given by other sources, the task force reported their findings at the next hearing, and the definition jointly developed by medicine and nursing was incorporated into the proposed legislation.

Process for Success

The leadership of the ArNA understood the monumental task and the many challenges and barriers to addressing the healthcare needs of Arkansans. The association decided that appointing a special task force to lead its efforts was the best strategy. This strategy provided a mechanism for focusing on the issue while ensuring that the health policy committee would continue to focus on broader policy issues.

The association selected a chair, included the chair in member selection by ArNA leadership, and established the first meeting. As the process evolved, two cochairs, a secretary, and a treasurer were named. The task force was representative of nursing broadly and included members of the Arkansas State Board of Nursing, advanced practice nurses with master's degrees (midwives, certified registered nurse anesthetists, nurse practitioners, and clinical nurse specialists), registered nurses, faculty from schools of nursing who prepared advanced practice nurses, and representatives from other nursing organizations. The task force met every other week during the first 6 months of the 2-year preparatory period, then weekly for the remaining year and a half.

The first order of business was to develop a strategic plan that included establishing a vision, mission, goals and objectives, strategies, and time line. The vision was critical as a means of keeping task force members focused on the vast needs of Arkansans, particularly those in rural areas. The vision statement also served to keep the broader ArNA membership focused. A literature search on advanced practice nursing and health policy issues was conducted, and articles were distributed to all task force members. The assumption was that all of the members needed information to expand their current knowledge. Subcommittees were developed based on goals and objectives and the operational needs of the task force. Chairs were assigned for each subcommittee, and thus began the 2-year journey.

The American Nurses Association (ANA) played a vital role in the process. The legal department was available to assemble and provide information, offer guidance, and identify potential barriers and challenges. The support provided by the ANA was pivotal to our success.

The work of the task force focused on external and internal strategies. External strategies focused on stakeholders, which included the Arkansas Medical Society, the Arkansas Medical Board, and the Pharmacy Association. Understanding the views of our colleagues in other disciplines and identifying the opposition to our plans were critical to our success. Many meetings focused on educating those disciplines about the legislation we were seeking. Often this was a balancing act, providing the right information but not too much of our strategy while attempting to keep our enemy close. We valued the process of negotiation and participated in many opportunities to negotiate with colleagues.

Throughout this process, the ArNA did have a line in the sand, defined as the point at which there was no negotiation. Our line in the sand included regulations of advanced practice nurses by the Arkansas State Board of Nursing and reimbursement paid directly to the nurses. These two points were never resolved until a vote on the legislation occurred.

The good news is that the advanced practice nurse legislation passed successfully in 1995. The legislation was successful in that the criteria for an advanced practice nurse to be licensed in the State of Arkansas were written by nursing, advanced practice nurses were to be regulated by nursing, and the legislation acknowledged national certification and educational requirements. Prescriptive authority was granted, and selected scheduled drugs could be ordered by an advanced practice nurse. Reimbursement to advanced practice nurses was lost at the last minute. For advanced practice nurses in the field of geriatrics, Medicare passed reimbursement regulations in 1997. Medicaid reimburses geriatric nurse practitioners according to national guidelines. Reimbursement is critical to meeting the needs of Arkansas citizens and is a topic that is still being discussed.

Many individuals participated in this successful campaign. A clear vision, legislation based on evidence and current literature, a comprehensive strategic plan, education of all parties (including those in opposition and those in support), and well-informed legislators were critical to success. Probably the most critical message in health policy legislation is to focus on the needs of the citizenry and what nursing needs to contribute.

Case Study Questions

- We suspect that most nursing professionals can expand on this case; however, the key question is, what was the nature of building a stakeholder network?

- Who were the critical first players in this movement, and why was their involvement critical?

- As the network expanded, which other professional groups were involved? Why were those groups, and not others, involved?

- Do you see why some professions were the logical next parts of the coalition for adopting change?

- Who was most likely to oppose advanced practice nursing? Obviously, you do not include likely opponents in the initial development of the network of stakeholders, but why?

- How did the coalition eventually succeed through this inclusive network?

- What would you have done differently in a different practice arena?

- What does this case study tell you about building stakeholders for advancing practice?

- What would you need to do to apply this policy to advancing roles in your healthcare setting?

Case Study

Internal Expertise Power: Expanding Newborn Screening in Arkansas

Ralph Vogel

Strides in technology have created great advances in how we can provide services to families and their children. A prime example is the expansion of newborn screening, which has dramatically increased the number and type of genetic conditions that can be detected immediately after birth. Historically, most states have screened for hemoglobinopathies (like sickle cell anemia), thyroid disorders, phenylketonuria, and galactosemia. These conditions, along with newborn hearing screening, were relatively easy to administer at a cost-effective rate. With advanced laboratory and computer technology, we can now add multiple genetic conditions that are identified during a single run. In 2004, the March of Dimes proposed expanding the genetic conditions for which newborns are screened to their List of 29, including several enzyme deficiencies and cystic fibrosis. The cost of the limited newborn screening had been approximately $15 per newborn, and it would increase to about $90 with the expanded list. Insurance companies would cover the cost of adding the additional conditions. The value of newborn screening is in identifying genetic conditions early and implementing treatment plans from birth. Over a life span, this greatly reduces the morbidity and mortality associated with later diagnosis. With some conditions, the care can be as simple as a dietary change that is implemented from birth. Early diagnosis also allows for genetic counseling with families about the risk that additional children will have the condition.

Many states adopted this recommendation quickly, although the process has been slower in others. In Arkansas, a committee, titled the Arkansas Genetics Health Advisory Committee (formerly Service), has existed for several years. Their mission is to monitor health care related to genetics in the state. This diverse committee includes several members of the Arkansas Department of Health (ADH) who are involved in the newborn screening program administration and laboratory testing, physicians from Arkansas Children's Hospital genetic clinic, and interested parties that either work in the area of genetics or are parents of children with genetic conditions.

The main purpose of the committee has been to coordinate care and to try to educate the public about genetic conditions and screening for newborns. The ADH receives samples from about 95% of the newborns in the state and does screening at their central location in Little Rock. When an infant is identified with a newborn genetic condition, the ADH notifies the community hospital and the assigned pediatrician, who counsels the family and develops a plan for care and follow-up.

Expanding the screening program to the existing March of Dimes List of 29 created several problems. The committee, however, felt strongly that it should take an advocacy role to address these concerns. The first problem was the cost of increased screening. Although most of the individual cost for each child could be absorbed by insurance or Medicaid reimbursement, as in other states, the initial financial support would need to be provided by the state. The ADH had no provision for increasing funding but estimated that the increased cost would be as follows:

- $2 million for equipment and supplies
- The addition of at least two laboratory technicians to do the increased testing
- The addition of at least one public health nurse to coordinate the increased number of identified genetic cases

- Training for new and current personnel on the new equipment
- Personnel time to develop and coordinate the expansion of the program
- Development of an education program to make parents and professionals aware of the changes

Overall, the estimated cost for start-up was approximately $3 million, some of which could be recouped after billing for the tests was established.

The committee and ADH decided that we would outline a plan for expansion with estimated costs and submit it to the director of the ADH, Dr. Faye Bozeman. With his approval, we would then approach legislators and ask for the needed funding to be included in the upcoming budget. Because the Arkansas state legislature convened only every 2 years, it would be critical to move forward over the next 6 months. We prepared a letter to Dr. Bozeman that the committee approved on a Friday with the intention of mailing it the following Monday. The next day, Saturday, Dr. Bozeman was killed in an accident on his farm; therefore, we were in a quandary about who should receive the letter and whose approval would be needed in the ADH. During the next 6 months, there was an interim head who was thrust into the position and did not want to approve anything at this level of expense. We were on hold until a permanent director was named. After about 3 months, we decided to take another tack and develop a plan to seek legislative approval for funding and then approach the new ADH director after the person was named. We developed a list of legislators to contact and identified members of the committee who had worked with the legislators in the past and could approach them.

By this time, we were 2 months from the legislature convening and knew that after it convened, nothing new would be introduced;

therefore, we had to get support ahead of time. We approached some legislators and received tacit support, but none were willing to introduce a new bill or request funding without a permanent head of ADH. We had lost the opportunity for funding until the next legislative session in 2 years.

The committee decided to continue to seek support from the legislators and ADH, with the idea of gaining funding in 2 years. Meanwhile, we began to look at other states and what newborn screenings they were currently doing to make sure that politicians were aware of national standards. We had identified that Arkansas was one of the last five states to not expand newborn screening, and all of the surrounding states in the region had incorporated all or a large part of the March of Dimes List of 29. Making legislators aware of this became one of our goals, and once they realized that the states surrounding Arkansas were already doing expanded screening of newborns, they were more receptive to our plan.

After we started to discuss funding with legislators during the legislative session, they seemed willing to support newborn screening. But we had a surprise: They said it did not require any special legislation or special funding; the ADH could expand newborn screening without their approval because this was already within their realm of responsibility. Funding could be obtained by submitting a budget request to cover the cost of expansion.

The interim head of ADH was willing to support this since the head of the newborn screening section was on our committee. By fall, we had the budget expansion approved and support for newborn screening expansion. The decision was then made to target July 1, 2008, as the date to start the expanded program.

After we knew the finances and political support were confirmed, we developed a time line that involved equipment acquisition, training for ADH staff, an education program for

the public, and a plan for making community hospitals and professional healthcare providers aware of the expansion. At this point, the ADH contacted members of the media that it had worked with in the past and developed a plan for public information advertisements to be run on television and radio. These began running in early May, 2 months before the July 1 start date. Because the media members had worked with ADH in the past, it was much easier to develop the advertisements. Print media advertisements were also started, and the local chapter of the March of Dimes provided funding and brochures that were distributed to OB/GYN physicians in the state to make expectant mothers aware of the testing to be done on their newborns. One of the members of the committee also wrote an article that appeared in the March issue of the *Arkansas State Board of Nursing Update* magazine, which is distributed to 40,000 healthcare providers in the state.

In July, the expanded screening began, and it has been continued with a relatively smooth transition, largely because of the preparation of the ADH staff in the laboratory and the outreach nurses. Because of the public awareness campaign, there has been little voiced concern from parents, and there seems to be an awareness of the value of the expanded screening.

Lessons learned from the process are as follows:

- Preparation is the key to a smooth transition.
- Know exactly what is required to proceed and who needs to approve new or expanded plans of action. If we had approached the legislature first to find out what they wanted, we could have saved time.
- Plan for the unexpected. We could not have anticipated Dr. Bozeman's death, but it did cause about a 6-month delay.
- Educate everyone who is going to be involved. This includes administrators, healthcare

providers, laboratory staff, parents, and professionals in the impacted communities.

- Discuss with the media exactly what they need and use their expertise in terms of length of announcements and the best ways to distribute information.

Although the entire process took more than 2 years, in the end, the transition has been very smooth, and few problems have been identified at any level. Having a diverse group on the committee was a strength because different members had different perspectives. This gave us much greater ability to anticipate problems and coordinate care, and in the end, the program will benefit newborns in Arkansas for years to come.

Case Study Questions

- This case is a good example of how the stakeholders adapted as the intended policy change moved from internal adoption of policy to legislation and back to internal adoption of policy within an existing organization. Can you see how the nature of the stakeholders defined for a legislative change is different from stakeholders for adaptation of existing policy?

- The initial group involved in this process was established primarily as an informational group, but it was modified to advocate change. How did the group evolve to influence policy differently? If the initial group had been more broadly defined at the start, would it have made the same mistake about requiring legislative change to adopt the policy? Why or why not?

Final Case Study

This final case study is presented to stimulate the reader's political thinking. We encourage you to read the case carefully and then consider how you would go about creating an environment for policy change.

Case Study

Workplace Violence

Steven L. Baumann and Eileen Levy

In the wake of the terrorist attack of September 11, 2001, and a series of tragic school shootings, workplace violence has gained national attention in the United States. Although nurses and other healthcare workers are generally well educated and regularly reminded to practice good handwashing and infection control, there is little attention given to the potential for violence in hospitals and other healthcare settings, even though it is common and can have devastating long-term consequences (Department of Health and Human Services, 2002; U.S. Department of Labor, 2004). According to Love and Morrison (2003), nurses who sustain injuries from patient assaults, in addition to suffering psychological trauma, are often out of work for periods of time, have financial problems, show decreased work productivity, make more errors at work, and report a decreased desire to remain a nurse. In addition to these problems, nurses who have been assaulted report feeling less able to provide appropriate care to their patients (Farrell, Bobrowski, & Bobrowski, 2006) and are reluctant to make formal complaints (Love & Morrison, 2003). As was the case with needlestick injuries in the past, many organizations do not openly discuss problems that increase the risk for violence, nor do they adequately prepare for episodes of violence, leaving nurses more likely to blame themselves for its occurrence.

The National Institute for Occupational Safety and Health (NIOSH), the same organization that requires hospitals to be attentive to infection control strategies and proper handling of hazardous materials, also provides clear definitions and guidelines to reduce the potential for violence in the workplace. According NIOSH, workplace violence includes acts of physical violence or threats of violence directed toward people on duty or at work (Department of Health and Human Services, 2002). NIOSH has recognized employer responsibilities in mitigating workplace violence and assisting employees who are victims (Love & Morrison, 2003). The U.S. government has required employers to provide safe workplaces since 1970 (U.S. Department of Labor, 2004). These federal guidelines call for hospitals and other organizations to incorporate written programs into the overall safety and health program for their facilities to ensure job safety and security. Violence prevention, they suggest, needs to have administrative commitment and employee involvement.

This case study is of a moderate-sized, non-profit community hospital in the New York metropolitan area. As in many parts of the United States, this hospital and the communities it serves are becoming increasingly crowded and diverse. In this environment of change and tension, the hospital is a meeting place of people, many not by choice but in crisis, bringing together dramatically different histories, backgrounds, educational attainment, and cultures. The hospital and its clinics have become increasingly stressful, unpredictable, and at times hostile places. For example, the use of hospitals as holding tanks for acutely disturbed and violent individuals, the release of mentally ill persons from public hospitals without adequate outpatient programs and follow-up services, and the accessibility of handguns and drugs in communities all contribute to hospital and community violence. A failure of leadership at various levels, as well as inadequate reimbursement from payers, has contributed to violence that can occur on its premises.

The case study hospital, like most in the United States, has dramatically reduced the number of public psychiatric beds. Many of these former psychiatric patients have to rely on outpatient mental health services supported by community hospitals with a limited number of beds on one or two psychiatric units. In addition, the case study hospital reduced inpatient and outpatient addiction services. New research suggests that actively psychotic patients with schizophrenia and patients with schizophrenia who had a premorbid conduct problem or exposure to violence are more likely to be violent than less acutely ill patients and those without substance abuse or antisocial personality comorbidity (Swanson et al., 2008). Nevertheless, it is a mistake to consider persons with mental illness or substance abuse as the only individuals who can become agitated or violent in healthcare settings. It is also shortsighted to solely blame any single policy, such as the deinstitutionalization of the chronically mentally ill, for workplace violence in the United States.

At the same time that the case study hospital has cut beds and programs for persons in distress, it has a clear mission/vision/value statement that puts professional nurses in leadership positions and has taken steps to address workplace violence. It has made efforts to reduce violence in high-risk areas, such as the emergency department and psychiatric unit, by restricting access to these areas, using surveillance equipment and panic buttons, and strictly requiring all staff to wear identification, as other hospitals have. Community hospitals, like the one in this case study, however, often do not provide the kind of ongoing self-defense and violence prevention education and training that many psychiatric hospitals provide. In addition, all hospitals should have a task force and regularly meeting committee consisting of management, human resources/employee relations, employee assistance program staff, security, and the office of chief counsel whose sole purpose is developing policies and procedures to prevent and address workplace violence.

Following The Joint Commission's (2008) lead, the case study hospital and nursing administration have hospital-wide discussions and training on behaviors that undermine a culture of safety. In addition, the hospital requires workplace violence risk assessment, hazard prevention and control, and safety and health training, as well as careful record keeping and program evaluation (U.S. Department of Labor, 2004). Hospitals need to keep in mind the malpractice crisis in this country. The move to put patients first does not turn over control of the hospital to patients or their families. Indeed, to understand Friedman (2007) correctly, to put patients' health and satisfaction first, the hospital needs effective leadership at the top and from its professional nurses. To prevent violence in the workplace, nurses need to strive to be as authentic in their patient contact as possible and to avoid detached, impersonal interactions (Carlsson, Dahlberg, Ekcbergh, & Dahlberg, 2006). The case study hospital provides considerable avenues of reward for individual nurses and other staff members to advance themselves and stand out as innovative, which helps mitigate the tendency for workers to herd—that is, to avoid developing themselves and improving the institution for the sake of togetherness with selected coworkers (Friedman, 2007).

The case study hospital does provide a psychiatric nurse practitioner on staff and on-site one day per week as an employee assistance provider. Having this person on-site provides an opportunity for hospital staff to be counseled on becoming less reactive to emotionally intense environments, as recommended by Friedman (2007). Healthcare organizations also need to provide referral information, such as to employee assistance programs or clinicians experienced in trauma care, for employees who may exhibit more serious and persistent reactions to perceived violence and aggression

(Bernstein & Saladino, 2007). Nurses and nursing organizations should become more familiar with national guidelines and recommendations and persuade their hospitals to adopt and implement them. The process for nurses is to focus more on taking responsibility for their own condition, practice self-regulation, and have a wide repertoire of responses to stressful situations. Although this does not guarantee that violence will be avoided, it does make it less likely to happen and makes nurses better able to keep it in perspective. Friedman (2007) described this as being able to turn down the dial or volume. Nurses need to be just as effective in managing toxic emotional environments as in handling toxic chemicals and infections. Nurses' interpersonal effectiveness is increased when they look for and support strengths in others. Postincident debriefing helps transform the experience into a team-building and learning opportunity. Leaders should involve all staff and review events, including what precedes and follows an incident.

Case Study Conclusion

A community hospital in the New York metropolitan area is presented as a case study of an organization struggling to carry out its mission in a way that facilitates the growth and well-being of its employees. The hospital is experiencing different pulls. On one hand, it has had to cut back on essential programs. On the other hand, the nurses and the central leadership in the hospital need to work together to avoid quick-fix solutions and suffer the failure of nerve that Friedman (2007) talked about. The busy hospital environment in a changing society is stressful and, at times, hostile and violent. Nurses need to be effective leaders to help protect the integrity of the hospital as an organization—to maintain its self-definition. They can best do this by becoming as self-defined as possible and by consistently implementing federal guidelines to prevent and manage workplace violence.

Case Study Questions

In this case, there is a need for policy change—the need for workplace violence policies. Here is our challenge to the reader. Can you take our two components, both an internal and external role, and define what needs to be done to accomplish this policy change? We suggest that you define the work in terms of your most likely environment, whether it is a psychiatric facility or a hospital or clinic. How would you go about creating an environment for policy change here?

Some core questions should guide you. First, what key stakeholders are in the initial stakeholder group (i.e., those most likely to feel the strongest need for the policy)? Remember, it is essential that stakeholders are identifiable and represent a clear position on this topic. Can you identify both internal and external stakeholders? Are they organized around various professional lines within your organization? How do you begin to create a shared view among these stakeholders? As you begin to broaden the network, which groups should be brought into the discussion? Let us give you an example: The human resource specialists in your organization will need to be involved at some point in creating a policy about the elimination and reduction of workplace violence. Should they, however, be in your initial set of stakeholders? Why or why not?

Now for the more difficult questions:

- What expertise is needed to make such a policy change?

- What kinds of facts (someone has to gather the data in a systematic way) need to be gathered?

- Are we discussing violence between patients and those providing medical services, or violence among fellow professionals within the organization?

- What kind of violence and danger are we discussing here—physical or verbal violence, or both?

- What about safety issues (including other types of danger to employees and patients)?

- Would you agree that an emergency room might see these questions a bit differently from those handling financial claims (although both have real needs)?

- How do you build expert power? Who shares it, and who might be expert in defining these issues over time?

As you create the case, think about developing it in two stages: the initial definition of the issues (expertise), and who needs a seat at the table (stakeholders) both inside and outside the organization. The second stage is writing and defining the policy. If the issue is defined well by all the stakeholders, the delineation of the necessary expertise of workforce violence will become a shared view among the stakeholders. Then, and only then, can one move to the writing of a policy about dealing with workplace violence. Do all the stakeholders need to be involved in writing that policy? We suggest that is not necessary for those involved to reach a broad agreement about the issues that define the policy itself.

Case Study References

Bernstein, K. S., & Saladino, J. P. (2007). Clinical assessment and management of psychiatric patients' violent and aggressive behaviors in general hospital. *Medsurg Nursing, 16,* 301–309.

Carlsson, G., Dahlberg, K., Ekcbergh, M., & Dahlberg, H. (2006). Patients longing for authentic personal care: A phenomenological study of violent encounters in psychiatric settings. *Issues in Mental Health Nursing, 27,* 287–305.

Department of Health and Human Services. (2002). *Violence: Occupational hazards in hospitals* (Document #2002-101). Cincinnati, OH: National Institute for Occupational Safety and Health.

Farrell, G. A., Bobrowski, C., & Bobrowski, P. (2006). Scoping workplace aggression in nursing: Findings from an Australian study. *Journal of Advanced Nursing, 55*, 778–787.

Friedman, E. H. (2007). *A failure of nerve: Leadership in the age of the quick fix.* New York, NY: Seabury.

Love, C. C., & Morrison, E. (2003). American Academy of Nursing Expert Panel on Violence policy recommendations on workplace violence (adopted 2002). *Issues in Mental Health Nursing, 24*, 599–604.

Swanson, J. W., Van Dorn, R. A., Swartz, M. S., Smith, M., Elbogen, E. B., & Monahan, J. (2008). Alternative pathways to violence in persons with schizophrenia. *The Role of Childhood Antisocial Behavior, 32*(3), 228–240.

The Joint Commission. (2008, July). *Behaviors that undermine a culture of safety.* Retrieved from http://www.jointcommission.org/assets/1/18/SEA_40.pdf

U.S. Department of Labor. (2004). *Guidelines for preventing workplace violence for health care & social service workers* (OSHA 3148-01R). Washington, DC: Occupational Safety and Health Administration.

Conclusion

Politics and policy requires an understanding of how to build support and adapt to change. If we are to be effective advocates, we must be responsive to broader societal needs. Building support is not done simply by presenting the facts. This toolkit is designed to help readers know what it takes in a political environment to build a case and adapt when necessary. A huge mistake in advocacy is to simply believe that the facts are on our side, and if we just continue to list the facts, everyone will believe! In reality, values and political issues are at the core of successful change. Our tasks as political advocates for change are as follows:

- Believe we can convince others to adapt
- Adapt ourselves to handle broader political value issues
- Learn to mobilize our expert power as one of the largest groups of stakeholders in the healthcare field

Discussion Questions

1. As you read through this chapter, describe the political environment of your own organization, both at the largest level and at a division or office level.

2. Internal and external stakeholders are important to any organization or policy. Describe your view about more reliance on internal stakeholders than on external stakeholders, and vice versa. Why do you think there are differences?

3. Expertise power is often difficult to define in detail, but how do we build a stronger perception of the importance of our expertise with those who work with our programs and agencies?

4. Looking at Figure 3-1, how do organizations overutilize the force component in organizational power? What kinds of evidence would you expect to see in an organization that is not using influence or authority well?

5. Given the need for greater collaboration in the health policy arena, how does improving your stakeholder relationships with other organizations and interests become even more important?

References

American Nurses Association. (2013). *Advocacy—becoming more effective*. Retrieved from http://www.nursingworld.org/MainMenuCategories/Policy-Advocacy/AdvocacyResourcesTools

American Nurses Credentialing Center. (2013). *ANCC Magnet Recognition Program*. Retrieved from http://www.nursecredentialing.org/Magnet.aspx

Buresh, B., & Gordon, S. (2000). *From silence to voice: What nurses know and must communicate to the public*. Ottawa, Ontario: Canadian Nurses Association.

Fottler, M. D., Blair, J. D., Whitehead, C. J., Laus, M. D., & Savage, G. T. (1989). Assessing key stakeholders: Who matters to hospitals and why? *Hospitals and Health Services Administration, 34*(4), 525–546.

Institute of Medicine. (2013). *The future of nursing*. Retrieved from http://www.thefutureofnursing.org/recommendations

National League for Nursing. (2013). *Faculty programs and resources: Public policy advocacy toolkit*. Retrieved from http://www.nln.org/facultyprograms/publicpolicytoolkit/publicpolicy-toolkit.htm

Wilson, J. Q. (1989). *Bureaucracy: What government agencies do and why they do it*. New York, NY: Basic Books.

CHAPTER 4

The Affordable Care Act: The Current Driver of Healthcare Reform

Elyse Berkman, Nancy Aries, and Barbara Caress

Overview

Despite strong public support for healthcare reform, the United States remains the only industrialized country without universal access to health care. The Affordable Care Act (ACA) is changing that landscape. It is a means to fill the gaps that currently exist through the provision of low-cost insurance and high-quality care. It aims to control costs through financial incentives that should improve care coordination and patient outcomes. Although the program met tremendous resistance since it was debated in Congress, it represents an important step to ensure access and quality care for all.

Objectives

- Understand the ideological debates that define the politics of national health insurance in the United States.
- Explain why President Obama made national health insurance a centerpiece of his first-term legislative program and how he succeeded in seeing the bill signed into law.
- Describe the features of the ACA, including the role of the individual mandate, adverse selection, cost control, and quality initiatives.
- Explicate how the ACA addresses problems of access, cost, and quality.
- Assess the status of implementation.

Introduction

Health reform is not a new topic on the public policy agenda. Despite strong public support for universal coverage, it has been an intensely debated issue for more than 100 years. The United States, however, remains the only industrialized country without universal access to health insurance that affords appropriate entry to the U.S. healthcare system (American Public Health Association, 2013). Lacking adequate health insurance means that upwards of 55 million persons have only limited access to this country's costly and complex system of health services (Schoen, Osborn, Squires, & Doty, 2013). This gap in health insurance coverage and access to care exists despite the fact that the United States spends almost twice as much as any other country on health care. In 2011, the World Bank reported that the United States spent 17.9% of its gross domestic product (GDP) on health care, while the average healthcare expenditure for the 13 highest-income countries, which includes the United States, was only 12% (Organisation for Economic Co-operation and Development, 2014; World Bank, 2013).

This chapter examines past efforts to create a program of national health insurance and the rejection of reform legislation. It then looks at how the policy lessons from these earlier efforts enabled President Barack Obama to craft a legislative program that garnered the support of the major healthcare lobbies and the majority of members of Congress. Consideration is then given to what is included in the ACA and what it is expected to achieve in terms of improved access, quality, and cost control. The last section reviews implementation and considers the persistence of opposition to the legislation.

History of National Health Insurance Initiatives

National health insurance is an issue that has come on and off the public agenda since the turn of the 20th century. There are always distinct economic, political, and social issues that shape the debate in each era, but there are also issues that remain constant over time. The first concern is access to affordable health care for all Americans and whether universal access requires some form of compulsory or national insurance. The second is cost and whether the rapidly escalating costs of health care are best contained through government intervention or the market. Both are tied to Americans' unfailing fear of government intervention. As a result, there is constant tension about whether government programs can be understood as advancing the cause of national health insurance or ensuring an adequate safety net for persons who cannot access the healthcare market.

Social Insurance and the American Context

More than 100 years ago, Germany's chancellor, Otto von Bismarck, led his country to adopt a system of social insurance that included compulsory sickness insurance to protect workers from lost wages due to illness (Steinmo & Watts, 1995). Similar systems were legislated in Austria, Hungary, Norway, Serbia, Britain, Russia, France, Switzerland, and the Netherlands. Social insurance was a political compromise between the business owners and the working class. It responded to the growing political discontent over industrialization by protecting the jobs and income of workers who became sick.

In the early 19th century, a program of national health insurance seemed politically feasible in the United States following passage of the workers' compensation laws between 1910 and 1913. Social reformers came to believe that a program of compulsory insurance against sickness, like the compulsory insurance against industrial accidents, was possible (Starr, 1982). Similar to the health insurance programs in Europe, it was seen as a way to offset wage losses and reduce the total cost of illness by providing medical care. The first model for a national proposal in 1915 was put forward by the American Association of Labor Legislation (AALL).

Despite high expectations for passage, no action was taken (Fein, 1989). Broad-based support for the proposal was missing because the two major interest groups were internally divided. Among physicians, the proposal was supported by the American Medical Association (AMA), which at the time was dominated by academics. They understood national health insurance as a way to advance the centralization of medical practice in hospital-based specialized group practices. The local medical societies, however, whose members feared that support of specialized group practices would undermine the role of solo practitioners, opposed the proposition. Labor also vacillated in its support of the AALL's proposal. Sickness funds would help build union membership, but they would result in higher dues.

Further undermining the cause was the absence of a clear mandate for federal intervention. The well-being of the population fell under state jurisdiction (Rich & White, 1996). This made it extremely difficult for the federal government to justify a role in protecting the social welfare of the population. Although Theodore Roosevelt supported the proposal, his defeat by Woodrow Wilson, who did not support social legislation, meant there was even

less political support to advance the program. When America entered World War I in 1917, national health insurance was essentially off the public agenda.

The Great Depression and the Reconsideration of National Health Insurance

Franklin Delano Roosevelt was the first president to support national health insurance while in office. The Social Security Act of 1935 initially included a program of compulsory insurance, which was among the most contested parts of the legislative debate. To avoid jeopardizing passage of a bill that would create a wide array of programs to protect the economic and social well-being of the American public, national health insurance was eliminated from the Social Security Act before the legislation was presented to Congress (Falk, 1977).

Both the proposal for national health insurance and its elimination from the legislation were grounded in the work of the Committee on the Cost of Medical Care (CCMC) (Fein, 1989). The CCMC was a commission supported by eight foundations charged with examining the rising cost of medical care. In forming its recommendations, the committee was split on the same issues that divided the medical profession 20 years earlier. There was no consensus as to whether medical services should be provided through organized group practices or through private doctors. In addition, the committee did not agree on whether there should be compulsory health insurance or a system of voluntary prepayment for medical care. To present a single report, the CCMC came out in favor of group practice and voluntary insurance (Fein, 1989). Because of the CCMC's support for voluntary health insurance, Roosevelt was comfortable taking national health insurance out of the Social Security Act. Health insurance was described as one aspect of income protection. For the neediest Americans, the payment for medical services could be built into the system of state-administered welfare programs. In addition, the Maternal and Child Health Program would provide ancillary services to pregnant women and children. The Social Security Act was considered by some to be the first step toward a comprehensive program of social insurance (Marmor, 1973). Many assumed national health insurance could be legislated later, when the economy improved.

Congress Debates National Health Insurance

National health insurance reemerged on the public agenda after World War II, when President Harry Truman proposed a program of compulsory health insurance whereby beneficiaries would have comprehensive medical benefits that included medical and dental care, 60 days of hospital care, nursing home care, and prescription drugs benefits. Doctors would have the option to be paid on a fee-for-service basis, per capita, or be salaried. The program would be financed by a 3% payroll tax (Quadagno, 2005).

The opposition's counterproposal was based on Senator Robert Taft's proposal for federal grants to participating states to help finance hospital and physician services for low-income and needy families. This approach was voluntary, and its impact would be limited to a small segment of the population. Taft's proposal was an extension of the social welfare system created under the Social Security Act that would ultimately be the predecessor of the Kerr-Mill Program and, later, Medicaid (Grogan & Patashnik, 2003).

The AMA became the central voice of opposition to Truman's proposal for compulsory health insurance. The AMA had coalesced in its opposition to national health insurance as it came under the control of private practice physicians (Quadagno, 2005). They feared that a program of universal care supported by the government would shift control over the practice of medicine from physicians to government bureaucrats. This would jeopardize what was considered the highest standard of medical care in the world because physicians would lose control over the practice of medicine. The AMA compared a government-sponsored program of national health insurance to socialism, and worse, communism, to convince Americans that the dangers of government control outweighed the advantages. By 1949, 61 million Americans had some form of insurance. They argued that the free market would continue to grow and serve all Americans, but it risked destruction with national health insurance.

Medicare, Medicaid, and National Health Insurance

The passage of Medicare and Medicaid are important to the discussion of national health insurance because of the role they played in advancing the argument for a national program that would create access to health services for all Americans (Ball, 1995). On one hand, proponents of national health insurance assumed that if they were successful, these programs could be expanded to more and more Americans (Cairl & Imerschein, 1977). On the other hand, the accommodations made to physicians, hospitals, and private insurance companies when these programs were developed meant there was no way for the government to control costs (Marmor, 1973).

Medical costs grew exponentially after the implementation of Medicare. As a consequence, costs emerged as an issue alongside access. The result was the reemergence of national health insurance on the federal agenda. The Kennedy-Griffiths bill called for a comprehensive, federally operated health insurance system similar to the Canadian single-payer system (Bodenheimer, 2003). As always, the question of equity remained the principal demand of national health insurance advocates. The Kennedy-Griffiths bill provided a way to rationalize the healthcare system and control costs through a regionalized system of planning, monitoring, and payment reform. It would set up a national budget, allocate funds to regions, and provide incentives for prepaid group practice, thus obligating private hospitals and physicians to operate within budget constraints.

The Nixon administration looked for alternatives that would use market forces and competition to bring healthcare costs down. He proposed the Health Maintenance Organization Act of 1973 as a conservative alternative to the Kennedy-Griffiths proposal. Health maintenance organizations (HMOs) promised to control costs through the rationalization of the delivery system (Starr, 1982). The Health Maintenance Organization Act required employers to offer an HMO option. It also provided financial assistance for start-up HMOs and overrode existing state legal barriers. Overall, the act conferred legitimacy on the HMO concept (Bodenheimer, 2003). In the long run, managed care did not extend access or decrease costs. As an alternative option, it added one more element to the fragmented system of care (Bodenheimer, 2003).

Clinton's National Healthcare Proposal

The possibility of national health insurance was dormant until Bill Clinton's election as president in 1992. Healthcare costs were skyrocketing. The framework for payment was shifting from indemnity to managed care. Individuals were becoming increasingly frustrated about their loss of provider choice. Clinton proposed a way to preserve the private and public insurance market and extend it to ensure universal coverage through managed competition. Under this framework, the federal government set the stage by guaranteeing all American citizens the right to a comprehensive set of health benefits while the states had the obligation for implementation through the organization of purchasing cooperatives. The cooperatives would neither deliver the healthcare services nor pay providers; instead, they would contract with varied private health plans, including HMOs and preferred provider organizations. The cost would be shared between individuals and employers in most instances. Managed competition was designed to control costs by encouraging consumers to make both quality-conscious and cost-conscious decisions. Incentives were built into the legislation to motivate insurers to serve both high-risk and low-risk populations (Starr & Zelman, 1993).

Clinton's national health reform may have offered a reasonable policy alternative to control healthcare costs and promote quality of care, but the politics of the policy-making process was among the reasons for its defeat (Skocpol, 1995). The first lady, Hillary Clinton, was appointed to chair the Task Force on National Health Care Reform. By crafting its bill in private, the task force's work was greeted with derision and suspicion. Original supporters, including the health industry and labor groups, changed their minds about managed competition. Other providers and stakeholders—such as the hospital industry, AARP, pharmaceutical companies, and the AMA—joined forces with the insurance companies to lobby against national healthcare reform

(Skocpol, 1995). Opposition was heavily funded and effectively reached their target market. Republicans were further able to play on the public's fear of large government and the possible loss of freedom that might ensue, and President Clinton did not defend accusations made about the bill. The legislation did not make it to a vote in either house.

Growth in the Number of Uninsured People

With the failure of the Clinton proposal, the number of uninsured people in the United States continued to grow. The U.S. population grew by 15% in the years between 1994 and 2009, while the number of uninsured people increased at more than double that rate. By 2009, the U.S. Census Bureau's Current Population Survey counted 50 million uninsured people—about one of every five U.S. residents younger than age 65. Had the mostly federally financed State Children's Insurance Program (SCHIP) not greatly expanded Medicaid's reach, the number of uninsured people would likely have hit 65 million by 2009 (Kaiser Family Foundation, 2009). At its creation in 1997, SCHIP was the largest expansion of taxpayer-funded health insurance coverage for children in the United States since the establishment of Medicaid in 1965. But the number of uninsured people remained high and could be described in the following ways (Kaiser Family Foundation, 2013a):

- Sixty percent of uninsured people live in families where at least one adult is a full-time worker. Fifteen percent also have a part-time worker in the family.
- Thirty-seven percent of uninsured people are very poor and live in families below the poverty threshold, which, in 2010, was $22,050 for a family of four. Low- to moderate-income families (below 400% of federal poverty standard) accounted for all but 10% of the uninsured population.
- Children are the least likely age group to be uninsured. Young adults are the most likely.
- The uninsured population varies greatly across the country. In 2012, 27% of Texans younger than age 65 were uninsured, as were 27% of Nevadans and 25% of Floridians. In contrast, only 4% of Massachusetts residents lacked coverage (as a result of the 2006 reform), as did 9% of Vermont and District of Columbia residents.
- A total of 8 in 10 uninsured people are U.S. citizens.

By the early 2000s, a great deal was known about the effect of being uninsured. First were health impacts. According to the Kaiser Family Foundation, "uninsured patients have increased risk being diagnosed in later stages of diseases, including cancer, and have higher mortality rates than those with insurance" (2013d). Although uninsured people are more likely to be admitted to a hospital when suffering from an avoidable health problem, they are less likely to receive needed services. (Kaiser Family Foundation, 2013b). In fact, a 2009 study conducted by faculty at the Harvard University School of Public Health attributed 45,000 deaths to the lack of health insurance (Wilper et al., 2009).

The growing number of uninsured people was also causing problems for safety-net institutions that served them (often in an emergency) and for other providers who were facing an increasing burden of uncompensated care (Holahan & Garrett, 2010). Most uninsured people did not have access to free or discounted care. They spent far more out of pocket than those with insurance. More than half of bankruptcies in the United States were associated with medical bills. While many in financial trouble had inadequate insurance, a disproportionate number of filings were made by uninsured people.

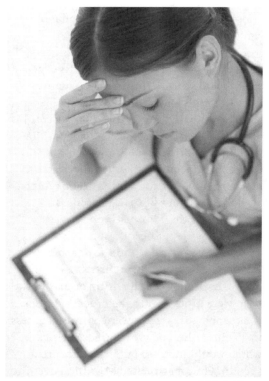

© Maridav/iStockphoto.com

Massachusetts Acts Alone

In 2005, about 10% of the Massachusetts population younger than age 65 was uninsured. The Massachusetts legislature chose to take action. Their reasons were the same as those that motivated the Clinton health plan and would greatly influence the development of the ACA: increasingly expensive health care and health insurance that fostered growth in the number of people who were uninsured and unable to receive regular care. The resulting stresses were apparent on

individuals and families as well as institutional providers (Symonds, 2006).

Between 2004 and 2006, the Affordable Care Today (ACT) coalition of community, labor, and political groups waged an energetic campaign that included collecting 75,000 signatures on a petition for state action to expand coverage. By April 2006, the Democrat-led state legislature and the Republican Governor Mitt Romney forged a compromise for a comprehensive one-state universal health insurance program. Its design and features presaged many of the elements incorporated into the ACA. Among the key features were the following (Kaiser Family Foundation, 2012a):

- Dependence on the continuation of employment-based coverage as the linchpin of coverage while using state programs to make insurance more affordable and accessible.

- The Commonwealth Health Insurance Connector, an exchange offering curated commercial products under the rubric of either the subsidized Commonwealth Care program for low- and moderate-income uninsured residents or nonsubsidized Commonwealth Choice plans.

- Insurance market reforms that required insurers to offer coverage to any eligible individual regardless of health status and health history. The state also created affordability standards in the commercial marketplace.

- Medicaid and SCHIP expansions to low-income families living below 300% of the federal poverty standard.

- Employer requirements to help pay the cost of coverage by any employer of 11 or more workers.

- Individual mandate to have insurance or pay a substantial penalty.

Obama and the Patient Protection and Affordable Care Act of 2010

The decade since the failure of the Clinton plan was marked by steeply increasing healthcare costs and declining levels of insurance coverage. Between 1999 and 2009, insurance premiums increased by 131% (Jacobs & Skocpol, 2012). The 2008 presidential election took place at the apogee of the 2008–2009 recession, during which, along with the loss of millions of jobs, loss of employment-based coverage accelerated. From its height in 2000, the percentage of people younger than age 65 who were covered through employment had declined each year. In 2009, employment-based insurance covered only 59% of U.S. residents younger than age 65 (U.S. Census Bureau, 2011). At the same time, the dip in the rate of economic growth further highlighted the effect healthcare spending had on the economy. In 2008, it was projected that health care would consume 15.2% of the GDP. It was difficult to imagine how the United States could restore a vibrant economy without finding some way to contain healthcare costs. Paradoxically, both Republican and Democratic candidates for major office argued for investment in national health insurance as a key mechanism to relieve the economic crunch.

As promised in his campaign, Barack Obama undertook health reform as the major initiative of his first term. The Obama administration's proposed health reform legislation was politically and programmatically modeled on the successful Massachusetts program (Kingsdale, 2009). His plan provided for the expansion of private insurance for moderate-income people who were uninsured and the Medicaid program for vulnerable populations. Central to the bill's intent were numerous provisions designed to control health spending through the eventual reorganization of the delivery system. The bill also included sections regarding regulation of the existing insurance market to make commercial insurance more affordable, more comprehensive, and more equitable.

Extrapolating on the 1993 debacle and replicating some of the Massachusetts experience, Obama reached out to representatives from Congress and healthcare stakeholders to build broad-based, nonpartisan support for his proposal. From the start, he faced opposition from the minority Republican party. But with enough Democratic strength in the Senate to prevent a filibuster, the administration forged ahead and sought a bipartisan proposal.

To bolster the administration's case, major lobbyists for hospitals, physicians, insurance companies, and the pharmaceutical and medical supply industries, who had been skeptical of health reform efforts in the past, were brought into the process (Jacobs & Skocpol, 2012). They were promised access to 25–30 million newly insured Americans, which would increase public healthcare spending by an estimated $1 trillion over the next decade. In addition, negotiations were held with each set of stakeholders to address their concerns regarding overregulation, the prohibition of price negotiations, and the reach of a public option.

The bills that would become the ACA passed the Senate in late December 2009 with no Republican votes. Then in January, the election of Scott Brown to fill the vacancy left by the death of Senator Ted Kennedy made it absolutely incumbent that the House accept the Senate bill so that it need not come back for Senate reconsideration. Despite repeated rebuffs from Democratic and Republican House moderates, Obama doggedly pushed ahead and kept the possibility of legislation alive. In the hopes of securing his Democratic base in the House of Representatives during the early winter of 2010, the administration conceded such key provisions as the creation of a public option and federal funding for abortion.

In the end, Obama's attempt to craft a bipartisan approach to health reform fell apart, and the legislation passed with the support of every Democrat in the Senate and 219 Democratic members of the House. No Republicans voted for the bill in either house. On March 23, 2010, President Obama signed the Patient Protection and Affordable Care Act (PPACA), and on March 30, 2010, he signed the Health Care and Education Reconciliation Act (HCERA) (Cannan, 2013). Together, these two pieces of legislation are called the *Affordable Care Act* or *ACA*. The term *Obamacare* is often used to refer to the legislation. It was a derogatory term coined by House Republicans, but Obama started using it as a way to destigmatize the expression.

The Affordable Care Act: What Is Included

The ACA was intended to move the United States incrementally closer to universal national health insurance. In doing so, it contained requirements regarding access, cost, quality, and organization and delivery of care that may, if implemented, transform much of the U.S. health system. As can be seen in Table 4-1, the legislation included a broad array of provisions (Kaiser Family Foundation, 2013b).

Table 4-1   ACA Provisions by Year

2010

Review of health plan premium increases

Changes in Medicare provider rates

Comparative effectiveness research

Prevention and Public Health Fund

Medicare beneficiary drug rebate

Small business tax credits

Medicaid drug rebate

Medicaid coverage for childless adults

Reinsurance program for retiree coverage

Preexisting condition insurance plan

New prevention council

Adult dependent coverage to age 26

(continued)

Table 4-1   ACA Provisions by Year (*continued*)

Consumer protections in insurance

Insurance plan appeals process

Health centers and the National Health Service Corps

Health Care Workforce Commission

2011

Minimum medical loss ratio for insurers

Closing the Medicare drug coverage gap

Medicare payments for primary care

Medicare prevention benefits

Center for Medicare and Medicaid Innovation

Medicare premiums for higher income beneficiaries

Medicare Advantage payment changes

Medicaid Health Homes

Chronic disease prevention in Medicaid

National quality strategy

Funding for health insurance exchanges

Nutritional labeling

Medicaid payments for hospital-acquired infections

Graduate medical education

Medicare independent payment advisory board

Medicaid long-term care services

2012

Accountable care organizations in Medicare

Uniform coverage summaries for consumers

Medicare Advantage plan payments

Medicare provider payment changes

Fraud and abuse prevention

Annual fees on the pharmaceutical industry

Medicaid payment demonstration projects

Data collection to reduce healthcare disparities

Medicare value-based purchasing

Reduced Medicare payments for hospital readmissions

2013

    State notification regarding exchanges

    Medicare Bundled Payment pilot program

    Medicaid coverage of preventive services

    Medicaid payments for primary care

    Flexible spending account limits

    Medicare tax increase

    Employer retiree coverage subsidy

    Tax on medical devices

    Financial disclosure

    Co-op health insurance plans

    Medicare disproportionate share hospital payments

    Medicaid disproportionate share hospital payments

2014

    Expanded Medicaid coverage

    Presumptive eligibility for Medicaid

    Individual requirement to have insurance

    Health insurance premium and cost-sharing subsidies

    Guaranteed availability of insurance

    No annual limits on coverage

    Essential health benefits

    Temporary reinsurance program for health plans

    Medicare Advantage plan loss ratios

    Wellness programs in insurance

    Fees on health insurance sector

    Medicare payments for hospital-acquired infections

2015

    Employer requirements

    Increase federal match for CHIP

2016

    Healthcare choice compacts

2018

    Tax on high-cost insurance

The Affordable Care Act: What Will Be Achieved?

More People Covered: The Individual Mandate

A central goal of the ACA is to extend affordable health insurance to uninsured American citizens and legal immigrants through a variety of mechanisms: Medicaid expansion for people with very low incomes and commercial products that would be affordable through sliding-scale tax subsidies for everyone else. The law requires near universality of participation through the individual mandate that, in 2014, requires all American citizens and legal immigrants to have basic health insurance or pay a tax penalty. Through these mechanisms, the framers of the ACA anticipated expansion of public and private health insurance to 30 million currently uninsured people.

Half of that expansion is to be through recalibration and federalization of Medicaid eligibility. The federal government is budgeted to pay virtually the full cost for all individuals and families with incomes under 138% of the federal poverty level. With the goal of helping young people with very low incomes to have coverage, the ACA has a special Medicaid entitlement provision for them (Jacobs & Skocpol, 2012). The impact of this provision, however, was limited by the Supreme Court decision in 2013 that upheld the constitutionality of the ACA but left the option of Medicaid expansion up the states. Twenty-four states have yet to opt in—leaving nearly 5 million adults ineligible for their home state's Medicaid program and too poor to qualify for federal assistance to purchase insurance on their own (Kaiser Family Foundation, 2013c).

Individuals younger than age 65 who are not eligible for Medicaid are expected to get health insurance either through their employer or by purchasing it through a health exchange. There are a variety of provisions to encourage employers to provide coverage for their employees and their dependents. Employers with more than 50 full-time employees must offer minimal affordable coverage or be subject to fines. In addition, the law provides for significant tax credits to incentivize small employers of low-wage workers and not-for-profit organizations to provide health benefits for their employees. The law also requires that employers who offer family coverage extend it to young adult children, and it sets certain minimum standards and coverage provisions (American Public Health Association, 2012). If the ACA succeeds in expanding coverage and lowering healthcare cost increases, employers and their workers will be among the primary beneficiaries of the law.

Most people who do not have employer-based plans can purchase insurance through state-run health insurance exchanges or marketplaces. The principle behind the exchanges is that by pooling many people, no individual or small group will have to bear a disproportionate share of the cost. In some ways, the exchange will act as a surrogate for a large employer, where insurance pooling happens naturally.

To address the issue of affordability, those with an income less than 400% of the poverty level can receive tax credits to reduce their premiums when they buy coverage through the exchange. To further enhance affordability, those who earn less than 250% of the poverty level can participate in cost-sharing programs. With cost sharing, the coverage has lower deductibles and copayments that are paid for by the federal government (Kaiser Family Foundation, 2012a).

The law also stipulates that insurance cannot be denied or cancelled because of anticipated health care utilization or cost (insurability). This is called guaranteed issue. In 2010, children and adults in some states who had previously been turned down for insurance because of preexisting conditions and had been uninsured for 6 months or longer were able to obtain coverage. In 2014, the ACA extended guaranteed issue to all adults in all states. Not covering people who are expected to use healthcare services makes insurance less costly. For insurance to be affordable and at the same time eliminate insurability requirements means that everyone—healthy or sick—must be in the pool. Without the individual mandate, some healthy people would opt out of insurance and pay for it only when they need it. The result would be ever-escalating premiums because only the sickest people would be in the pool (Alliance for Health Reform, 2012).

The exchanges are intended to simplify much of the complexity of health insurance by allowing consumers to comparison shop for the best affordable option. They have an overview of premiums versus deductibles, copays versus network size, and so forth. The theory is that the information available on the mostly online exchanges will provide an incentive for higher quality treatment at a lower cost. In some ways, the exchange model is a return to Clinton's managed competition idea.

States had the option of building their own state-based exchange or entering into a partnership with the federal government, or defaulting to a federally run exchange. As of January 2014, 17 states had created their own exchanges, 7 had opted for a joint program with the federal government, and 27 had refused to participate.* Residents of those 27 states were serviced by the federal exchange, which listed state-specific offerings presented through a federal template (Kaiser Family Foundation, 2014).

More Benefits and Protections

Public and private insurance companies must now provide 10 essential health benefits to participate in state exchanges: outpatient (ambulatory) care; emergency services; hospitalization; maternity and newborn care; mental health and addiction services, including behavioral health treatment; prescription drugs; rehabilitative and habilitative services and devices; laboratory services; preventive services, such as vaccines and chronic disease management; and pediatric services, including oral and vision. In addition, many preventive services—such as mammograms and colonoscopies; flu, mumps, and measles vaccinations; and blood pressure and cholesterol screenings—are included for free; neither copays nor deductibles can be charged.

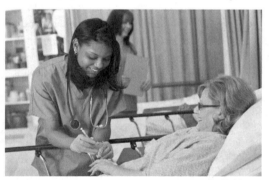

©asiseeit/iStockphoto.com

*State-specific exchanges: California, Colorado, Connecticut, District of Columbia, Hawaii, Idaho, Kentucky, Maryland, Massachusetts, Minnesota, Nevada, New Mexico, New York, Oregon, Rhode Island, Vermont, Washington. Partnership exchanges: Arkansas, Delaware, Illinois, Iowa, Michigan, New Hampshire, West Virginia. Federal exchange: Alabama, Alaska, Arizona, Florida, Georgia, Indiana, Kansas, Louisiana, Maine, Mississippi, Missouri, Montana, Nebraska, New Jersey, North Carolina, North Dakota, Ohio, Oklahoma, Pennsylvania, South Carolina, South Dakota, Tennessee, Texas, Utah, Virginia, Wisconsin, Wyoming.

The exchanges offer four tiers of coverage plus a limited catastrophic plan. The tiers are based on the percentage of costs (actuarial value) that the health plan can be anticipated to cover based on a typical group of enrollees. The coverage options ranges from the bronze tier, which covers 60% of expected costs, to the platinum tier, which covers 90% of costs. In between are gold (80%) and silver (70%) tiers. Every enrollee's out-of-pocket expenses are capped at $6,250 in 2014. The caps in subsequent years will be adjusted for inflation. Regardless of tier or plan design, the plan is responsible for all covered expenses in excess of the out-of-pocket maximum. Within these broad limits, insurance companies are free to invent plans with widely different features— networks, coinsurance, deductibles, and copays. They are required only to explain their offerings in a common prescribed format that was developed to allow consumers to compare one plan with the next (Levitt, Claxton, & Pollitz, 2012).

The ACA does not regulate insurance company premiums—that job is left to state insurance agencies—but it does impose some restrictions on rate setting. First, insurance companies may not charge higher premiums for individuals due to preexisting conditions, use of health services, or gender. Depending on preemptive state law, insurance companies are permitted to charge a predetermined additional percentage for individuals who smoke, are older, and reside in high-cost medical areas (Kaiser Family Foundation, 2012b). Insurance companies are required to spend at least 80 or 85% of insurance premiums on medical services depending on group size. This is called the medical loss ratio. In the year after the ACA was passed, many Americans received payments from their insurance companies because a greater percentage of their premiums was being spent on administrative support than was allowed by law.

There are a number of new transparency requirements, including annual reports that track quality improvement efforts. To a large extent, the areas that are being tracked align with the National Quality Strategy. Measures include strategies to improve health services, patient outcomes, and population health. These include harm reduction, promotion of patient-centered care, and the proper use of electronic records, among others. A new not-for-profit organization, the Patient-Centered Outcomes Research Institute, will identify, research, and compare clinical effectiveness treatments (Kaiser Family Foundation, 2012a).

Cost Control through Medicare Reconfiguration

The implementation of all health insurance subsidies built into the ACA was projected to cost $1 trillion between 2013 and 2022. None of the money will be paid from the government's tax-generated general fund. Instead, all the money is expected through reductions in federal spending on Medicare and Medicaid, additional revenue from taxes on insurance companies and other parts of the healthcare industry, higher premiums from higher income Medicare beneficiaries, an increase in Medicare tax from people who earn $200,000 or more, and a general slowdown in healthcare spending over what was projected prior to enactment of the ACA. In other words, the ACA is premised on reducing the rate of growth of healthcare costs. The largest reduction in the rate will come from changes in the way Medicare pays for care. Embedded in the ACA are plans to reduce Medicare payments to providers by $716 billion over a 10-year period.

Among the first actions designed to contain Medicare spending was a permanent reduction in the special allowance the government paid to the Medicare Advantage plans. There are numerous provisions related to provider payments to reduce the growth in future Medicare payments, including smaller annual adjustments and reducing special payments to hospitals that currently serve the uninsured population. Most of the details were to be designed by a new Independent Payment Advisory Board, whose 15 members were to be appointed by the president and confirmed by the Senate. Although the ACA contains the legislative authority to create the board, its establishment has been caught in the web of partisan politics, and as of June 2014, no appointments had been made.

Among the most promising payment reform initiatives is Accountable Care Organizations (ACOs), in which groups of doctors and hospitals or other healthcare providers take responsibility for the care of 5,000 or more Medicare beneficiaries. The federal government will share savings with an ACO if, at the end of a period, costs are contained and care is not compromised. Quality standards must be met. If, on the other hand, costs rise more than expected or quality is not maintained, the federal government may penalize the ACO. On January 1, 2014, there were 366 federally qualified Medicare ACOs across the country (Muhlestein, 2014).

The ACA also addresses the problems of persons who receive both Medicare and Medicaid or are dually eligible (McDonough, 2011). There are 9 million people who are dually eligible. On average, they are far less healthy than other Medicaid or Medicare beneficiaries and account for a disproportionate share of both Medicare and Medicaid payments (Coughlin, Waidmann, & Phadera, 2012). The ACA

created the federal Coordinated Health Care Office, another new entity within the Centers for Medicare and Medicaid Services, which is responsible for coordination between the federal government and the states to improve access and care coordination for this population. Improving care coordination is essential to reduce hospital and nursing home admissions, improve outcomes, and lower costs.

Increasing Primary Care Capacity

By expanding access to health insurance, it is important that there is the capacity to serve people who are newly insured. Several initiatives have been put into place. The ACA aims to induce more MDs and nurse practitioners to practice primary care by increasing reimbursement for their services. Medicare provider payments are increasing 10% for primary care services and for general surgeons who practice in underserved communities from 2011 through 2015. Medicaid will increase provider payments for primary care services to be equal to Medicare Part B. States will receive 100% matching funds from the federal government to fund the payment increase (Centers for Medicare and Medicaid Services, 2014).

Grants are available for primary care residencies in underserved areas and teaching hospitals that help low-income students become physicians, as well as graduate-level nursing education, under Medicare. The loan repayment program is offering primary care professionals, such as nurses and physicians, funds to repay student loans in exchange for 2 years of service working in underserved areas. Grants for nurse practitioners who are providing primary care in federal health centers and clinics are also available (Kaiser Family Foundation, 2012a).

Through the ACA, new funding has been allocated for community health centers and school-based health centers. The funds will be used to create centers in underserved areas and expand preventive and primary care services at existing centers.

Improved Public Health

The United States healthcare delivery system is often referred to as *disease care*. The ACA endorses an evolution toward a system that is grounded in prevention and health promotion. A number of initiatives have been put forth in support of this shift in thinking and practice. The Prevention and Public Health Fund (PPHF) was created "to provide for expanded and sustained national investment in prevention and public health programs to improve health and help restrain the rate of growth in private and public health care costs" (Patient Protection and Affordable Care Act, 2010). Over 10 years, $15 billion will be spent on state and local public health initiatives (American Public Health Association, 2013). This is the first mandatory public health fund. The PPHF supports the work of the Centers for Disease Control and Prevention and the Health Resources and Services Administration, which includes community and clinical prevention, public health infrastructure and training, and research and tracking (American Public Health Association, 2013).

Community Transformation Grants (CTGs) will be awarded to fight chronic disease on the community level. These grants are part of a larger initiative to link the findings of biomedical researchers to the practice of medicine. The grant recipients will focus on promoting smoke-free, active, and healthy lifestyles; prevention and maintenance of high blood pressure and cholesterol; promoting safe environments; and reducing health disparities in underserved populations (Centers for Disease Control and Prevention, 2012). CTGs are cross-sector collaborations that bring healthcare delivery systems to the population.

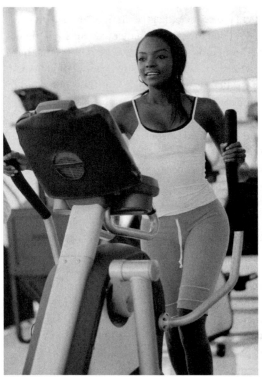

©Andres Rodriguez/Dreamstime.com

Broad public education campaigns have been designed to improve the health of the population by focusing on preventable diseases such as heart disease, cancer, and diabetes. These campaigns will focus on behavioral change (Shearer, 2010). Hospitals, government health agencies, and various stakeholders must engage in community health improvement strategies and meet the requirements of a Community Health Needs Assessment (CHNA) to keep their tax exempt status (Centers for Disease Control and Prevention, 2013). Restaurants with more than 20 locations must provide calorie labeling on menu boards, drive-through windows, and vending machines. Additional nutritional information must be available at the customer's request (McDonough, 2011).

Politics of the Transition

Court and Medicaid Expansion

The opposition to the ACA has been strong. Not a single Republican member of the House or Senate voted for the law in 2009–2010. Since then, thousands of business, political, religious, and community groups have lobbied and demonstrated against the law. Approximately once per month, the Republican-controlled House passes a defunding bill that has no hope of passage in the Democratic Senate.

The most significant challenge to the law came through the courts. Twenty-five Republican governors, together with the National Federation of Independent Business and a number of related organizations, challenged the constitutionality of the individual mandate and the Medicaid expansion. On the last day of the 2011–2012 term, the Supreme Court found the individual mandate to be constitutional but issued a complicated decision on the Medicaid issue. A majority of the justices found that states did not have adequate notice to voluntarily consent, therefore the secretary of Health and Human Services could not make payment of all Medicaid funds contingent on agreeing to expand. The court's majority did not invalidate the expansion section of the law, but it eviscerated the federal government's ability to enforce it. Medicaid expansion has now become a state option (Liptak, 2012).

The Disaster of Going Live

Political opposition to the ACA gathered momentum after October 1, 2013, when the much-anticipated exchanges opened for business. Despite many heartwarming stories about persons who did not have health insurance for 6, 8, or 10 years due to preexisting conditions, the process of purchasing insurance through the exchanges proved more difficult than anyone imagined (Cohn, 2013). While some people were easily able to purchase insurance, others made multiple failed attempts. Somewhat fewer problems were reported by the states that opted to run their own exchanges. Correcting these problems has been a top priority for the Obama administration.

Many people were disappointed by what they were offered on the exchanges—plans that were too costly, too few providers, deductible or copays that were too high. One person reported looking for a family plan but could not find one that had a pediatrician within 20 miles of her home. Another found that her life-sustaining prescription drugs would not be covered. Even with the significant technological and information difficulties, the exchanges reached more than 100% of their target enrollment by March 31, 2014, the official end of the open enrollment period. As of that date, 8 million people had enrolled in an exchange plan, and another 4.8 million had been found eligible for Medicaid and CHIP (Assistant Secretary for Planning and Evaluation, 2014).

Conclusion: Change the American Way, an Incremental Step

The ACA is changing the landscape of the healthcare delivery system in the United States. Designed to fill insurance gaps that currently exist, the legislation's aim is to provide coverage through low-cost insurance and high-quality care. These problems are broad, and so are their solutions. Success is not guaranteed. It is hard to predict exactly what the impact of the policies will be on the health of Americans and the healthcare delivery system. "Every citizen deserves the right to a healthy and productive life. That's the politics of health care" (Nickitas, 2013, p. 265).

The fact remains that the United Sates is the only developed country without universal access to health care or health insurance. Not every state is participating in Medicaid expansion, and funding has not increased for safety-net services. Approximately 30 million individuals living in the United States are not American citizens and will remain uninsured. The ACA is an amazing accomplishment for the Obama administration. It is a step closer to a cohesive national system. The next administration that proposes health system reform will use Obama's successes and failures as a guide to achieving the next step. Strong political leadership will be imperative.

Discussion Questions

1. How would you explain the political and cultural resistance to national health insurance in the United States?
2. How does the ACA move the United States closer to providing health insurance coverage to all Americans?
3. How will the ACA help control costs and improve the quality of care?
4. Given the limits of the ACA and the difficulties encountered in implementing the exchanges, what policy changes would you recommend to provide health insurance to those who remain uninsured?

References

Alliance for Health Reform. (2012). *Covering health issues* (6th ed.). Retrieved from http://www. allhealth.org/sourcebookcontent.asp?CHID=121

American Public Health Association. (2012). *Affordable care act overview.* Retrieved from http://www.apha.org/NR/rdonlyres/26831F24-882A-4FF7-A0A9-6F49DFBF6D3F/0/ACAOverview_Aug2012.pdf

American Public Health Association. (2013). *Prevention and public health fund.* Retrieved from http://www.apha.org/APHA/CMS_Templates/ChannelDefault.aspx?NRMODE=Published&NRNODEGUID=%7bD71F6AD2-E25B-460E-AFC0-2984BF741331%7d

&NRORIGINALURL=%2fadvocacy%2fHealth%2bReform%2fPH%2bFund%2f&NRCACHEHINT=NoModifyGuest#PPHFFAQ

Assistant Secretary for Planning and Evaluation. (2014). *Profiles of Affordable Care Act coverage expansion enrollment for Medicaid/CHIP and the health insurance marketplace,10-1-2013 TO 3-31-2014. (May 1, 2014).* Retrieved from http://aspe.hhs.gov/health/reports/2014/MarketPlaceEnrollment/Apr2014/Marketplace_StateSum.cfm

Ball, R. (1995). What Medicare's architects had in mind. *Health Affairs, 14*(4), 62–73.

Bodenheimer, T. (2003). The movement for universal health insurance: Finding common ground. *American Journal of Public Health, 93*(1), 112–115.

Cairl, R., & Imershein, A. (1977). National health insurance policy in the United States: A case of non-decision-making. *International Journal of Health Services, 7*(2), 167–178.

Cannan, J. (2013). A legislative history of the Affordable Care Act: How legislative procedure shapes legislative history. *Law Library Journal, 105*(2), 2013–2017. Retrieved from http://www.aallnet.org/main-menu/publications/llj/llj-archives/vol-105/no-2/2013-7.pdf

Centers for Disease Control and Prevention. (2012). *Community transformation grants (CTG).* Retrieved from http://www.cdc.gov/communitytransformation/

Centers for Disease Control and Prevention. (2013). *Resources for implementing the community health needs assessment process.* Retrieved from http://www.cdc.gov/policy/chna/

Centers for Medicare and Medicaid Services. (2014). *Affordable Care Act.* Retrieved from http://www.medicaid.gov/affordablecareact/affordable-care-act.html

Cohn, J. (2013). *The truth about the Obamacare rollout: The feds botched the website but the states are doing much better.* Retrieved from http://www.newrepublic.com/article/115230/obamacare-implementation-what-feds-got-wrong-states-got-right

Coughlin, T. A., Waidmann, T. A., & Phadera, L. (2012). Among dual eligibles, identifying the highest-cost individuals could help in crafting more targeted and effective responses. *Health Affairs, 31*, 1083–1091.

Falk, I. S. (1977). Proposals for national health insurance in the USA: Origins and evolution, and some perceptions for the future. *The Milbank Memorial Fund Quarterly: Health and Society, 5*(2), 161–191.

Fein, R. (1989). *Medical care, medical costs: The search for a health insurance policy.* Cambridge, MA: Harvard University Press.

Grogan, C., & Patashnik, E. M. (2003). Universalism within targeting. *Social Service Review, 77*(1), 51–71.

Holahan, J., & Garrett, B. (2010). *The cost of uncompensated care with and without health reform.* Washington, DC: Urban Institute. Retrieved from http://www.urban.org/UploadedPDF/412045_cost_of_uncompensated.pdf.

Jacobs, L. R., & Skocpol, T. (2012). *Health care reform and American politics: What everyone needs to know.* New York, NY: Oxford University Press.

Kaiser Family Foundation. (2009). *The impact of Medicaid and SCHIP on low-income children's health.* Retrieved from http://kaiserfamilyfoundation.files.wordpress.com/2013/01/7645-02.pdf

Kaiser Family Foundation. (2012a). *Focus on health reform, explaining health care reform: Questions about health insurance subsidies.* Retrieved from http://kaiserfamilyfoundation.files.wordpress.com/2013/01/7962-02.pdf

Kaiser Family Foundation. (2012b). *Focus on health reform; health insurance market reforms: Rate restrictions.* Retrieved from http://kaiserfamilyfoundation.files.wordpress.com/2013/01/8328.pdf.

Kaiser Family Foundation. (2013a). *Key facts about the uninsured population.* Retrieved from http://kaiserfamilyfoundation.files.wordpress.com/2013/01/7962-02.pdf.

Kaiser Family Foundation. (2013b). *Summary of the Affordable Care Act.* Retrieved from http://kaiserfamilyfoundation.files.wordpress.com/2011/04/8061-021.pdf

Kaiser Family Foundation. (2013c). *The coverage gap: Uninsured poor adults in states that do not expand Medicaid.* Retrieved from http://kff.org/health-reform/issue-brief/the-coverage-gap-uninsured-poor-adults-in-states-that-do-not-expand-medicaid/

Kaiser Family Foundation. (2013d). *The uninsured: A primer: Key facts about health insurance on the eve of coverage expansions.* Retrieved from http://kff.org/report-section/the-uninsured-a-primer-2013-4-how-does-lack-of-insurance-affect-access-to-health-care/

Kaiser Family Foundation. (2014). *State decisions for creating health insurance marketplaces.* Retrieved from http://kff.org/health-reform /state-indicator/health-insurance-exchanges/

Kingsdale, J. (2009). Implementing health care reform in Massachusetts: Strategic lessons learned. *Health Affairs, 28*(4), 588–594.

Levitt, L., Claxton, G., & Pollitz, K. (2012). *Private insurance benefits and cost-sharing under the ACA.* Retrieved from http://kff.org/health-reform/perspective/private-insurance-benefits-and-cost-sharing-under-the-aca/

Liptak, A. (2012, June 28). Supreme Court upholds health care law, 5–4, in victory for Obama. *The New York Times.* Retrieved from http://www.nytimes.com/2012/06/29/us /supreme-court-lets-health-law-largely-stand.html?pagewanted=all&_r=0

Marmor, T. (1973). *The politics of Medicare.* Hawthorne, NY: Aldine.

McDonough, J. E. (2011). *Inside national health reform.* Berkeley: University of California Press.

Muhlestein, D. (2014). *Accountable care growth in 2014: A look ahead.* Retrieved from http: //www.cap.org/apps/docs/advocacy/aco /ac_growth_2014.pdf

Nickitas, D. M. (2013). The politics of health care: Congress vs. consumers. *Nursing Economics, 31*(6), 265.

Organisation for Economic Co-operation and Development (OECD. (2014). *OECD Factbook 2014: Economic, Environmental and Social Statistics,* OECD Publishing. http://dx.doi.org/10.1787/factbook-2014-ed

Patient Protection and Affordable Care Act, Public Law 111-148, Section 4002: Prevention and Public Health Fund (2010).

Quadagno, J. (2005). *One nation uninsured: Why the US has no national health insurance.* New York, NY: Oxford University Press.

Rich, R. F., & White, W. D. (1996). Health care policy and the American states: Issues of federalism. In R. F. Rich & W. D. White (Eds.), *Health policy,* federalism and the American states. Washington, DC: Urban Institute Press.

Schoen, C., Osborn, R., Squires, D., & Doty, M. M. (2013). Access, affordability, and insurance complexity are often worse in the United States compared to ten other countries. *Health Affairs, 32.* Retrieved from http://www.commonwealthfund.org /publications/in-the-literature/2013/nov /access-affordability-and-insurance.

Shearer, G. (2010). *Prevention provisions in the Affordable Care Act* (Issue brief). American Public Health Association. Retrieved from http://www.apha.org/NR/rdonlyres/763D7507-2CC3-4828-AF84-1010EA1304A4/0/FinalPreventionACAWeb.pdf.

Skocpol, T. (1995). *Boomerang: Health reform and the turn against government.* New York, NY: W. W. Norton.

Starr, P. (1982). *The social transformation of American medicine.* New York, NY: Basic Books.

Starr, P., & Zelman, W. A. (1993). A bridge to compromise: Competition under a budget [Suppl.]. *Health Affairs,* 7–23.

Steinmo, S., & Watts, J. (1995). It's the institutions, stupid! Why comprehensive national health insurance always fails in America. *Journal of Health Politics, Policy and Law, 20*(2), 329–372.

Symonds, W. C. (2006, April 3). In Massachusetts, health care for all? *Bloomberg Business Week.*

U.S. Census Bureau. (2011). *Current population reports: Income, poverty, and health insurance coverage in the United States: 2011.* Washington, DC: Author. Retrieved from http://www.census.gov/prod/2012pubs/p60-243.pdf

Wilper, A., Woolhandler, S., Lasser, K., McCormick, D., Bor, D., & Himmelstein, D. (2009). Health insurance and mortality in U.S. adults. *American Journal of Public Health, 99*(12), 2289–2295.

World Bank. (2013). *World development indicators: Health systems.* Retrieved from http://wdi.worldbank.org/table/2.15

The Health Labor Force: Understanding the Distribution of Power and Influence

CHAPTER 5

Nurses: Leading Change to Improve Health and Health Care

Donna M. Nickitas

Overview

Nurses comprise the largest segment of the healthcare workforce in the United States, and they are the professionals who spend the most time providing direct care to patients. They play an essential role in helping to advance the nation's health. "Registered Nurses represent the largest profession within the U.S. health workforce, with over 2.7 million RNs employed in 2010 (U.S. Bureau of Labor Statistics [BLS], 2012). The BLS forecasts demand for RNs will result in 3.5 million nursing jobs by 2020, marking a 26% increase over 10 years" (Spetz, 2014). Nurses are indispensable to a patient's overall quality of health, safety, and satisfaction with care delivery. They are well positioned to improve health and health care, and to influence policy. This ability to drive health policy emerges from the recommendation of the Institute of Medicine's report titled *The Future of Nursing: Leading Change, Advancing Health* (2010) to promote nurses for appointments to governing boards, commissions, task forces, and other policy-related entities.

As hospitals begin to submit new data to the Centers for Medicare and Medicaid Services on patient satisfaction, nursing will be one of the most important factors in how patients rate their hospital experiences and whether they would recommend their hospital to a family member or friend (Centers for Medicare and Medicaid Services, 2006). In fact, several studies have demonstrated a relationship between patient satisfaction and nurse staffing levels, a higher proportion of registered nurse (RN) skill mix, RN–physician collaboration, and nurses' work environments (Bolton et al., 2003; Cramer, 2014; Daley, 2014; Larrabee et al., 2004; McGillis Hall et al., 2003; Roberts, 2014; Seago, Williamson, & Atwood, 2006; Sovie & Jawad, 2001; Tervo-Heikkinen, Kiviniemi, Partanen, & Vehvilainen-Julkunen, 2009; Tervo-Heikkinen, Kvist, Partanen, Vehviläinen-Julkunen, & Aalto, 2008; Vahey, Aiken, Sloane, Clarke, & Vargas, 2004). Today's healthcare environment is exceedingly complex and requires that nurses be exceptionally prepared to provide quality health care and that they support healthcare reform.

The Institute for Healthcare Improvement (IHI) has developed a framework that describes an approach to optimizing health system performance (2014). IHI says new designs must be developed to simultaneously pursue three dimensions, which they call the Triple Aim:

- Improving the patient experience of care (including quality and satisfaction)
- Improving the health of populations
- Reducing the per capita cost of health care

It is important that nurses focus on excellent patient care outcomes and identify nursing practices that align with the Triple Aim. Policy makers and healthcare stakeholders must be informed about the education–quality relationship of nurses and how the nursing profession adds value to the overall healthcare delivery system. This chapter will focus on ways in which nurses lead change to improve health and health care that drive economic and social policies that effectively promote the health of populations.

Objectives

- Explain the critical role nurses play in leading change to improve health and health care.
- Inform nurses about how healthcare reform will achieve the Triple Aim of better care for individuals, better health for populations, and lower per capita costs.
- Identify the challenges and opportunities for addressing the nation's shortage of nurses and nurse faculty.
- Describe various approaches and solutions to the nursing shortage.

Origins of the Nursing Profession

From its beginning, nursing was defined as having "charge of the personal health of somebody . . . and what nursing has to do . . . is to put the patient in the best condition for nature to act upon him" (Nightingale, 1860, p. 126). This early definition of nursing was written by Florence Nightingale and included many of the concepts still considered important today; this was remarkable considering how undeveloped professional nursing was in the mid- to late-1800s. Nightingale was strategic in her thinking about the importance of the observational skills of nurses and the impact of the environment on health. She clearly recognized health promotion and health maintenance as important responsibilities of nursing.

Until the late 19th century, nursing was seen as common employment for women, and nurses were viewed as second-class citizens with ill morals and poor character. To overcome the negative societal views of nursing and to improve the qualities of potential nurse recruits, efforts were made to establish proper preparation for nurses. A physician, Ann Preston, organized in 1861 the first training program for nurses in the United States at Philadelphia's Woman's Hospital. This training program was open to women "who wished greater proficiency in their domestic responsibilities" (Stevens, 1989, p. 17).

The choice to use hospitals as the site for training nurses expanded rapidly in the late 1800s as hundreds of new hospitals were built under the aegis of religious orders, ethnic group industrialists, and elite groups of civic-minded individuals who looked for efficient ways to staff their wards. Because student nurses were a constantly renewable source of low-cost workers to staff the wards, even some of the smallest hospitals maintained nursing schools (Stevens, 1989). Hospital nursing school programs, therefore, were primarily sequences of on-the-job training rather than academic courses.

World War I had a profound affect on the nursing profession. Before the war, nursing was divided into three domains: public health, private duty, and hospital. Public health nursing was an elite pursuit and was recognized as instrumental in the campaign against infectious diseases, such as tuberculosis, and in promoting population health, such as infant welfare. By 1920, more than 70% of nurses worked in private duty; about half of those worked in patients' homes and half worked for private patients in hospitals. Hospital nurses were primarily those in training. The war emphasized the drama and effectiveness of hospitals, and it soon codified hospitals as the center of nursing education in the increasingly specialized acute care medical environment. The war experience established nurses as dedicated associates in hospital science. Nursing

leaders promoted the idea of upgrading nursing through high-quality hospital nursing schools, preferably associated with universities. The choice to idealize the role of nurses as dedicated and deferential to physician specialists in the hospital marginalized the independent role of nurses in social medicine and public health. The social medicine and public health aspects of nursing were subjugated to the image of nursing as a symbol of patriotism, national sacrifice, and efficiency.

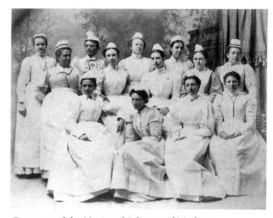

Courtesy of the National Library of Medicine

As World War II brought increased specialization to the field of nursing and ultimately funding for the educational preparation of nurses, they began to specialize during the 1950s. Because of the short supply of nurses after World War II, hospitals began to group the least physiologically stable patients in one nursing unit for intensive care, where the more competent nurses cared for the sickest patients. This arrangement did not lower the need for nurses but instead created the need for a critical care nurse specialty as the need for staff nurses continued to grow. To increase manpower, Congress passed the Nurse Training Act of 1964 and the Health Manpower Act of 1968. The Nurse Training Act of 1971 added substantially to the federal support of nursing education (Lamm, 1996). Nevertheless, state funding provided the largest support for nursing schools, 80% of which are in colleges and universities.

Nursing Definitions: Past and Present

The definitions of nursing in the early 20th century focused on nursing functions and were holistic. Virginia Henderson wrote one of the most widely accepted definitions of nursing in this era: "Nursing may be defined as that service to an individual that helps him to attain or maintain a healthy state of mind or body" (Harmer & Henderson, 1939, p. 2). She later refined her definition into one that is perhaps best known in the world because of its adoption by the International Council of Nurses:

> The unique function of the nurse is to assist the individual, sick or well, in the performance of those activities contributing to health or its recovery (or to a peaceful death) that he would perform unaided if he had the necessary strength, will or knowledge. And to do this in such a way as to help him gain independence as rapidly as possible. (Henderson, 1960, p. 3)

In 1952, Hildegard Peplau added an important dimension to the definition of nursing by expressing it in interpersonal terms. Peplau stated that "the goals of nursing are currently in transition; it's major concerns fifty years ago had to do with getting sick people well; today, nursing is more concerned with ways for helping people to stay well" (1992, p. 6). Nursing

theory development during the 1950s and 1960s continued to refine the definition of nursing.

In the contemporary sphere of nursing, the current definition emerges from the 2003 edition of the American Nurses Association's (ANA) Nursing's Social Policy Statement:

> Nursing is the protection, promotion, and optimization of health and abilities, prevention of illness and injury, alleviation of suffering through the diagnosis and treatment of human response, and advocacy in the care of individuals, families, communities, and populations. (American Nurses Association [ANA], 2010, p. 41)

This definition of nursing provides a framework for nursing practice and curriculum development, and it defines the boundaries, functions, and purpose of the profession. It includes the four essential characteristics of nursing: human responses or phenomena, theory application, nursing actions or interventions, and outcomes (ANA, 2010.) A clear understanding of the boundaries of nursing is needed as more allied health professions and unlicensed assistive personnel are added to the patient care arena. Policy makers need to understand the role of nursing to make the best decisions on healthcare policy. With this goal in mind, nurses must work with key policy makers to promote crucial conversations about economic and social policies that can cost-effectively promote the health of communities. The profession is well positioned to play a leadership role in helping the government address the $2.7 trillion spent on health care annually (Hartman, Martin, Benson, Catlin, & National Health Expenditure Accounts Team, 2013).

Nursing Regulation

Nursing regulation is provided by government oversight through administrative and legislative bodies within each state. Nursing as a health profession must be regulated because it may pose risk of harm to the public if it is practiced by someone who is unprepared and incompetent. As a rule, the public may not have sufficient information and experience to identify an unqualified healthcare provider and is vulnerable to unsafe and incompetent practitioners; therefore, to protect the public's health and interest, each state establishes its own board of nursing, which is responsible for the regulation of nursing practice, including the scope of practice. Boards of nursing are authorized to enforce the Nurse Practice Act (NPA) and develop administrative rules, regulations, and other responsibilities in accordance with the act. The definition in the NPA acts as the legal definition of nursing in that state. The legislatures of all states and territories have enacted an NPA. The NPA itself is insufficient to provide the necessary guidance for the nursing profession; therefore, each NPA establishes a board of nursing that has the authority to develop administrative rules or regulations to clarify the law or make it more specific. Rules and regulations must be consistent with the NPA and cannot go beyond it. These rules and regulations undergo a process of public review before enactment. After they are enacted, rules and regulations have the full force and effect of law (National Council of State Boards of Nursing, 2014a).

The specific details of the NPA differ among states; however, they all must include the following (National Council of State Boards of Nursing, 2014b):

- Authority, power, and composition of a board of nursing
- Education program standards
- Standards and scope of nursing practice
- Types of titles and licenses
- Requirements for licensure
- Grounds for disciplinary action, other violations, and possible remedies

Every nurse must be informed and educated about the practice of nursing in his or her state. It is a right granted by a state to protect those who need and require nursing care. The guidelines of the NPA and its rules provide safe parameters within which to work, and they protect patients from unprofessional and unsafe nursing practice. The act is a dynamic document that evolves and is updated or amended as changes in scope of practice occur.

Licensure

State boards of nursing regulate nursing practice, including the scope of nursing practice. In each state, the model NPA describes the scope of practice for RNs, licensed practical/vocational nurses, and advanced practice nurses (APRNs). Licensure is one type of regulation. It is the process by which boards of nursing grant permission to an individual to engage in nursing practice after determining that the applicant has attained the competency necessary to perform a unique scope of practice safely (National Council of State Boards of Nursing, 2011). Licensure is necessary when the regulated activities are complex; it requires specialized knowledge and skills, as well as independent decision making. The National Council of State Boards of Nursing includes the following in the intent of licensure:

- A specified scope of practice may be performed legally only by licensed individuals.

- Title protection is granted to those individuals who meet the legal and educational standards of the profession. Licensed individuals adhere to professional codes of conduct.
- The authority to take disciplinary action is granted to protect the public if the licensee violate the laws or rules.

"The mission of the National Council of State Boards of Nursing is to provide education, service, and research through collaborative leadership to promote evidence-based regulatory excellence for patient safety and public protection" (National Council of State Boards of Nursing, 2010).

Certification

Certification is another type of credential that affords title protection and recognition of accomplishment, but it does not include a legal scope of practice. The federal government has used the term *certification* to define the credentialing process by which a nongovernmental agency or association recognizes individuals who have met specified requirements. Many state boards of nursing use professional certification as one requirement toward granting authority for an individual who obtained advanced or specialized training in an area of practice, as with RNs.

Although specialty certification was found to be associated with better patient outcomes, such outcomes were associated only when care was provided by baccalaureate-educated nurses (Kendall-Gallagher, Aiken, Sloane, & Cimiotti, 2011). The authors concluded that no effect of specialization was seen in the absence of baccalaureate education.

Some state government agencies have also used the term *certification* for governmental credentialing. Confusion may occur because regulatory agencies and professional membership associations may use the same term in a different context. Certification is the regulating process under which a state or voluntary professional organization, such as a national board, attests to the educational achievements and performance abilities of persons in a healthcare field of practice. This certification provides practitioners with an additional sense of personal and professional accomplishment beyond an academic degree and licensure.

Certification is a much less restrictive regulation than licensing. It allows the public, employers, and third-party payers to determine which practitioners are appropriately qualified in their specialty or occupation. It generally has no provision for regulating impaired or misbehaving practitioners other than putting them on probation or dropping their certification. Unlike licensure, certification has no legal basis for preventing an impaired or professionally delinquent individual from practicing (National Council of State Boards of Nursing, 2011).

Nursing's Professional Status

Recognition

From the very beginning, the nursing profession struggled with the challenge of being recognized as a valuable contributor to health care in settings such as hospitals, nursing homes, schools, health departments, and industry. In part, much of this lack of recognition was because nursing was, and still is, a female profession, with only 9.1% of the workforce represented by men (Health Resources and Services Administration, 2013). While the increases in enrollment are a positive indicator, the representation of men in nursing education programs remains low. Current estimates show that men are approximately 9–11% of the nursing workforce (National Advisory Council on Nurse Education and Practice [NACNEP], 2013). Men accounted for 8.8% of all baccalaureate degree graduates, 10.6% of master's degree graduates, and 4% of doctoral program graduates in the fall of 2004 (NACNEP, 2008).

As a female-dominated profession, society views caring by nurses as natural to their gender role and not within the scope of a professional role that requires education and licensure, like law and medicine. This is evidenced in the education of nurses. During the latter part of the 19th century, much of nursing education and preparation was hospital-based apprenticeships. Nurses learned by doing and were dominated by hospital administrators and the medical profession, who were university trained. Nurses were expected to carry out the orders of physicians. With this subservient position, along with the increasing demands of hospitals, nurses quickly became discouraged and turned to collective bargaining and union representation for expanded access to decision making, higher wages, and improved job security.

With hospital training programs now accounting for less than 5% of new graduates, nurses have been able to professionalize their educational preparation (Aiken, Cheung, & Olds, 2009). From hospital training in the early 19th century to university-based schools of nursing in the beginning of the 20th century to the present and the emergence of associate's degree programs of the mid-20th century, nursing has slowly begun to lift the quality and quantity of the workforce. In October 2010, the Institute of Medicine released its landmark report, *The Future of Nursing*, initiated by the Robert Wood Johnson Foundation, which called for increasing the number of baccalaureate-prepared nurses in the workforce to 80% and doubling the population of nurses with doctoral degrees (Institute of Medicine [IOM], 2010).

Leading Change to Advance the Nation's Health

Nurses are essential to the healthcare system, serving on the front lines at the bedside and in the board room. The U.S. Bureau of Labor Statics forecasts that demand for RNs will result in 3.5 million nursing jobs by 2020, suggesting a marked increase of 26% from 2010 levels. This will shift RN employment away from acute care to the outpatient or ambulatory care setting, particularly to physicians' offices and home care services. Additionally, the Affordable Care Act (ACA) will impact where RNs will work and the skills that will be needed within those settings. For example, nurses will be expected to focus on roles that include care coordination, case management, patient educators, and chronic care specialists (Spetz, 2014).

The demand for RNs will continue to grow at a higher rate, driven largely by population growth due to the increased number of older adults who require more healthcare services. To meet this demand, nurses must demonstrate leadership by becoming more effective in political advocacy to advance nursing and nurse workforce issues to the national health agenda. Only by active participation will the professional status and recognition of nursing improve. Nurses at all levels of practice must articulate in a clear and succinct way the reasons that nursing matters to the overall health and well-being of the nation. As *The Future of Nursing* suggests, nurses should be full partners with other healthcare professionals in redesigning health care in the United States (IOM, 2010).

Recommendation 7: Prepare and enable nurses to lead change to advance health. Nurses, nursing education programs, and nursing associations should prepare the nursing workforce to assume leadership positions across all levels, while public, private, and governmental health care decision makers should ensure that leadership positions are available to and filled by nurses. (IOM, 2010, p. 5)

Having strong leadership skills and competency to lead change will empower nurses at all levels; however, full recognition of nursing as a profession requires nurses themselves to take initiatives to negotiate that kind of dramatic shift in order to break the perceptions of physicians and other healthcare administrators. To claim leadership, nurses have strategized about the need to extend their education from the lowest level allowed for licensure to a higher level, such as a master's or doctorate degree. It is argued that the highest level of education will gradually raise the image of nursing as a profession and better prepare nurses in this highly complex and evolving healthcare environment. With a higher education, nurses increase their capacity beyond direct patient care to other roles that qualify them to teach and to conduct healthcare services and related research.

Expanding nursing's influence through the academy and in research provides influence and leadership by giving the nursing profession a voice to exercise knowledge in patient care and public health issues. Nursing research contributes to the discipline of nursing science and improves the nation's health. For example, research funded by the National Institute of Nursing Research (NINR) provides new opportunities to integrate physical, social, and behavioral sciences and design new technology and

tools that add new knowledge of care across the life span. This knowledge is essential to the present and future health of the nation.

Additionally, nursing research seeks to address care management of patients during illness and recovery, reduce risks for disease and disability, promote healthy lifestyles, enhance the quality of life for those with chronic illness, and promote care for individuals at the end of life. It is through funding from NINR that nursing research helps to advance nursing practice, improve patient care, eliminate health disparities, and attract new students to the profession. It is important to note that for nearly 30 years, NINR has been part of the future of the nation's healthcare system by providing grants, research training, and interdisciplinary practice and education.

Physically Challenging

Nursing is a physically challenging occupation that has impacted nurse morale and nurse retention. Since the mid-1980s, minimizing inpatient hospital stays has been increasingly emphasized, with a commitment to reduce hospital lengths of stay and support continued hospital downsizing; however, because hospitals now treat much sicker patients than before, more nurses are needed per unit, and their work has become more intensive. In fact, the current shortage has burdened the nurse workforce with extended work hours and shifts and has exacerbated occupational injuries and related disabilities. Nelson and Baptiste (2004) identified that patient handling and movement tasks are physically demanding, performed under unfavorable conditions, and often unpredictable in nature. Caring for today's patients, regardless of setting, offers multiple challenges, including variations in size, physical disabilities, cognitive function, and level of cooperation, and fluctuations in condition, all of which cause greater risk for nursing personnel.

It is estimated that each year, 12% of nursing personnel will consider a job transfer to decrease risk, and another 12–18% will leave the nursing profession because of chronic back pain (Moses, 1992; Ovayolu, 2014; Owen, 1989). The cost of work-related musculoskeletal disorders in nursing is quite high and includes indirect costs associated with temporary hires for replacement personnel, overtime to absorb the duties of an injured worker, legal fees, production losses for time spent on claim processing and witnessing, decreased output after a traumatic event, and training for temporary or replacement personnel (Charney, Zimmerman, & Walara, 1991; Ovayolu, 2014; U.S. Department of Labor, Occupational Safety and Health Administration, 2009). The physical difficulty of high-risk patient handling tasks varies by clinical setting. It is critical to understand the specific high-risk tasks in each setting because solutions must be specifically applied to address each high-risk task. Nurses must gain additional and extended education in evidence-based solutions for high-risk patient handling tasks in complex medical and patient care settings. Various types of interventions are being implemented in an attempt to reduce high-risk patient handling tasks. An ergonomic approach has been used, with supporting evidence for solutions that have proved effective. In 2004, the ANA developed a program called Handle with Care that supports safe practices for patient handling. The ANA recently issued a position statement supporting actions and policies that result in the elimination of manual patient lifting to promote a safe environment of care for nurses and patients (ANA, 2014). The ANA is advocating in support of Safe Patient Handling & Mobility (H. R.

2480). The bill is designed to decrease the potential for injury to all who provide and receive care while reducing work-related healthcare costs and improving the safety of patient care delivery. Nurses are encouraging the secretary of labor to issue an occupational safety and health standard to reduce injuries to patients and nurses by establishing a prevention standard.

All nurses must be informed and educated about the use of patient handling equipment, with proper body mechanics emphasized, including evidence-based solutions such as the use of patient handling devices, patient care ergonomic assessment protocols, no-lift policies, and patient lift teams. There are remarkable growth opportunities, and burdens, for nursing employment. The challenge is to promote a safe environment of care for nurses and patients that reduces the risk and physical demands on nurses, ensuring greater coordination and continuity of care.

Pathways to Nursing as a Career Choice

As healthcare needs grow more complex, the career pathway of nursing has evolved into the following career choices: RNs, APRNs, clinical nurse specialists, and clinical nurse leaders. Each of these professional roles requires unique educational preparation and training.

Registered Professional Nurses

RNs are typically prepared for professional practice through different levels of nursing education. To achieve the RN title, an individual must graduate from a state-approved school of nursing—either a 4-year university program or a 2-year associate's degree program—and pass a state RN licensing examination called the National Council Licensure Examination (NCLEX) for Registered Nurses. The 4-year university-based bachelor of science in nursing (BSN) degree provides the nursing theory, sciences, humanities, and behavioral science preparation necessary for the full scope of professional nursing responsibilities. It also provides the knowledge base necessary for advanced education in specialized clinical practice, research, or primary health care. A 2-year program granting an associate's degree in nursing (ADN) prepares individuals for a defined technical scope of practice. Set in the framework of general education, the clinical and classroom components prepare ADN graduates for nursing roles that require nursing theory and technical proficiency. Many RNs whose first degree is an ADN return to school during their working life to earn a bachelor's degree or higher.

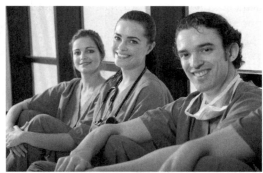

©michaeljung/Shutterstock, Inc.

Advanced Practice Registered Nurses

APRNs have expanded in numbers, and their responsibilities and capabilities have developed over the past several decades. Currently, there is no uniform model of regulation of APRNs across the states. Each state independently determines the APRN legal scope of practice, the roles that are recognized, the criteria for entry into advanced practice, and the certification examinations accepted for entry-level competence assessment. Many licensing exams—such as those for RNs, clinical nurse specialists (CNSs), and clinical nurse leaders (CNLs)—offer a license title without distinguishing between those who graduated from a diploma program and those who graduated from a BSN, master's, or doctorate program.

APRNs are highly valued and are an integral part of the healthcare system. They include certified nurse practitioners (NPs), certified nurse–midwives (CNMs), CNSs, and certified registered nurse anesthetists (CRNAs). Each APRN has a unique history and context. The title distinguishes one's academic achievement and the profession level of one's practice. Although education, accreditation, and certification are necessary components of an overall approach to preparing an APRN for practice, the licensing boards governed by state regulations and statutes are responsible for setting practice within a given state.

The types of APRNs include the following:

- Nurse practitioners deliver front-line primary and acute care in community clinics, schools, hospitals, and other settings, and they perform such services as diagnosing and treating common acute illnesses and injuries; providing immunizations; conducting physical exams; and managing high blood pressure, diabetes, and other chronic problems.

- Certified nurse–midwives provide prenatal and gynecological care to normal healthy women; deliver babies in hospitals, private homes, and birthing centers; and continue with follow-up postpartum care.

- Clinical nurse specialists provide care in a range of specialty areas, such as cardiac, oncology, neonatal, pediatric, and obstetric/gynecologic nursing.

Table 5-1   Medicare Approved Charges

	2011	2012	Percentage increase
APRNs total	$2,412,898,300	$2,718,521,734	12.7
NPs	$1,452,958,877	$1,677,842,316	15.5
CRNAs	$899,995,592	$978,973,321	8.8
CNSs	$56,838,086	$58,189,376	2.4
CNMs	$3,105,746	$3,516,721	13.2
All Part B providers	$126,576,996,112	$128,081,437,867	1.2

Source: Data from McMenamin, P. (2014). QuickStats—2012 APRNs in Medicare Part B. ANA NurseSpace. http://www.ananursespace.org/blogsmain/blogviewer/?BlogKey=b9e87d7e-57a1-4c93-b9b9-e48874a-2be0c

- Certified registered nurse anesthetists administer more than 65% of all anesthetics given to patients each year and are the sole providers of anesthesia in approximately one-third of U.S. hospitals.

The use of APRNs in healthcare settings is increasing. Peter McMenamin, senior policy fellow–ANA health economist at the ANA, reported on the *One Strong Voice* blog that national data reveal the utilization statistics of APRNs enrolled as Medicare Part B providers for 2012 (Table 5-1).

In the aggregate, the Medicare-approved charges for all Part B providers increased by 1.2% from 2011 to 2012. NPs showed the largest increase at 15.5%. CNMs experienced an increase of 13.2%, also above the APRN average (McMenamin, 2014).

All four APRN roles increased their Medicare persons served statistics by more than proportionate amounts. In 2012, APRNs (billing under their own Nurse Practitioner Identification number) provided one or more services to 11.4 million fee-for-service Medicare Part B beneficiaries, just more than 1 million additional patients compared with 2011. This was an increase in persons served of 9.7%. NPs led the

pace, with a 12.4% increase in persons served, or 718,660 additional patients (McMenamin, 2014).

The number of persons eligible for Medicare increased by 2 million in 2012, resulting in an increase of 3.3% in the Part B population, compared with increases of 2.5% experienced in the 3 preceding years.

Specialization and the Evolution of Nursing Roles

The increasing specialization of nurses is demonstrated in the evolving role of CNSs and CNLs. Just as the role of NPs evolved over several decades to meet demands for increased access to primary health care, the role of the CNS was developed in response to the specialized nursing care needs of increasingly complex medical needs. Like a physician specialist, CNSs are advanced practice specialists with in-depth knowledge and skills that make them valuable adjunct practitioners in specialized clinical settings. In today's healthcare system, nurses are critical caregivers who have a profound effect on the lives of patients and their families. They play an essential role in the quality of care patients receive; CNSs play a unique role in the delivery of high-quality nursing care. In addition to direct patient care, CNSs also engage in teaching, mentoring, consulting, research, management, and systems improvement. Able to adapt their practice across settings, these clinicians greatly influence outcomes by providing expert consultation to all care providers and by implementing improvements in healthcare delivery systems. Furthermore, the growing body of research on CNS outcomes shows a strong correlation between CNS interventions and safe, cost-effective patient care. CNS practice has been directly linked to reducing hospital costs and lengths of stay, reduced frequency of emergency room visits, improved pain management practices, increased patient satisfaction with nursing care, and fewer complications in hospitalized patients (Fulton & Baldwin, 2004; National Association of Clinical Nurse Specialists, 2013). Unfortunately, the constraining forces of today's practice environment of mounting financial pressure, limited nursing resources, and changing technology, along with greater patient acuity and shorter lengths of stay, have tested the very core of the profession's values and contributions to quality care.

A CNL is a master's-prepared generalist who puts evidence-based practice into action and serves as a central liaison between the patient and all other healthcare providers. CNSs play an important role in the provision of nursing care that does not duplicate the emerging role of the CNL. In terms of focus, CNLs are educated as generalists, whereas CNSs are prepared for specialty practice. To understand the role of CNLs, it is important to differentiate the duties of CNLs and CNSs. A CNL coordinates and implements client care, whereas a CNS designs and evaluates patient-specific and population-based programs. A CNL evaluates and implements evidence-based practice,

whereas a CNS has the added responsibility of generating new evidence. The CNS and CNL roles are distinct and complementary (Spross et al., 2004). The American Association of Colleges of Nursing (AACN) envisions that these clinicians will work collaboratively to ensure that patients receive the best possible care. Nurses are needed both at the point of care and in advanced practice roles to deliver care that is growing intensely more complicated.

Current State of the Profession

Demand

In 2006, there were 2.4 million nurses in the workforce, comprising the largest segment of professionals (28%) working in the healthcare industry (Mee, 2006; U.S. Bureau of Labor Statistics, 2007). According to the U.S. Bureau of Labor Statistics Monthly Labor Report for January 2012, RNs are projected to add the largest number of new jobs (more than 711,900) to the healthcare practitioners and technical occupations group from 2010 to 2020. Healthcare and technical occupations are projected to add 2 million new jobs from 2010 to 2020, the second most of any major group. This follows an increase of 601,700 jobs from 2006 to 2010, more growth than any other occupational group (Lockard & Wolf, 2012).

Despite job growth, Buerhaus, Potter, Staiger, and Auerbach (2008) project a shortage of 500,000 nurses by 2020. As health care continues to shift from acute care hospitals to more community-based primary care and other outpatient sites, and because of the rising complexity of acute care, the demand for RNs in hospitals will continue to climb by 36% by 2020 (NACNEP, 1996). Nurses as front-line caregivers provide ongoing vigilance to reduce bad things that may happen to patients, such as medication errors, patient falls, and pressure ulcers. The shortage of RNs, in combination with an increased workload, poses a threat to quality of care.

The long-term supply of RNs relies on the student pool that is currently enrolled or interested in nursing education programs. Economic factors, such as tuition requirements and financial aid availability, duration of the academic program, wages of the markets upon graduation, and the number of nursing education programs, will also influence an individual's decision to become a nurse.

> At all [educational] levels, professional-level nursing programs reported increases in the number of students from minority backgrounds over the past year. While the percentage of students from underrepresented backgrounds in entry-level baccalaureate nursing programs increased to 28.1%, the proportion of minority students in master's programs increased to 29.3%, in research-focused doctoral programs to 27.7%, and in practice focused doctoral programs to 24.3%. (American Association of Colleges of Nursing [AACN], 2013)

The AACN survey data from 2012 to 2013 shows that enrollment in entry-level baccalaureate nursing programs increased by 2.2%. The organization's fall 2013 annual survey reveals that enrollment in all types of professional registered nursing programs increased from 2012 to 2013, including increases in baccalaureate (2.2%), RN to baccalaureate (15.2), master's (6.7%), PhD (1.3%), and doctor of nursing practice (DNP) (27.4%). This is not adequate to meet the demand. The problem is not found with the number of persons interested in pursuing a nursing career. According to new survey data released by the AACN, fewer than half of all qualified applicants to entry-level baccalaureate nursing programs were admitted and enrolled last year despite calls to increase the number of well-educated RNs in the U.S. workforce. However, the shortage of faculty, insufficient clinical education sites, and budget cuts continue to act as barriers to future growth in undergraduate education (AACN, 2014).

"According to a 2013 survey conducted by the National Council of State Boards of Nursing and The Forum of State Nursing Workforce Centers, 55% of the RN workforce is age 50 or older" (AACN, 2014). According to Berlin and Sechrist (2002), the average age of nurse faculty at retirement is 62.5 years.

Although the percentage of people entering a university program for graduate-level education who have a BSN degree is rising, nurses with graduate education will likely not choose a faculty position that combines teaching and research. Most clinical care and administration roles offer a higher and more competitive salary than academic positions while still affording opportunities to teach and carry out research.

> The AACN survey found that total enrollment in all nursing programs leading to the baccalaureate degree is 276,946, an increase from 259,100 in 2011. Within this population, 174,644 students are enrolled in entry-level baccalaureate nursing programs. In graduate programs, 101,616 students are enrolled in master's programs, 5,110 are enrolled in research-focused doctoral programs, and 11,575 are enrolled in practice-focused doctoral programs in nursing. (AACN, 2013)

DNP programs account for the largest share of growth in this student population, with a 40.9% increase in enrollments reported this year (85 schools reporting). In 2009, the number of students enrolled in research-focused doctoral programs (i.e., PhD or DNSc) increased by 4.1%, according to preliminary estimates. See Figure 5-1 for the numbers of master's and doctoral graduates from 2007 to 2011.

A second factor is wages, which are a way to attract nurses to the field and retain them after they are in practice. RNs are among the highest paying occupations; registered nursing continues as the top occupation in terms of the largest job growth from 2006 to 2016 (Dohm & Shniper, 2007). This job projection growth suggests that more than 587,000 new jobs will be created through 2016. Nearly 57% of RNs worked in general and medical and surgical hospitals, where RN salaries averaged $60,970 per year. The increase in nurses' wages over the past 30 years accounts for the increase in persons who are interested in applying to baccalaureate nursing programs.

Solutions to the Nursing Shortage

Solutions to the nurse shortage crisis focus on recruiting and training more students to choose nursing as a career, but they neglect to raise the education level of the current nursing workforce or promote the teaching faculty position. In academic institutions, raising faculty salaries and using new teaching models, such as distance learning and simulation, are common strategies to attract more faculty members or use fewer faculty in existing programs. Nonetheless, the true solution may rely on education policy to realign the workforce educational composition to the real demand of nursing with graduate-level education:

- Expand programs
- Implement accelerated programs
- Provide funding support

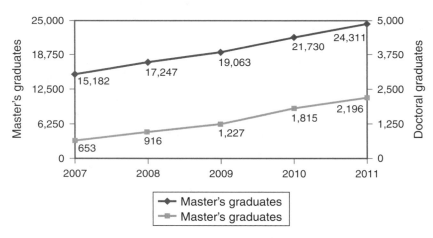

Data Source: HRSA compilation of data from the AACN Research and Data Center, 2012

FIGURE 5-1 Master's and doctoral graduates, 2007-2011

Reproduced from Health Resources and Services Administration (HRSA). Bureau of Health Professions. National Center for Health Workforce Analysis. (2013). The U.S. Nursing Workforce: Trends in Supply and Education. Retrieved from http://bhpr.hrsa.gov/healthworkforce/supplydemand/nursing/nursingworkforce/nursing-workforcefullreport.pdf

Policy as a Tool to Influence Nursing Professionalism and Nursing

Healthcare policy, whether it is created through governmental actions, institutional decision making, or organizational standards, creates a framework that can facilitate or impede the delivery of healthcare services. Thus, engagement in the process of policy development is central to creating a healthcare system that meets the needs of its constituents. Political activism and a commitment to policy development are central elements of professional nursing practice; therefore, the nursing profession and master's and doctoral graduates must assume a broad leadership role on behalf of the public and the profession (Ehrenreich, 2002). Health policy influences multiple care delivery issues, including health disparities, cultural sensitivity, ethics, the internationalization of healthcare concerns, access to care, quality of care, healthcare financing, and issues of equity and social justice in the delivery of health care. Nurses must stand ready to design, implement, and advocate for healthcare policy that addresses issues of social justice and equity in health care. Nurses can become potent influencers in policy formation. They have the capacity to analyze the policy process and the ability to engage in politically competent action. This capacity includes the ability to engage proactively in the development and implementation of health policy at all levels, including institutional, local, state, regional, federal, and international levels. Professional nurses must be seen as leaders in the practice arena and provide a critical interface among practice, research, and policy.

Preparing nurses with the essential competencies to assume a leadership role in the development of health policy requires opportunities to contrast the major contextual factors and policy triggers that influence health policy making at various levels. For example, nurses can take the following actions:

- Critically analyze health policy proposals, health policies, and related issues from the perspective of consumers, the nursing profession, other health professions, and other stakeholders in policy and public forums.
- Demonstrate leadership in the development and implementation of institutional, local, state, federal, or international health policy.
- Influence policy makers through active participation on committees, boards, or task forces at the institutional, local, state, regional, national, or international levels to improve healthcare delivery and outcomes.
- Educate others, including policy makers at all levels, regarding nursing, health policy, and patient care outcomes.
- Advocate for the nursing profession within the policy and healthcare communities.
- Develop, evaluate, and provide leadership for healthcare policy that shapes healthcare financing, regulation, and delivery.
- Advocate for social justice, equity, and ethical policies within all healthcare arenas.

The goal is to create a healthcare delivery system that ensures high-quality care at the exact time when the patient needs it. Nurses are creating model programs in acute care, primary care, and public health settings that are improving the health status of individuals while reducing costs (Hassmiller, 2009). These programs promote the goals that policy makers seek for health reform, including expanding access, improving quality and safety, and reducing costs (Robert Wood Johnson Foundation, 2009). They address problems related to both the supply and demand for nursing services that may be solved with educational, professional, and institutional remedies.

Educational Remedies (Increase Number of Schools and Accelerated Programs)

To meet the more complex demands of today's healthcare environment, academic nurse leaders across all schools of nursing are working together to increase the proportion of nurses with a baccalaureate degree from 50 to 80% by 2020. These leaders are beginning to partner with education accrediting bodies, private and public funders, and employers to ensure funding, monitor progress, and increase the diversity of students to create a workforce prepared to meet the demands of diverse populations across the life span.

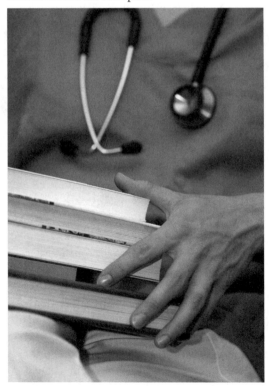

©Carlos Arranz/Shutterstock, Inc.

Accelerated nursing programs continue to be an important pathway into nursing for individuals with degrees in other fields who are looking to change careers. Accelerated nursing programs are available in 46 states plus the District of Columbia and Puerto Rico. In 2012, there were 255 accelerated baccalaureate programs and 71 accelerated master's programs available at nursing schools nationwide. In addition, 25 new accelerated baccalaureate programs are in the planning stages, and 7 new accelerated master's programs are also taking shape (AACN, 2012). Accelerated baccalaureate programs offer the quickest route to licensure as an RN for adults who have already completed a bachelor's or graduate degree in a nonnursing discipline. Fast-track baccalaureate programs take between 11 and 18 months to complete, including prerequisites. Fast-track master's degree programs generally take about 3 years to complete. Graduates of accelerated programs are prized by nurse employers who value the many layers of skill and education these nurses bring to the workplace. Employers report that these graduates are more mature, possess strong clinical skills, and are quick studies on the job.

In 2004, 13% of the nation's RNs held either a master's or doctoral degree as their highest educational preparation. The current demand for master's- and doctoral-prepared nurses for advanced practice, clinical specialties, teaching, and research roles far outstrips the supply. The focus must remain on four key areas: establishing strategic partnerships and resource alignment, formulating policy and regulation, increasing faculty capacity and diversity, and redesigning educational curricula. Despite the increased interest in nursing programs, limited clinical placements for students and a dearth of nurse educators to teach courses are making it difficult for many schools to expand enrollment in their programs. Increasing enrollment in baccalaureate nursing programs is a critical first step to correcting an imbalance in the nursing student population and reversing our nation's diminishing supply of nurse educators. In almost all jurisdictions, nursing faculty must possess a graduate degree to assume a full-time teaching role. Because the overwhelming majority of nurses with master's and doctoral degrees began their education in baccalaureate programs, efforts to alleviate the faculty shortage must focus on expanding enrollments in 4-year nursing programs.

Professional Remedies (Change Status of Nurses)

The role of nursing leadership is fundamental to overturning the misconception that nurses act as subordinates in providing patient care. This misconception is based on the traditional nurses' role of taking physicians' orders. This view of nursing has not been overturned completely in the public eye because of a lack of nursing leadership. Recruitment efforts focus mainly on the role of nurses in helping sick patients, assisting physicians, and bringing direct care to patients, but nothing is mentioned about the role of nursing as a leadership profession to improve our healthcare administration, develop healthcare policy, and influence medical practice. To change the general opinion of nursing, nurses must understand the multiple career choices they have and the meaning of their education.

Nursing is no longer a profession that merely follows physicians' orders; rather, it has nurses on the front line participating in initiatives to lead healthcare reform and suggest ways to improve access, cost, and quality. For example, advanced practice

nurses have developed initiatives around new infrastructure care models that focus on primary care, chronic care management, care coordination, and wellness. These include the Transition Care Model (TCM) designed by Mary Naylor, director of the Robert Wood Johnson Foundation Interdisciplinary Nursing Quality Research Initiative and professor at the University of Pennsylvania School of Nursing. Under this model, APRNs serve as primary care coordinators to help older patients avoid hospitalizations and promote longer term positive health outcomes. The nurse meets with a hospitalized patient to coordinate service, evaluate medications, and establish a postdischarge plan of care that meets with the patient's and caregiver's goals. Within a day of being released from the hospital, the nurse visits the patient's home. The TCM focuses on continuity, evidence-based practice, coordination across the board, and improved outcomes. In this model, a transitional care nurse, who is an advanced practice nurse, is assigned to a patient upon admission into the hospital. This nurse immediately conducts an in-depth assessment of the patient's and the family's goals and initiates communication and collaboration with the patient's care providers, including the primary care physician. Additionally, this nurse visits the patient daily while he or she is admitted and develops an appropriate evidence-based transition care plan with the rest of the care team. Upon discharge, the nurse and other members of the healthcare team will work with the patient to implement the care plan, reassess the patient, and collaborate with the patient's other caregivers. This model has been shown to increase patient satisfaction and improve patient physical function and quality of life (Naylor et al. 2009).

Another example of expert care coordination and meeting the needs of special populations is that of Ruth Watson Lubic. She has founded certified birth centers, the Maternity Center Association in New York City, and the Family Health and Childbirthing Center in Washington, DC. These programs offer prenatal and labor and delivery care for women who have low-risk pregnancies. The care provided at these birth centers has demonstrated significant cost savings for childbearing women, reduced the Cesarean rate in 2005 compared with the rest of New York City (15% versus 28%), and significantly lowered the rates of premature and low birth weight babies, resulting in $1.2 million in cost savings. If this nurse-driven innovation were converted to a nationwide model, the potential savings could be almost $13 billion for Medicaid-funded deliveries.

Finally, the newest model of care on the healthcare landscape will be funded by the federal government. President Obama has pledged $8.6 billion over 20 years for the Nurse–Family Partnership. This partnership pairs a nurse with a low-income first-time mother. Over 2 decades, the program has shown significantly better pregnancy outcomes, reductions in high-risk and subsequent pregnancies, fewer injuries among children, reduced child abuse, and fewer language delays among children. The program has generated a $5.70 return for every dollar invested and a net benefit to society of $17,000 to $34,000 per family served (Lee, Aos, & Miller, 2008).

Institutional Remedies (Recruitment from Overseas)

Healthcare providers have sought their own solution to the shortage of nurses by recruiting nurses from abroad. The growth of foreign-born RNs averaged 6% per year, compared with 1.5% of all RNs between 1994 and 2001. Nonetheless, the growth of foreign-born RNs doubled to 12.5% in 2002 (Buerhaus, 2009). Overall, the growth of foreign-born RNs has accounted for more than one-third of the growth of total RN employment in the United States since 2002 (Buerhaus, Staiger, & Auerbach, 2003). After a temporary decline in 2005 because of the expiration of work visas, foreign-born nurse employment has increased again, surpassing growth in employment among nurses born in the United States (Huston, 2013).

The major factor that impacts the inflow of foreign-born or foreign-educated RNs is the availability of the employment-based visa. Because the recruitment of foreign nurses is usually conducted in less developed countries, the possibility of residing in the United States permanently with an income higher than they earn at home is very attractive.

Although some hospitals may find it faster to employ already educated RNs from other countries than to wait for an increase in enrollment and graduation in U.S. nursing programs (Zachary, 2001), internationally educated RNs may create a liability for the quality and safety of patient care. Some internationally educated RNs have difficulty with communication because of language or culture differences, which causes lapses in patient safety and quality of care. There is also a gap in comparative assessments on care outcomes and safety between those who are educated in the United States and those who are internationally educated. More research is needed to investigate these relationships. The demand for foreign-educated RNs will likely continue or increase; interventions developed to improve communication skills among all nurses across borders are necessary.

Increasing foreign labor in nursing may have a long-term effect on our immigration policy, the wages of future nurses, and the labor composition for RNs. Importing more foreign-born or foreign-educated nurses will increase our long-term domestic nursing supply; however, we will likely shift our shortage problem to another part of the world, thus affecting the quality of care in those countries by depleting their nursing staffs. The potential problem or benefit is still unknown; the best solution to solve our nursing shortage might be to break current domestic barriers that prevent men or underrepresented races, such as Hispanics, from entering the field.

Advocacy as a Tool to Influence Nursing Policy and Programs

Contemporary nursing practice requires that nurses be well prepared to engage healthcare consumers, their families, and others about nursing's contributions to health care. Every patient care encounter is an opportunity for nurses to demonstrate their critical thinking, compassion, and professional expertise. These encounters allow the public to understand better "just how nurses save lives, alleviate suffering and even keep down healthcare cost" (Buresh & Gordon, 2006, p. 21). Nurses have a professional obligation to articulate how intellectually demanding and complex nursing care is and to demonstrate the ways in which they have developed and implemented innovative models of care that promote the goals of health reform: expanding access, improving quality and safety, and reducing costs. When nurses provide thoughtful insight and passion about nursing, the public gains an accurate image of nurses. It is only through compelling and complete descriptions of the work of nurses that others come to value and appreciate that work. Changing the status of nursing means making the profession more visible to the public and policy makers. It requires that nurses inform and educate policy makers and leaders of healthcare delivery organizations about how patient-centered, safe, and efficient care contributes to slowing the rate of total healthcare expenditures. Nurse leaders must take responsibility to educate nurse clinicians so they can take advantage of changes in payment policies by making sure the contributions of nurses are visible. This requires using pay-for-performance measures and bundling hospital payments to patient-centered practices of its nursing staff. By linking hospital performance to nurse performance, nurses demonstrate increased understanding of the economic implications of their clinical and administrative practice. The time has come to fully recognize nursing's social relevance as the nation addresses healthcare reform legislation. The economic, political, and social forces behind healthcare reform favor the interests and advancement of the nursing profession.

Conclusion

This chapter is dedicated to preparing the next generation of nursing advocates who can purposefully and effectively contribute to shaping public policy at the national, state, and local levels. Nurses play an essential role in supporting and realizing the vision for health care in the United States. As the largest segment of the healthcare workforce, nurses need to be full partners with other health professions to achieve significant improvements at the local, state, and national levels in both the delivery and health policy arenas. As a professional partner, nurses understand and have demonstrated expertise and experience with innovative models of care delivery, as well as the financial, technical, and political savvy to close clinical and financial gaps within a healthcare delivery system (Nickitas, 2010).

There are a variety of ways for nurses to engage in grassroots opportunities, professional development, and networking that can ensure they are well prepared to participate in healthcare and public policy reform and the policymaking process. Buerhaus, Potter, Staiger, and Auerbach (2008) suggested that nurses must intensify efforts to "increase the capacity of nursing education programs so that the aging RNs who will retire from the workforce during 2015–2020 can (a) be replaced, and (b) the total supply of RNs can be increased to meet the increasing demand for health care" (p. 249). This increased effort will mean a commitment to a better prepared workforce where nursing education curricula place greater emphasis on evidence-based nursing practice and where quality, safety, geriatrics, chronic conditions, and nursing care extend beyond the acute hospital setting into nonacute care settings.

With the adoption of information technologies, the expanded use of care delivery models (including care coordination and transitional care), and a better prepared nursing workforce, society will benefit from increased nurse autonomy, productivity, and satisfaction.

Discussion Questions

1. Describe how nurses can use their knowledge, perspective, experiences, and skills as communicators to change public policy at all levels of government.
2. What are the most critical questions facing nursing for which policy makers need evidence to inform their decision making?
3. What is the role of government in advancing the impact of nursing on performance improvement and patient outcomes?
4. Discuss how nurses can position themselves to lead change to improve health and health care and drive policy.

Legislative Resources

- Congress.gov: Summaries and status of bills, and text of congressional bills and public laws. http://beta.congress.gov/
- Congressional Budget Office (CBO): Reports and analyses of congressional budget and cost issues. http://www.cbo.gov/
- Office of Management and Budget (OMB): Information about the president's budget proposals and management policies. http://www.whitehouse.gov/omb/
- The White House: Information about executive branch initiatives and policies. http://www.whitehouse.gov/
- U.S. Government Accountability Office (GAO): Studies and reports about how to ensure accountability of the federal government and improve its performance. http://www.gao.gov/

- U.S. House of Representatives: Information about members of the House of Representatives, house committees, and legislation. http://www.house.gov/
- U.S. Senate: Information about members of the Senate, senate committees, and legislation. http://www.senate.gov/

Federal Agency Sites

- Agency for Healthcare Research and Quality (AHRQ): Information about grants available for colleges of nursing. http://www.ahrq.gov/
- Bureau of Health Professions: Information about grants available from the Division of Nursing. http://bhpr.hrsa.gov/nursing/
- Bureau of Labor Statistics: Economic and labor statistics of the U.S. workforce. http://www.bls.gov/home.htm
- Centers for Disease Control and Prevention (CDC): Information about protecting the health and safety of people, and credible information to enhance health decisions. http://www.cdc.gov/
- Centers for Medicare and Medicaid Services (CMS): Information about the agency that administers Medicare and Medicaid. http://cms.hhs.gov/
- Department of Homeland Security: Information about the mission and purpose of homeland security. http://www.dhs.gov/
- Federal Register: Rules, proposed rules, and notices of federal agencies and organizations, as well as executive orders and other presidential documents. http://www.gpo.gov/fdsys/browse/collection.action?collectionCode=FR
- Health Care 411: Weekly audio and video programs featuring the latest research findings from the Agency for Healthcare Research and Quality. http://www.healthcare411.ahrq.gov/
- Indian Health Service (IHS): Information about grants available for colleges of nursing, scholarships, and loan repayment programs for nursing students. http://www.ihs.gov/
- National Institute of Nursing Research (NINR): Information about extramural research programs, training opportunities, the advisory council and *The Outreach* newsletter. http://www.nih.gov/about/almanac/organization/NINR.htm
- National Institutes of Health (NIH): Information about grants available to colleges of nursing, links to various NIH institutions, and the latest health information. http://www.nih.gov/
- NIH Guide: The NIH Guide is available on the NIH's Office of Extramural Research (OER) website. http://grants.nih.gov/grants/oer.htm
- U.S. Department of Education: Information about projects sponsored by the Department of Education and student financial assistance. http://www.ed.gov/
- U.S. Department of Health and Human Services (HHS): Information about grants available for colleges of nursing and current HHS research. http://www.hhs.gov/
- U.S. Department of Labor: Information about workforce issues and policies. http://www.dol.gov/
- U.S. Department of Veterans Affairs: Information about the veterans' health system and services. http://www.va.gov/

Other Related Sites

- Access Healthcare Services: Leading nurse staffing agency, servicing healthcare facilities in all 50 states. http://www.accesshealthcareservices.com

- American Council on Education (ACE): Represents broad higher education policy concerns, regulatory issues, budget, appropriations, student aid, and testimony. http://www.acenet.edu/Pages/default.aspx
- Congressional Quarterly (CQ): Information and insight about government and politics. http://www.cq.com
- Institute of Medicine (IOM): Information and advice concerning health and science policy. http://www.iom.edu/
- Johnson and Johnson Campaign for the Future of Nursing: Information about careers in nursing. http://www.discovernursing.com/
- Library of Congress: Information about how to research at the Library of Congress. http://www.loc.gov/
- MEDLINE: This site, sponsored by the National Library of Medicine, is one of the most comprehensive bibliographic databases online. It contains bibliographic citations and author abstracts from the past 4 years from biomedical journals published in the United States and foreign countries. The database covers many fields, including nursing and the healthcare system. More than 33,000 records are added each month with material from special list journals, like the *International Nursing Index*. http://www.nlm.nih.gov/pubs/factsheets/medline.html
- National Library of Medicine (NLM): Information about grants available to colleges of nursing, research activities, and NLM services. http://www.nlm.nih.gov/
- Nursing Jobs: Offers permanent, per diem, or travel nursing jobs. http://www.nursing-jobs.us/
- Robert Wood Johnson Foundation (RWJF): Information about research grants to study health care issues. http://www.rwjf.org/en/about-rwjf.html

- Roll Call: News about Capitol Hill and politics in Washington. http://www.rollcall.com/
- The Joint Commission: Information about the safety and quality of care provided to the public due to health care accreditation. http://www.jointcommission.org/
- *The Washington Post*: News about Washington, national politics, and policy. http://www.washingtonpost.com/

References

Aiken, L. H., Cheung, R., & Olds, D. (2009). Education policy initiatives to address the nurse shortage. *Health Affairs, 28*(4), w646–w656.

American Association of Colleges of Nursing. (2012). *Schools that offer accelerated baccalaureate programs for nonnursing college graduates, fall 2011.* Retrieved from http://www.aacn.nche.edu/Education-Resources/APLIST.PDF

American Association of Colleges of Nursing. (2013). *Annual report, advancing higher education in nursing.* Washington, DC: Author.

American Association of Colleges of Nursing. (2014). *Nursing shortage fact sheet.* Retrieved from http://www.aacn.nche.edu/media-relations/fact-sheets/nursing-shortage

American Nurses Association. (2010). *Nursing's social policy statement: The essence of the profession* (3rd ed.). Washington, DC: Nursesbooks.org.

American Nurses Association. (2014). *Safe patient handling and mobility.* Retrieved from http://www.nursingworld.org/MainMenuCategories/WorkplaceSafety/Healthy-Work-Environment/SafePatient

Berlin, L. E., & Sechrist, K. R. (2002). The shortage of doctorally prepared nursing faculty: A dire situation. *Nursing Outlook, 50*(2), 50–56.

Bolton, L. B., Aydin, C. E., Donaldson, N., Brown, D. S., Nelson, M., & Harms, D. (2003). Nurse staffing and patient perceptions of nursing care. *Journal of Nursing Administration, 33*(11), 607–614.

Buerhaus, P. (2009). Avoiding mandatory hospital nurse staffing ratios: An economic commentary. *Nursing Outlook, 57,* 107–112.

Buerhaus, P., Potter, V. Staiger, D. O., & Auerbach, D. (2008). *The future of the nursing workforce in the United States: Data trends and implications.* Sudbury, MA: Jones and Bartlett.

Buerhaus, P., Staiger, D., & Auerbach, D. (2003). Is the current shortage of hospital nurses ending? Emerging trends in employment and earnings of registered nurses. *Health Affairs, 22*(6), 191–198.

Buresh, P., & Gordon, S. (2006). *Find from silence to voice.* New York, NY: Cornell University Press.

Centers for Medicare and Medicaid Services. (2006). Medicare program; hospital outpatient prospective payment system and CY 2007 payment rates; CY 2007 update to the ambulatory surgical center covered procedures list; Medicare administrative contractors; and reporting hospital quality data for FY 2008 inpatient prospective payment system annual payment update program—HCAHPS survey, SCIP, and mortality. *Federal Register, 71*(226), 67960–68401.

Charney, W., Zimmerman, K., & Walara, E. (1991). The lifting team: A design method to reduce lost time back injury in nursing. *AAOHN Journal, 39*(5), 231–234.

Cramer, E. (2014, January). Improving the nursing work environment. *American Nurse Today,* 55–57.

Daley, K. (2014). Numbers alone are not enough: Work environment and optimal staffing together matter for patients. *The American Nurse,* 3.

Dohm, A., & Shniper, L. (2007). *Occupational employment projections to 2016.* Washington, DC: U.S. Department of Labor, Bureau of Labor Statistics.

Ehrenreich, J. H. (2002). *A guide for humanitarian, health care, and human rights workers.* New York, NY: State University of New York.

Fulton, J. S., & Baldwin, K. (2004). An annotated bibliography reflecting CNS practice and outcomes. *Clinical Nurse Specialist, 18*(1), 21–39.

Harmer, B., & Henderson, V. (1939). *Textbook of the principles and practice of nursing 1939* (4th ed.). New York, NY: Macmillan.

Hartman, M., Martin, A. B., Benson, J., Catlin, A., & National Health Expenditure Accounts Team. (2013). National health spending in 2011: Overall growth remains low, but some payers and services show signs of acceleration. *Health Affairs, 32*(1), 88–99.

Hassmiller, S. (2009). *Six questions on health reform with Susan Hassmiller.* Retrieved from http://www.rwjf. org/pr/product.jsp?id=41749

Health Resources and Services Administration. (2013). *The U.S. nursing workforce: Trends in supply and education.* Retrieved from http://bhpr.hrsa.gov/healthworkforce/supplydemand/nursing/nursingworkforce/nursingworkforcefullreport.pdf

Henderson, V. (1960). *Basic principles of nursing care.* Geneva, Switzerland: International Council of Nurses.

Huston, C. (2013). *Professional issues in nursing: Challenges & opportunities.* New York, NY: Lippincott Williams & Wilkins.

Institute for Healthcare Improvement. (2014). *The IHI Triple Aim.* Retrieved from http://www.ihi.org/engage/initiatives/TripleAim/Pages/default.aspx

Institute of Medicine. (2010). *The future of nursing: Leading change, advancing health.* Retrieved from http://www.iom.edu/Reports/2010/The-future-of-nursing-leading-change-advancing-health.aspx

Kendall-Gallagher, D., Aiken, L., Sloane, D. M., & Cimiotti, J. P. (2011, January). Nurse Specialty certification, inpatient mortality and failure to rescue. *Journal of Nursing Scholarship, 43*(2), 188–194.

Lamm, R. D. (1996). The coming dislocation in the health professions. *Healthcare Forum Journal, 39*(1), 58–62.

Larrabee, J. H., Ostrow, C. L., Withrow, M. L., Janney, M. A., Hobbs, G. R., Jr., & Burantet, C. (2004). Predictors of patient satisfaction with inpatient hospital nursing care. *Research in Nursing and Health, 27*(4), 254–268.

Lee, S., Aos, S., & Miller, M. (2008). *Evidence-based programs to prevent children from entering and remaining in the child welfare system: Benefits & cost for Washington.* Olympia: Washington State Institute for Public Policy. Document No. 08-07-3901.

Lockard, C. B., & Wolf, M. (2012). *Occupational employment projections to 2020.* Washington, DC: U.S. Department of Labor, Bureau of Labor Statistics.

McGillis Hall, L., Doran, D., Baker, G. R., Pink, G. H., Sidani, S., O'Brien-Pallas, L., & Donner, G. J. (2003). Nurse staffing models as predictors of patient outcomes. *Medical Care, 41*(9), 1096–1109.

McMenamin, P. (2014). *QuickStats—2012 APRNs in Medicare Part B.* Retrieved from http://www.ananursespace.org/blogsmain/blogviewer/?BlogKey=b9e87d7e-57a1-4c93-b9b9-e48874a2be0c

Mee, C. (2006). Nursing 2006 salary survey. *Nursing, 36*(10), 46–51.

Moses, E. B. (Ed.). (1992). *The registered nurse population: Findings from the national sample survey of registered nurses.* Washington, DC: U.S. Department of Health and Human Services, U.S. Public Health Service, Division of Nursing.

National Advisory Council on Nurse Education and Practice. (1996). *First report to the secretary of the Department of Health and Human Services on the basic registered nurses workforce.* Rockville, MD: U.S. Department of Health and Human Services.

National Advisory Council on Nurse Education and Practice. (2008). *Meeting the challenges facing the nurse workforce in a changing health care environment of the new millennium.* Retrieved from ftp://ftp.hrsa. gov/bhpr/nursing/sixth.pdf

National Advisory Council on Nurse Education and Practice. (2013). *Achieving health equity through nursing workforce diversity.* Retrieved from http://www.hrsa.gov/advisorycommittees/bhpradvisory/nacnep/Reports/eleventhreport.pdf

National Association of Clinical Nurse Specialists. (2013). *Impact of the clinical nurse specialist role on the costs and quality of health care.* Retrieved from http://www.nacns.org/docs/CNSOutcomes131204.pdf

National Council of State Boards of Nursing. (2010). *Mission and values.* Retrieved from https://www.ncsbn.org/182.htm

National Council of State Boards of Nursing. (2011). *The 2011 uniform licensure requirements.* Retrieved from https://www.ncsbn.org/11_ULR_table_adopted.pdf

National Council of State Boards of Nursing. (2014a). *Boards of nursing.* Retrieved from https://www.ncsbn.org/boards.htm

National Council of State Boards of Nursing. (2014b). *Nurse practice act, rules and regulations.* Retrieved from https://www.ncsbn.org/1455.htm

Naylor, M. D., Feldman, P. H., Keating, S., Koren, M. J., Kurtzman, E. T., Maccoy, M. C., & Krakauer, R. (2009). Translating research into practice: Transitional care for older adults. *Journal of Evaluation in Clinical Practice, 15,* 1164–1170. doi: 10.1111/j.1365-2753.2009.01308.x

Nelson, A., & Baptiste, A. (2004). Evidence-based practices for safe patient handling and movement. *Online Journal of Issues in Nursing, 9*(3). Retrieved from www.nursingworld.org/MainMenuCategories/ANAMarketplace/ ANAPeriodicals/OJIN/TableofContents/Volume92004/No3Sept04/EvidenceBasedPractices.aspx

Nickitas, D. M. (2010). A vision for the future health care: Where nurses lead the change. *Nursing Economic$, 28*(6), 361, 385.

Nightingale, F. (1860). *Notes on nursing: What it is and what it is not.* New York, NY: Dover.

Ovayolu, O. (2014, January/February). Frequency and severity of low back pain in nurses working in intensive care units and influential factors. *Pakistan Journal of Medical Sciences,* 70–76.

Owen, B. (1989). The magnitude of low-back problems in nursing. *Western Journal of Nursing Research, 11,* 234–242.

Peplau, H. E. (1992). *Interpersonal relations in nursing*. New York, NY: Springer.

Robert Wood Johnson Foundation. (2009). *Charting nursing's future: Nursing's prescription for a reformed health system*. Princeton, NJ: Author.

Roberts, D. (2014, January). Nurses are driving quality in all care settings. *American Nurse Today*, 54.

Seago, J. A., Williamson, A., & Atwood, C. (2006). Longitudinal analyses of nurse staffing and patient outcomes: More about failure to rescue. *Journal of Nursing Administration*, *36*(1), 13–21.

Sovie, M. D., & Jawad, A. F. (2001). Hospital restructuring and its impact on outcomes: Nursing staff regulations are premature. *Journal of Nursing Administration*, *31*(12), 588–600.

Spetz, J. (2014). How will health reform affect demand for RNs? *Nursing Economic$ of Health Care and Nursing*, *32*(1), 42–44.

Spross, J., Hamric, A., Hall, G., Minarik, P., Sparacino, P., & Stanley, J. (2004). *Working statement comparing the clinical nurse leader and clinical nurse specialist roles: Similarities, differences and complementarities*. Washington, DC: American Association of Colleges of Nursing.

Stevens, R. (1989). *In sickness and in wealth: American hospitals in the twentieth century*. New York, NY: Basic Books.

Tervo-Heikkinen, T., Kiviniemi, V., Partanen, P., Vehvilainen-Julkunen, K. (2009). Nurse staffing levels and nursing outcomes: A Bayesian analysis of Finnish-registered nurse survey data. *Journal of Nursing Management*, *17*(8), 986–993.

Tervo-Heikkinen, T., Kvist, T., Partanen, P., Vehviläinen-Julkunen, K., & Aalto, P. (2008). Patient satisfaction as a positive nursing outcome. *Journal of Nursing Care Quality*, *23*(1), 58–65.

U.S. Bureau of Labor Statistics. (2007). *Occupational employment and wages for 2006*. Retrieved from http://stats.bls.gov/oco/ocos083.htm

U.S. Bureau of Labor Statistics. (2012). *National employment matrix*. Retrieved from http://data.bls.gov/oep/nioem/empiohm.jsp

U.S. Department of Labor, Occupational Safety and Health Administration. (2009). *Guidelines for nursing homes. Ergonomics for the prevention of musculoskeletal disorders*. Retrieved from https://www.osha.gov/ergonomics/guidelines/nursinghome/final_nh_guidelines.html

Vahey, D. C., Aiken, L. H., Sloane, D. M., Clarke, S. P., & Vargas, D. (2004). Nurse burnout and patient satisfaction. *Medical Care*, *42*(Suppl. 2), II57–II66.

Zachary, G. (2001, May 24). Labor movement: Shortage of nurses hits hardest where they are needed the most. *The Wall Street Journal*, pp. A1, A12.

CHAPTER 6

Physicians: From Solo Practitioners to Team Leaders

Nancy Aries and Barbara Caress

Overview

When medicine works, it can be very good, but when it fails, it can be very bad. The challenge of this chapter is to describe more fully how physicians function within the larger arena of the healthcare system to understand what factors reinforce the practice of medicine, thus leading to the best possible results. By understanding who becomes physicians, what their areas of medical expertise are, where they practice, and how they are paid, it is possible to look in more detail at the problems associated with medical practice and how to ensure that physicians provide the best possible care. The chapter refers to many of the ways the practice of medicine is changing in terms of the location and content of care and the ways these changes are supported and reflected in the Affordable Care Act.

Objectives

- Understand both the centrality and limits of physicians in defining how the health system functions.
- Appreciate the changes in physician practice in the late 20th and early 21st century and how they impact access, quality, and cost of care.
- Understand how the organization of the healthcare system influences physician behavior and vice versa.
- Recognize that healthcare reform is meant to increase access to health care and control healthcare costs, as well as influence physician practice to improve the quality of care.

Medical Professionalism

Cystic fibrosis is a genetic disease that is characterized by the body's inability to manage chloride, a chemical needed to turn food into energy. The result is a thickening of body secretions or mucus, which prevents the body from absorbing food. If untreated, a child with cystic fibrosis will fail to grow. Ultimately, the secretions block the passageways in the lungs, leading to death. Although there is no cure for cystic fibrosis, the treatment protocols are well documented and standardized. Patients receive nutrients and follow strict diets to ensure their growth. They have medicated nebulizers and are percussed (thumped on the chest) twice a day to break up and expel mucus. Close monitoring by physicians and other health professionals to ensure adherence to the treatment plan can mean that a person with cystic fibrosis will live well beyond childhood.

Warren Warwick was director of the Fairview-University Children's Hospital cystic fibrosis center in Minneapolis for almost 40 years. This treatment center has some of the best outcomes in terms of patient longevity in the United States. Given the standardization of the treatment protocol, the range of outcomes cannot be explained by chance. Warwick attributes his program's success to the advice of doctor Leroy Matthews: "You do whatever you can to keep your patients' lungs as open as possible" (Gawande, 2005).

Atul Gawande (2005) described Warwick's appointment with Janelle, a 17-year-old with cystic fibrosis. Janelle's lung capacity had dropped from better than 100% to 90% in a little over 3 months. This is not a bad level of functioning for a 17-year-old. It is a higher level of functioning than many other persons her age. Dr. Warwick, however, was not satisfied. With time and patience, he got Janelle talking about the changes in her life that led her to stop taking medications and being percussed daily. She had a boyfriend and was not spending as much time at home. Having no adverse signs of the disease, even though she was failing to comply with the medical regimen, reinforced her sense that she was not doing tremendous harm to herself. Dr. Warwick continued to talk to Janelle about the kinds of accommodations they could jointly make to increase her compliance. They needed to find a strategy that was mutually acceptable. Gawande concluded that flexibility and the pursuit of new ways to achieve better functioning of the lungs resulted in excellence.

Janelle's story stands in sharp contrast to that of Lia Lee (Fadiman, 1997). Lia was a Hmong child who was diagnosed with epilepsy before her first birthday. Lia's family had recently immigrated to the United States. They barely spoke English and were unfamiliar with Western medical practice. Lia's condition, however, was tremendously tenuous. Given the difficulty that the doctors had controlling the disease, her medication regimen was complex and constantly changing. Her parents' failure to adhere to the regimen led one physician to report her family to Child Protective Services. As a result, Lia was removed from her home and placed in foster care. Although the foster family was loving and made sure that Lia followed the prescribed medical regimen, the placement was exceptionally stressful for Lia. She was returned home with the parents' agreement to comply with the doctors' orders, but her condition continued to deteriorate. She continued to have seizures until one seizure, a grand mal, did not stop. Lia was taken to the hospital, where doctors found her to be in septic shock. The doctors stopped the seizures and cured the sepsis, but Lia was brain dead. For the next 26 years she lived at home, comatose (Fox, 2012).

Although Lia's story can be told as one of medical noncompliance, that is too simple an explanation for her brain death. Lia's parents, recently arrived Hmong refugees, spoke practically no English. The first times they took Lia to the emergency department, there were no interpreters who spoke Hmong; thus, her condition was misdiagnosed. A correct diagnosis was made only when Lia arrived at the emergency room during an epileptic seizure. With only limited means of communication, there was no way to bridge what the doctors understood to be a disease best managed with anticonvulsant medications and her parents' belief that Lia's soul had left her body and needed to be brought back. Each acted in good faith. Each cared for Lia's well-being. Lia's medications were changed 23 times over 4 years in an attempt to stabilize her condition. The Lees engaged shamans to treat her soul, which they thought was being hurt by all of her medications. The divide between the two resulted in what her doctors considered her death on the night she had her grand mal seizure. In retrospect, everyone involved agreed that adherence to what was perceived as the best possible treatment regimen for epilepsy most likely resulted in a worse outcome than would have happened if the doctors and Lia's parents jointly devised a plan that would accommodate the cultural divide between Lia's parents and the physicians' understanding of health and disease.

These two stories have so many similarities, yet they describe such different perceptions of what constitutes good care. In both cases, the care of the children was managed by physicians. In addition to the physicians, these diseases required a team of caregivers who could work together to ensure compliance. The physicians based the children's care on evidence about which treatments resulted in the best possible outcomes. Both children's conditions were extremely complex, and any backsliding in treatment could result in a worsening of the condition.

However, there are also differences that can be found between these stories. The first is the episodic versus chronic approach to the treatment of complex conditions. Implicit in the telling of these two stories is the episodic nature of Lia's care. She was seen in the emergency department by different doctors who, in some cases, had not even read her medical record. In contrast, Janelle's care was managed by a team that was informed about all aspects of the progression of the disease and her psychosocial condition. The second is the differences in the parents' role in the care process. In Janelle's case, her parents were not only involved but primary caregivers. It was not the case for Lia, whose parents, Foua and Nao Kao, were treated dismissively throughout most of her course of treatment. The last, and most subtle, is the changing nature of the physicians' role as caregiver. For Janelle, the physician is truly part of a team where the role of other clinical professionals and nonprofessional caregivers is instrumental. To keep Janelle's lungs at such a high level of functioning required more than her periodic visits with Dr. Warwick. What is not related in the telling of her story is the importance of nurses, nutritionists, physical therapists, respiratory therapists, and social workers to support her and her family at all times during her treatment. Such team-based care is the lynch pin of many of the system changes promoted in the Affordable Care Act (ACA).

In this chapter, we examine the role of physicians in this system of care that is capable of providing high-quality care, as epitomized by Janelle's experience, and is also capable of providing cutting-edge treatment that fails to meet the patient's needs, as in the case of Lia. To do so, the chapter is organized in three parts. We begin by explaining who makes up the physician labor force, where physicians practice, and how they are paid. In the second part, we review the literature on medical errors because it provides a window for understanding how the organization of medical practice can undermine the best intents of those who practice medicine. Finally, we consider a number of initiatives that are designed to address the structural limits of physician practice and to encourage changes in physician practice.

Who Are the Doctors? Physician Supply

There are approximately 1 million physicians in the United States (Association of American Medical Colleges, 2013). Is this enough to meet healthcare needs in the United States? How many physicians are enough? The answer depends on how the delivery of health care is organized and the services available to prevent, treat, and ameliorate health conditions. The greater the reliance on physicians in the provision of primary care, the greater the need for physicians. Inversely, the more the roles of advanced practice nurses and physician assistants are extended, the lower the physician-to-population ratio can be. Likewise, advances in medical technology impact physician-to-population ratios. For the past 40 years, there has been a steady growth not only in the number of physicians but also in physician-to-population ratios (Goodman & Fisher, 2008).

Starting in the 1950s, the demand for medical services increased for three interrelated reasons. First, more patients had access to employer-based health insurance and could afford to purchase services. Between 1940 and 1950, the number of Americans with such coverage grew from 21 million to 142 million (Pentecost, 2007). The number with insurance grew exponentially with the passage of Medicare and Medicaid in 1965 (Marmor, 1973). Finally, technological innovation began to quicken, which directly impacted the possibilities of medicine and the array of services that patients could receive (Stockburger, 2004). As a result, by 1970, the Carnegie Commission called for expanding the supply of doctors by 50%. The commission proposed that the number of students educated at each school and the number of medical schools be increased (Knowles, 1970).

Government intervention made both possible. Many states funded the building of new medical schools. As Table 6-1 indicates, the number of physicians per 100,000 in population increased from 142 to 319 by 2010, and the number of medical schools increased from 79 to 141. In addition, Medicare made funds available to pay for graduate medical education (Ludmerer, 1999). It got to the point where more residency slots were available than there were American-trained physicians to fill them. These slots started to be filled by international medical graduates (IMGs) (Mullan, 1997). The demand for new doctors continues to grow. Several provisions of the ACA are designed to encourage growth in the physician complement by funding new residency training programs (Heisler, 2013).

Even with the dramatic growth of the medical profession, every recent study has concluded that we face an impending shortage of physicians, particularly in primary care specialties. The Health Resources and Service Administration (HRSA) expects a shortage of between 55,000 and 150,000 physicians by 2020 (Health

Table 6-1   Physician Supply and Number of Medical Schools, 1950–2005

Year	Number of Physicians	Physicians per 100,000 Population	Number of Medical Schools	Number of Medical Graduates
1950	219,997	142	79	5,553
1960	260,484	142	86	7,081
1970	334,028	160	103	8,367
1980	467,679	202	126	15,113
1990	631,830	249	126	15,398
2000	813,770	291	125	15,712
2005	844,464	293	125	15,761
2010	985,375	319	141	16,836

Sources: Data from http://bhpr.hrsa.gov/healthworkforce/reports/factbook02/FB201.htm, http://bhpr.hrsa.gov/healthworkforce/reports/factbook02/FB109.htm, and http://www.aamc.org/data/facts/2008/gradraceeth0208.htm

Resources and Services Administration [HRSA], 2008). The Association of American Medical Colleges pegged the number at 125,400 by 2025 (Dill & Salsberg, 2008). To meet the demand that will be created by population growth and an aging population, we need to train an additional 3,000 doctors per year (Council on Graduate Medical Education, 2005). The Council on Graduate Medical Education's estimates were based on the assumption of the status quo in terms of how medical care is currently organized and delivered to a growing and aging population. Newer studies predict a worsening of shortages due to increased demand as a result of expanded health insurance coverage under the ACA and the aging physician workforce (Association of American Medical Colleges, 2010b). Fully one-quarter of the active physician workforce is 60 years or older, and another 24.5% are between 50 and 60 years of age.

A 2013 report issued by the Congressional Research Service summarized it this way: "The current and future physician supply may be inadequate. Some experts suggest that there are too few physicians overall, too few primary care physicians specifically, and that physicians are inadequately distributed throughout the United States" (Heisler, 2013).

Race and Gender

Despite the fact that the number of minorities in the general population is increasing more rapidly than the number of whites, the percentage of minority physicians is still exceedingly low (Association of American Medical Colleges, 2010a). In the early 1970s, the percentage of minority physicians increased from about 3% to 8% of all physicians. It reached its height of about 14% in the mid-1990s but has decreased slightly since then. When the numbers are broken out by racial and ethnic group, Asians have seen the greatest increase in number and percentage, making up 22% of enrolled medical students in 2011 (Association of American Medical Colleges, 2012). Blacks and Hispanics still struggle to see substantial growth in their numbers. Black enrollment peaked at 9% in 1995, and Hispanic enrollment peaked at just over 7% in 1996.

Although an argument could be made that the percentage of minority physicians in the labor force should be equal to the percentage of minorities in the population on the grounds of social equity, this is not the sole basis for concern about the low percentage of minorities trained as physicians. Minority physicians help increase access to health services. Black and Hispanic physicians are more likely to practice in minority communities that are otherwise underserved (Association of American Medical Colleges, 2010a; Komaromy et al., 1996). Minority physicians also help advance cultural competence and reduce cultural barriers to care in medical practice and research by advancing issues that are not always seen by the white majority.

Women have fared much better than underrepresented minorities. In 1970, there were just over 25,000 female physicians. By 2010, women comprised almost 30% of the physician labor force (Young, Chaudhry, Rhyne, & Dugan,

2013). The dramatic increase in the number of women is best understood by examining medical school enrollments where women now make up almost 50% of the entering classes (Table 6-2). Although women are achieving equity in terms of their numbers, women's participation in the physician labor force is important because women are more likely than men to engage in primary care practice, an area where there are severe physician shortages. In 2007, 45% of women physicians were primary care physicians (Association of American Medical Colleges, 2008).

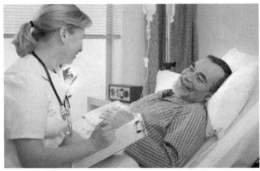

© Alexander Raths/ShutterStock, Inc.

Table 6-2   Women's and Minority Participation in Medical School

Academic Year	Medical School First-Year Enrollment	Female First-Year Enrollment		Minority First-Year Enrollment (Underrepresented Minorities)	
	Number	Number	Percentage	Number	Percentage
1970–1971	11,348	1,256	11.1	808	7.1
1980–1981	17,186	4,966	28.9	1,548	9.0
1990–1991	16,876	6,550	38.8	1,470	8.7
2000–2001	16,699	7,659	45.9	1,739	10.4
2010–2011	18,665	8,756	46.9	1,504	8.1

Underrepresented minority: African Americans, Latinos/Hispanics, and Native Americans.

Sources: Data from http://www.aamc.org/data/facts/2008/women-count.htm (Retrieved April 18, 2009), http://books.nap.edu/openbook.php?record_id=729&page=178 (Retrieved April 18, 2009), http://content.nejm.org/cgi/content/full/331/7/472?ijkey=c0848499053c96554e68195c4d8d158ef09434c&keytype2=tf_ipsecsha, and http://www.aamc.org/data/facts/archive/famg72001a.htm (Retrieved April 18, 2009).

International Medical Graduates

The supply of physicians is augmented by the growing number of physicians who are trained in countries outside the United States and Canada. The demand for IMGs is due in part to the fact that the population of the United States has grown more rapidly than the number of medical school graduates. IMGs now comprise about a quarter of practicing physicians in the country. It is estimated that slightly more than 10% of the IMGs are American citizens who study abroad. The rest are foreign nationals who chose to move to the United States to practice medicine; the dominant countries of origin are India, the Philippines, Mexico, and Korea. The IMGs, as underrepresented minorities and women, play a particularly important role because they tend to be primary care physicians who often practice in underserved areas (Hart et al., 2007).

What Do Physicians Do? Physician Practice Patterns

Specialization

It is important to understand how the increasing complexity of medical practice directly impacts access to and the cost of care. The more specialized the practice of medicine, the more difficult it is to obtain cost-effective primary care (Goodman & Fisher, 2008). At the same time, research indicates that the greater the supply of primary care physicians, the better the patient outcomes (Starfield, Shi, Grover, & Macinko, 2005). Over the past 40 years, however, there has been an overall decline in the percentage of physicians going into primary care. The growth of managed care in the 1990s heightened concern over the decreasing percentage of primary care physicians because managed care relied more heavily on generalists than did private medical practice (Wennberg, Goodman, Nease, & Keller, 1993). Federal and state policies designed to increase the number of primary care physicians resulted in a slight increase during the 1990s. By 2000, the percentage of primary care physicians had increased to 38%. Primary care demand is expected to increase 14% between 2010 and 2020, but HRSA projects only an 8% increase in primary care full-time equivalent physicians during the decade (HRSA, 2008).

The underlying issue is how best to provide integrated and continuous care, such as Janelle receives for her cystic fibrosis. The prevailing belief is that a primary care physician is more able to manage a patient's care than is a specialist who treats a specific condition. There are two models worth considering that sought to advance this organizational premise. In the 1960s, a new specialty in family practice medicine was developed. The intent was to provide advanced training for physicians who were interested in providing primary care but felt that a 1-year internship did not adequately train them for the complexity of medicine. Although family practice has shown some traction, the number of physicians currently choosing this residency option is declining (Colwill, Cultice, & Kruse, 2008). Alternatively, some argue that this is not a problem of merely increasing the supply of primary care physicians; rather, the problem is seen as structural. The healthcare delivery system is highly fragmented, and this mitigates the type of coordination that is held as an ideal. The current articulation of this concept is that patients need a medical home where every effort can be made to provide continuous and coordinated care (R. A. Berenson et al., 2008). Medical or healthcare homes improve health outcomes and lower the costs of care by creating a long-term stable and trusting relationship between the patient and his or her healthcare provider and the provider's team (Reid et al., 2010). The homes are designed to guide patients through the complex healthcare system and seek to integrate patients as active participants in their own health and well-being (Nickitas, 2009). Janelle's care takes place in such a medical home.

Where Do Physicians Practice?

Geographic Distribution

The growing physician supply has not resulted in equalization in the distribution of physicians across geographic areas. The Bureau of Health Professions estimated that 20% of the population lives in an area that carries the designation of medically underserved based on the availability of primary care physicians (Rosenbaum, Jones, Shin, & Ku, 2009). Physicians prefer to practice in urban and suburban communities, leaving inner cities and rural communities underserved. Despite the presence of two academic medical centers, Harlem, a New York City neighborhood in northern Manhattan, is designated as medically underserved (Healthcare Association of New York State, 2009).

Rural and inner city communities find it hard to attract physicians for several reasons. First, rural and inner-city practices tend to be primary care practices. There are fewer opportunities to practice the type of medicine for which most physicians were trained during their residencies and fellowships. Second, although just about everyone needs primary care, specialists need a certain population density to ensure they will have an adequate number of patients to make up a full-time practice. Third, there is an income differential between primary care physicians and specialists. Primary care physicians have lower incomes than specialists (U.S. Bureau of Labor Statistics, 2013). Furthermore, the incomes of physicians practicing in medically underserved communities are lower still than the incomes of physicians who care for urban middle-income patients (Schroeder, 1992). The same issues related to the content of practice and income can be applied to physicians who choose to work in public health programs.

In the 1960s and 1970s, it was assumed that government programs, such as the National Health Service Corps, would incentivize physicians to practice in medically underserved areas. By creating a loan forgiveness program for doctors who practiced in rural areas and, later, medically underserved areas, it was hypothesized that some physicians would choose to remain in these communities for the long term. Although it was successful in recruiting physicians to rural and inner-city neighborhoods, the program was largely disassembled during the Reagan administration (Sardell, 1988). In the 1980s and 1990s, with the growth of managed care, it was assumed that market forces would influence more young physicians to choose primary care practice in underserved communities. Faced with the possibility of closed physician panels, economic theory suggested that physicians would opt to practice in geographic areas where there were physician shortages. This did not prove to be the case. The rate of increase of physicians practicing in areas with high physician population ratios is occurring more rapidly than in underserved areas (Goodman, 2004).

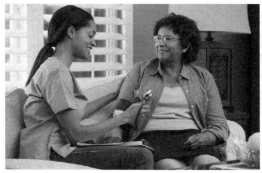

© monkeybusinessimages/iStock/Thinkstock

Organizational Setting

Where physicians are practicing, how those practices are organized, and the ways physicians are being compensated are changing rapidly. As Table 6-3 indicates, physicians can no longer be described as independent entrepreneurs. Thirty years ago, solo practice was the most common arrangement. Forty percent of active MDs were solo practitioners. A decade later, the number had fallen to 3 in 10. By 2012, according to an American Medical Association (AMA) survey, about 18% were working alone (Kane & Emmons, 2013). And among the youngest cohort of doctors (younger than age 40), only 5% were in solo practice (Welch, Cuellar, Stearns, & Bindman, 2013).

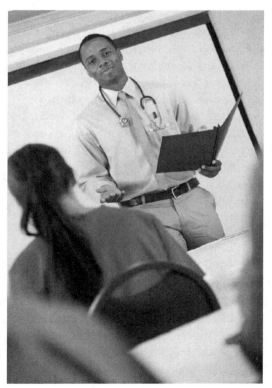

© asiseeit/iStockphoto.com

Historically, physicians worked alone or in partnership with another physician. They saw patients either in their offices or through home visits. Technological advances required more sophisticated delivery sites. Services such as X-rays, surgery, and pathology were best provided in larger spaces where conditions could be monitored. Physicians in most cases chose not to own hospitals or become hospital employees (Starr, 1982). Rather, they developed collaborative relations whereby they received privileges to admit and treat patients at a particular hospital with the understanding that they would maintain the integrity of the medical services through an autonomous committee structure.

Two interrelated changes impacted this organizational model. The first is the growth of group practice. Multispecialty group practices, such as the Mayo Clinic, provide a rational organizational model because they can ensure the coordination of complex patient care. These plans depend on a primary care gatekeeper who would be responsible for the management of a patient's care. With patient access to specialists controlled by primary care physicians, specialists are pressured to become part of a group practice. As the reliance on gatekeeping lessened in the late 1990s, there was decreased pressure on physicians, particularly specialists, to join multispecialty groups; however, the trend continues. Small- to moderate-sized groups have replaced solo practice as the most common practice setting. There has also been an expansion of very large multispecialty groups. In 2011, 27% of all active MDs worked in settings with 100 or more other physicians (Welch et al., 2013).

The second change to affect physicians' relations with hospitals is financial. An

Table 6-3   Distribution of U.S. Physicians by Age and Practice Size, 2011

	Younger than 40	40-59	60 or older	Age missing
Total	125,170	316,259	120,411	18,733
Percent	21.6	54.5	20.7	3.2
Practice size (number of physiciams)				
1	5.4%	17.9%	32.3%	30.3%
2-10	21.3	25.5	24.5	24.3
11-50	25.2	21.8	17.3	17.7
51-100	10.7	8.4	6.3	6.8
>100	37.4	26.4	19.7	21

Source: Data from http://content.healthaffairs.org/content/32/9/1659.full (Retrieved January 12, 2014)

increasing number of physicians are working either as direct employees of hospitals or in practices owned in whole or in part by hospitals. This is particularly true of primary care physicians whose practices are most likely to be hospital owned. A 2012 AMA survey showed that 45% of internal medicine practices were at least partially owned by hospitals (Kane & Emmons, 2013). One possible explanation is that hospitals seek control of primary care practices because they are valued as referral sources for specialized inpatient and outpatient care and are relatively inexpensive to maintain. Another explanation involves the increased ability to provide services in ambulatory care settings so that specialist physicians do not need to rely as heavily on hospitals to provide complex patient care. As a result, the diagnosis and treatment of patients is moving out of the hospital into ambulatory settings. This means hospitals are competing with physicians for patients. Unlike their primary care brethren, internal medicine subspecialty practices are among the least likely to be hospital owned (Kane & Emmons, 2013).

Physicians who are employed by hospitals fall into three general categories. A large and growing subgroup are hospitalists, who coordinate the services of specialists and other healthcare providers and services to hospitalized patients. Hospitalists were first employed in 1995, and there are an estimated 30,000 physicians who trained in primary care and are working as hospitalists in the United States. Many younger physicians are opting for this type of practice, which has been shown in some cases to transform the way inpatient care is delivered. The Association of American Medical Colleges reports that 30% of general internists younger than age 45 are working as hospitalists (2012).

The other significant category of hospital-employed physicians consists of specialists working at academic medical centers that provide state-of-the-art health services, educate healthcare practitioners, and undertake research to advance health and well-being. These physicians hold faculty appointments at the medical school and have teaching responsibilities. They are members of faculty practice plans and care for patients at the affiliated hospital, and they are typically engaged in research. Last, there is a growing trend for community hospitals to employ physicians

(Casalino, November, Berenson, & Pham, 2008). These hospitals are seeking to ward off the competition and stabilize the provision of services. Physicians in their employ are making lifestyle choices to have more regular work hours and greater job security.

Two groups of physicians do not show up in those percentages. A small number of physicians are engaged in public health activities. These physicians are typically employed in federal and state public health programs and are responsible for ensuring the health of populations. A small number of physicians also work in clinics that are organized to provide services to persons who cannot readily access the private practices of physicians previously described. In some instances, the physicians who have worked at these clinics are full time. In other instances, they work at these clinics on a part-time basis. The clinics may be operated as part of an academic medical center, by a public health department, or by a community group. These centers often provided the kind of medical home that patients in private settings hope to use.

How Are Physicians Paid?

Physician Income

Physicians have the highest median income of all occupational groups in the United States (U.S. Bureau of Labor Statistics, 2013). They are also among the occupation groups with the most dissimilar earnings. Although physicians' reported average income was $241,000, the average for men was 30% greater than for women ($259,000 versus $199,000). Even among primary care physicians, women earned less than their male colleagues ($161,000 compared with $189,000). A 2012 survey of physician income by specialty found that physicians who specialized in caring for people with HIV had

the lowest average income of $170,000, and orthopedic surgeons reported average incomes of $405,000 (Medscape, 2013). Physicians in the United States are the most highly paid group of medical practitioners in the world. On average, U.S. physicians earn three times more than their counterparts who work in countries that belong to the Organisation for Economic Co-operation and Development (Bodenheimer, 2005).

Physician Payment

Physicians derive their income from several sources. The most common way in which physicians are paid is fee for service. In its simplest form, this means that patients pay physicians for the services they receive. The concept of fee for service is complex because physicians do not charge or receive the same payment from all patients for the same service. For older patients, they usually accept the fee established by the Medicare fee schedule. If physicians participate in a managed care panel or in a preferred provider organization, they agree to accept a discounted fee for their services. It is assumed that access to a patient population offsets the possible loss of revenue from the discount. Managed care organizations and preferred provider organizations are not the only payers with fee schedules. Medicaid also has a fee schedule that is substantially below what physicians charge for services to private patients.

A growing percentage of physicians are salaried. Physicians who work for the government in departments such as Public Health or the Veterans Administration have always been paid an annual salary. Doctors who worked for health maintenance organizations were among the first practicing physicians who were salaried. These precursors to accountable care organizations employed a group of physicians to assume contractual responsibility for ensuring the delivery of a range of services, including hospitalization and ambulatory care, to its members. A growing number of physicians are employed by medical schools and hospitals, in addition to interns and residents. Rather than follow a patient based on disease, they work in the hospital to ensure the management of complex cases (Wachter & Goldman, 2002).

In reality, most physicians' incomes come from hybrid arrangements. Medical school faculty members provide one of the best examples. The physicians receive a base salary from the medical school. This salary ostensibly covers the cost of their teaching and other service to the school. In addition, faculty members derive income from the revenues they generate by participating in practice plans at the hospital. Although the payment for their services goes to the medical center, physicians receive some portion of the fee. Another example includes physicians in private practice who derive the better part of their incomes from fee-for-service practice. These same physicians might also cover clinic sessions at an emergency room or neighborhood health center. The physician would be paid a fixed amount for the session even though the patients would be charged on a fee-for-service basis.

The Impact of Financial Arrangements on Physician Practice and Physician Income

Physician income has become a major policy issue because physicians purportedly control close to 70% of healthcare costs. The ways physicians are reimbursed influences the ways that they practice medicine (Hillman,

Pauly, & Kerstein, 1989); therefore, there is a quest to advance a payment scheme that incentivizes physicians to act in ways that are both economic and ensure quality patient care. Many factors can influence physicians' judgments about patient care plans. Patient mix, for example, is one factor that can impact physician practice under fee-for-service medicine (Town, Wholey, Kralewski, & Dowd, 2004). If physicians see a large number of private-pay patients, the incentive may to be to overtreat because physicians are well paid for these services. The same physicians may be incentivized to undertreat patients with similar conditions who are covered by managed care companies, given the discounted fee. Physician ownership of equipment, such as X-ray and EKG machines, and organizations like laboratories and rehabilitation centers can also influence practice patterns. Physicians who own equipment are more apt to use it during a routine office visit than their counterparts who do not own such equipment (Schroeder & Showstack, 1978). A similar dynamic exists where physicians have an ownership stake in ancillary services, such as hospitals and laboratories (Stensland & Winter, 2006).

The structure of payment not only affects the ways in which physicians provide services, it also impacts physician compensation. The ways services are identified on bills can impact the total charges to a patient. An example is the practice of unbundling services. Rather than providing patients with an all-inclusive bill, physicians have discovered that by billing for each component of a visit, they receive a higher rate of pay for the same level of service. The last way that financial structures can influence physician pay is through the substitution of services. Physicians direct patient treatment by deciding what diagnostic tests, treatments, and follow-up care will be prescribed. Often the more expensive alternative is chosen despite the lack of evidence associated with its efficacy (Kassirer, 2005).

Physician Payment Reform

What has evolved is a cat-and-mouse system of financial reward for physicians. The largest payers of health services, the government and private insurance companies, are looking at payment methods that will encourage physicians to provide cost-effective care. In return, physicians are looking to manipulate the payment system to protect and increase their incomes. Physicians' income, however, has not kept pace with the rate of inflation. The decline in income is attributed to the failure of fees from Medicare and private health insurance to keep pace with inflation (Tu & Ginsburg, 2006). There is an assumed association between this finding and the fact that the percentage of physicians who provide charity care has declined from 76% to 68% between 1996–1997 and 2004–2005 (Cunningham & Hadley, 2008).

While there is agreement about the need to reform physician payment, there is no agreement about the best methods (R. E. Mechanic & Altman, 2009). Early efforts such as Relative Value Scales did not have the intended consequences of rewarding primary and chronic care providers (Bodenheimer, Berenson, & Rudolph, 2007).* A range of options are currently being considered. Closest to the status quo, the recalibration of fee-for-service medicine would minimize the types

*Relative Value Scale is a system of physician payment developed by Medicare based on the value of a medical service relative to other medical services.

of financial incentives that currently exist to overtreat or undertreat patients depending on the reimbursement. Similarly, the use of global payments would build on the model of capitated payments used by managed care organizations. To overcome the incentive to undertreat, payment would be linked to performance measures. A third alternative is to bundle physician payments based on an episode of care. The alternative receiving the greatest attention is pay for performance, a system of payment that rewards physicians and providers for meeting performance measures (Werner & Dudley, 2009). Although there are several hundred pay-for-performance programs, there are few good outcome measures and no certainty about how much of a physician's pay should be related to performance or improvement. Under the auspices of the ACA, a number of physician payment reforms are being tested, including bonuses or penalties based on quality and efficiency standards (RAND, 2013).

Physician Accountability

Historically, physicians have been responsible for regulating the practices of their colleagues (Freidson, 1970). Their expertise is, in part, the basis of their autonomy to define both the content of their work and the ways in which health services are organized. Physicians, for example, not only set the standards of care but also determine who will provide the care and in what setting. As a result, physicians control both the supply of and demand for health services. Their power, however, is moderated by their fiduciary relationship to their patients—meaning that they are obligated to do everything in their power to ensure the well-being of their patients.

Self-regulation is carried out in multiple ways. The first point of control is the system of medical education. Physicians are responsible for all facets of this endeavor. They determine the size and composition of medical school classes, and they control decisions related to medical school curricula through their participation on medical school faculty and accrediting bodies (Ludmerer, 1999). Medical education is just the beginning of the accountability structure.

A second point of control is government regulation of physicians (Field, 2007). The government is concerned with the public's safety; therefore, the right to practice medicine is limited to those persons who have demonstrated a mastery of the field. All physicians are required to pass national boards and licensure examinations that fall under the auspices of state governments. In addition, states guarantee that physicians keep up with the field by setting standards for continuing medical education. Authority over the government regulation relies heavily on the medical profession. The standards used by the states are set, implemented, and overseen by physicians. Likewise, the professional review boards that evaluate physicians for malpractice fall under the auspices of physicians who are employees of the states.

Finally, hospitals have a stake in ensuring that physicians with hospital privileges are held to the highest standards of practice. Institutional providers also defer oversight to medical professionals. All physicians' credentials are reviewed and presented to the hospitals' boards of trustees before they are awarded hospital privileges. Each hospital also maintains medical boards that review all deaths that occur in the hospital. This is an opportunity for physicians to determine whether a physician's practice adhered to accepted standards of care. Beginning in the 1980s, under pressure from the government, hospitals instituted utilization review to assess physician practice relative to their peers.

Medical Errors

Theoretically, a system of self-governance, such as utilization review, should lead to high-quality care. A review of the literature on medical errors indicates that this is not necessarily the case. Complications are a natural result of medical practice that intervenes in complex human processes, and mistakes are the normal consequence of human activity. The challenge is to describe complications that are preventable—to understand the causes of medical error and document its prevalence.

The Institute of Medicine defines medical error as "the failure to complete a planned action as intended or the use of a wrong plan to achieve an aim." An adverse event is defined as "an injury caused by medical management rather than by the underlying disease or condition of the patient" (2000, p. 28). The types of medical errors include the following:

- Diagnostic error, such as misdiagnosis leading to an incorrect choice of therapy; failure to use an indicated diagnostic test; misinterpretation of test results; and failure to act on abnormal results

- Equipment failure, such as a monitor that fails to function during a procedure

- Infections, such as nosocomial and postsurgical wound infections

- Blood transfusion-related injuries, such as giving a patient the incorrect blood type

- Misinterpretation of other medical orders, such as failing to give a patient a salt-free meal, as ordered by a physician

Frequency of Medical Errors

Although dramatic malpractice awards capture the headlines, medical errors and complications are far more systematic. A November 1999 report of the Institute of Medicine indicated that as many as 44,000 to 98,000 people die in hospitals each year as the result of medical errors (Institute of Medicine, 2000). A more recent evaluation of premature deaths associated with preventable harm set the number at 400,000 and the number of nonlethal serious harm incidents at 10 to 20 times that number. This would make medical errors (preventable adverse events) the third leading cause of death in this country, after heart disease and stroke (Jones, 2013).

Causes of Medical Errors

Observers and scholars have offered an array of explanations for why preventable mistakes happen. These range from malfeasance resulting from personal impairment or greed to a systematic critique of the way U.S. medical professionals are trained and health care is organized.

Impaired Providers The simplest explanation for medical mistakes is provider impairment. Physicians, nurses, and other practitioners are no less likely to have substance abuse problems than other Americans. There are no recent large-scale studies of substance abuse among physicians, but the best available estimates are that during their practice lifetimes, 8–12% of physicians will experience a substance-related problem (Baldiserri, 2007):

- 112,000 will have an alcohol-related disorder
- 64,000 will have a drug-related disorder

Substance abuse is the most common reason for disciplinary action by state medical and nursing boards. Like physicians, nurses report significant levels of substance abuse. A 1998 survey of RNs found that 3.6% used marijuana and/or cocaine, 5.6% abused prescription drugs, and 16.0% reported binge drinking (Trinkoff & Stor, 1998).

Another source of impaired judgment is more subtle: the effect of industry–physician relationships. Under the headline "Doctors Reap Millions for Anemia Drugs," *The New York Times* reported how drug companies paid physicians to prescribe expensive anemia drugs. "Critics, including prominent cancer and kidney doctors, say the payments give physicians an incentive to prescribe the medicines at levels that might increase patients' risks of heart attacks or strokes" (A. Berenson & Pollack, 2007). The prescription drug industry spent $20 billion on direct marketing to physicians in 2007. In fact, 94% of all practicing physicians received some gift from the medical device, biological, or pharmaceutical industries (Wazana, 2000).

System-Induced Errors Much more complicated than errors made by impaired physicians are errors that occur as a part of the usual practice of medicine. Take, for example, *New Yorker* author Dr. Atul Gawande's report on himself (Gawande, 1999). He describes what happened when, as a surgical resident, he treated a semicomatose car crash victim. She was having difficulty breathing, and Gawande intubated her; however, he missed the mark, and the woman's oxygen level fell dangerously. Instead of assisting her breathing, his actions actually blocked her airways. At this point, an experienced anesthesiologist arrived and managed to slip a tube through the vocal cords and reestablish oxygen flow to the heart. The woman recovered and was discharged several days later. According to

Gawande, the root cause of his error was inexperience. As Gawande commented, "Mistakes do happen. We think of them as aberrant. They are anything but" (1999, p. 40). Could it have been prevented? Yes, with fundamental change in the way surgical residents are trained and emergency care is delivered, it could have been prevented—that is possible but extremely difficult to achieve.

Dr. Jerome Groopman goes further in his critique arguing that errors occur because there is a flaw that undermines much of contemporary medicine: "Why do we as physicians miss the correct diagnosis? It turns out that the mistakes are rarely due to technical factors, like the laboratory mixing up the blood specimen of one patient and reporting another's result. Nor is misdiagnosis usually due to a doctor's lack of knowledge about what later is found to be the underlying disease" (Groopman, 2007).

As we saw with the case of Lia Lee, cultural differences complicate medical care and can lead to tragic errors. In Lia's case, many of the problems occurred because Lia's family did not speak English; however, in the case of Willie Ramirez, fluency in English was not the problem. The meaning of words, however, in different cultures was. Willie Ramirez was 18 years old. He collapsed outside his girlfriend's house after complaining of a severe headache and was taken to the hospital. His family and friends reported to the doctors in the emergency room that Willie was "intoxicado." The physician understood this to mean that Willie had overdosed. To Cubans, however, the word is all encompassing. If they had pursued his case further and called in a neurosurgeon, they would have found that Willie was having a brain hemorrhage. He would not have become a quadriplegic (Price-Wise, 2008).

Medical Errors and Malpractice

Mr. Ramirez was awarded $71 million to pay for full-time medical care for the rest of his life and to compensate him for the severe avoidable injury. Whether this is an excessive settlement is unknown, but it raises two concerns, neither of which is supported by the data. The first is that the threat of malpractice litigation will lead to the excessive practice of defensive medicine and an increase in healthcare costs. A study of the effects of liability insurance found a modest increase in the use of screening procedures but no overall increase in expenditures (Baicker & Chandra, 2004). The second concerns the impact of malpractice litigation on rising healthcare costs. Medical liability accounted for only $55 million or 2.4% of healthcare spending in 2008. A study of the relationship between malpractice awards and medical error conducted by physicians at the Harvard School of Public Health found that "the vast majority of expenditures go toward litigation over errors and payment of them" (Studdert et al., 2006, p. 2033). While some litigation might be without merit, it would not have a major impact on overall health care spending (Mello, Chandra, Gawande, & Studdert, 2010). Another study estimated that claims not involving errors accounted for only 13–16% of the total cost of malpractice payments (Thomas et al., 2000).

Medical Errors, Physician Practice, and the Barriers to Quality Care

By examining the problem of medical errors, one gets a window on the problems that flow from the system of care as it is currently organized. First, there is an overreliance on the biomedical or physician-oriented model of care (Mishler, 1981). Although many people seek care on an annual basis and hope to prevent disease through immunizations or early detection, the overall system is designed to address illness. Little effort goes into prevention, which is considered a matter of public health, or for the management of chronic conditions, such as heart disease and diabetes. Provisions in the ACA are intended to change this by incenting physicians to provide and patients to seek preventive services.

The second consequence that follows from the first is the mismatch between patient need and physician supply. The physician workforce is highly specialized and heavily located in urban areas. Underrepresented communities, including both racial and ethnic minorities and those with lower socioeconomic status, have more difficulty getting care due to the specialization of physicians and their choice to practice in middle-class or wealthy urban or suburban settings—class matters. The lack of access contributes to tremendous disparities in health outcomes (Schoen et al., 2013). Persons from higher socioeconomic classes have better outcomes than persons from lower socioeconomic classes.

The third consequence is the inconsistent quality of care. Inconsistent quality results first from the effects of inequitable distribution of physicians by geographic location and specialty. Inconsistent quality is further affected by the organizations where physicians work. Health outcomes are better in settings that have high volume and good oversight. When New York State began to publish data on outcomes for cardiac catheterization and bypass surgery, it was assumed the data would be used by patients to select a physician and hospital that were known to have better outcomes. It was found was that hospitals used the data to improve the delivery of care to ensure better outcomes (Chassin, 2002).

Overcoming the Barriers to Quality Care

With growing recognition of medical errors and unequal access to care and inequitable outcomes have come increased efforts to overcome the historic, structural, and organizational barriers to good-quality care. The medical profession has become increasingly concerned that it has not adequately held itself to professional standards (D. Mechanic, 1996; Rothman, 2000).

In 2002, several societies representing internal medicine physicians published a physician charter that asserted three principles that underpin the doctor–patient relationship (ABIM Foundation, ACP-ASIM Foundation, & European Federation of Internal Medicine, 2002). The first was the primacy of patient welfare. This commitment calls on physicians to uphold patients' interests. Second is the principle of patient autonomy. The doctor–patient relationship is being redefined as consultative. Doctors have the expertise to share with patients, but patients have concerns that extend beyond biomedicine and may influence the course of medical care they select. The last is the principle of social justice. The charter asserts that physicians must promote the fair distribution of healthcare resources. Physicians should actively work to eliminate discrimination in health care, whether based on race, gender, socioeconomic status, ethnicity, religion, or any other social category.

Doctors are also moving to reform the education system and the overall organization of care. There is growing interest in the ways professionalism can be taught and modeled (Branch et al., 2001; Kao, 2003). It is also the case that physicians are increasingly coming to understand and value the importance of the medical team. Health services are too complex to be provided by a single person. It takes a team with broad-ranging expertise to provide necessary treatment (O'Malley, Tynan, Cohen, Kemper, & Davis, 2009). Only a team can ensure the continuity of care within and across care settings. What is being described is the importance of a patient having a medical home where there are high levels of coordination among all providers who interact with patients (Enthoven, Crosson, Stephen, & Shortell, 2007).

Institutional providers are also looking for ways to provide their own oversight of physicians. As hospitals are pressured to control costs, they have tried to influence physicians' practices without compromising quality. In addition to utilization review, hospitals have also sought to create greater alignment of physician and hospital interests through the creation of physician hospital organizations and the employment of hospitalists. There is also a movement for more evidence-based practice. Organizations like Leapfrog, an employer-based group, seek to improve quality of health care, making data available about hospital care and working to develop incentives to reward quality care (Leapfrog Group, 2009).

The government has also sought greater accountability from physicians given its financial interest in the healthcare system. With the recognition that physicians' financial interests could be in conflict with patients' interests, the government has imposed regulations around self-dealing (Mitchell, 2007). Physicians cannot be reimbursed by Medicare and Medicaid for the treatment of patients who are being referred to facilities where that physician has an ownership stake. Likewise, the government has begun to impose minimum practice standards to prevent physicians from potentially jeopardizing patient well-being. There is greater pressure for mistake reporting and suspension of licensure in cases of malpractice.

There is also a growing movement for private payer regulation of physician practice that has been motivated by the desire to control costs but now recognizes the delicate relationship between cost and quality. This began nearly 25 years ago with such practices as requiring patients to receive a second opinion before undergoing an expensive medical procedure. These efforts did not achieve their desired end of controlling costs or limiting unnecessary care. Physicians were reticent to make judgments about their colleagues. This led insurers to implement programs requiring prior authorization by the insurers before treatment occurred. What followed was the utilization of physician panels by managed care organizations to control physician practice. This was more complicated to implement than originally assumed. Efforts to create limited pools led to challenges by patients and doctors related to freedom of choice, but it was harder to have a panel of any willing provider adhere to fixed practice guidelines. Efforts to shift financial risk onto doctors also had limited success in terms of shifting physician practice. The evolution of payer regulation has now taken the form of pay for performance and performance networks. Under pay for performance, physician reimbursement will be linked to patient outcomes. Performance networks seek a similar end in terms of rewarding healthcare networks that achieve high quality of care at lower costs through the redesign of the ways health care is delivered (Pham, Ginsburg, McKenzie, & Milstein, 2007).

Conclusion: Choices and Interests

This chapter asks questions about the ways physicians impact the provision of health care and patient outcomes. The answer, in a nutshell, is that it depends. It depends on who become physicians, how they are trained, where they practice, how they are paid, and what exactly they do. The analytic challenge is in understanding and interpreting all these combinations and their permutations.

Do physicians matter as much today as they did during the mid- and late 20th century? Yes, physicians still drive much of the organization and delivery of health care. Our system of care is defined by physician expertise and, as a result, is heavily biased toward the type of care most physicians are trained to provide. Given their dominance over the healthcare professions, physicians have been given the legal authority to ensure the standard of care.

However, due to the complexity of care and the greater need for care coordination, the balance of power is shifting toward a transdisciplinary approach where the patient is the center. This requires shared power among all health providers, with the patient's choice for treatment first and foremost. Lapses and compromises in how this is being done are excellent windows into how our health system functions.

How should the job of physicians be changed in our 21st-century environment? The policy lessons to be derived from this chapter go back to the place where we started: Decisions have winners and losers. In this case, highly specialized care has produced enormous advances in the effectiveness of medicine. At the same time, it has limited access to low-income and minority populations and rural populations. The pressure now is to create a more equitable system. Health reform will succeed if it supports systems that can ensure the type and quality of care that Janelle receives for her treatment of cystic fibrosis. Such care is highly dependent on involving patients and their families and on involving the team of providers who all hold a piece to understanding the complexity of what is needed. It requires physicians to willingly engage in this process, which an increasing number of physicians are ready to do.

Discussion Questions

1. Why do primary care physicians earn so much less than specialists?
2. What accounts for the decline of solo practice?
3. Why do doctors make mistakes?
4. Is self-regulation of physicians good enough?
5. How can care be improved?

References

ABIM Foundation, ACP-ASIM Foundation, & European Federation of Internal Medicine. (2002). Medical professionalism in the new millennium: A physician charter. *Annals of Internal Medicine, 136*(3), 243–246.

Association of American Medical Colleges. (2008). *Physician specialty data.* Retrieved from https://www.aamc.org/download/47352/data/specialtydata.pdf

Association of American Medical Colleges. (2010a). *Diversity in the physician workforce: Facts and figures 2010.* Retrieved from https://members.aamc.org/eweb/upload/Diversity%20in%20the%20Physician%20Workforce%20Facts%20and%20Figures%202010.pdf

Association of American Medical Colleges. (2010b). *The impact of health care reform on the future supply and demand for physicians updated projections through 2025.* Retrieved from https://www.aamc.org/download/158076/data/updated_projections_through_2025.pdf

Association of American Medical Colleges. (2012). *Matriculants to U.S. medical schools by race, selected combinations within Hispanic or Latino ethnicity, and sex, 2009–2012.* Retrieved from https://www.aamc.org/download/321474/data/2012factstable9.pdf

Association of American Medical Colleges. (2013). *2013 state physician workforce databook.* Retrieved from https://members.aamc.org/eweb/upload/State%20Physician%20Workforce%20Data%20Book%202013%20%28PDF%29.pdf

Baicker, K., & Chandra, A. (2004). *The effect of malpractice liability on the delivery of health care.* NBER Working Paper No. 10709. Retrieved from http://www.nber.org/papers/w10709.pdf

Baldiserri, M. (2007). Impaired healthcare professional. *Critical Care Medicine, 35*(2). Retrieved from http://66.199.228.237/boundary/boundary_violations_and_physician_impairment/impaired_physicians.pdf

Berenson, A., & Pollack, A. (2007). Doctors reap millions for anemia drugs. *The New York Times.* Retrieved from http://www.nytimes.com/2007/05/09/business/09anemia.html?pagewanted=print&_r=0

Berenson, R. A., Hammons, T., Gans, D. N., Zuckerman, S., Merrell, K., Underwood, W. S., & Williams, A. F. (2008). A house is not a home: Keeping patients at the center of practice redesign. *Health Affairs, 27*(5), 1219–1230.

Bodenheimer, T. (2005). High and rising health care costs. Part 3: The role of health care providers. *Annals of Internal Medicine, 142*(12), 996–1002.

Bodenheimer, T., Berenson, R. A., & Rudolph, P. (2007). The primary care-specialty income gap: Why it matters. *Annals of Internal Medicine, 146*(4), 301–306.

Branch, W., Kern, D., Haidet, P., Weissman, P., Gracey, C. F., Mitchell, G., & Inui, T. (2001). Teaching the human dimensions of care in clinical settings. *Journal of the American Medical Association, 286*(9), 1067–1074.

Casalino, L. P., November, E. A., Berenson, R. A., & Pham, H. H. (2008). Hospital–physician relations: Two tracks and the decline of the voluntary medical staff model. *Health Affairs, 27*(5), 1305–1314.

Chassin, M. (2002). Achieving and sustaining improved quality: Lessons from New York State and cardiac surgery. *Health Affairs, 21*(4), 40–51.

Colwill, J. M., Cultice, J. M., & Kruse, R. L. (2008). Will generalist physician supply meet demands of an increasing and aging population? *Health Affairs, 27*(3), w232–w241. Retrieved from http://content.healthaffairs.org/cgi/content/full/27/3/w232?maxtoshow=&HITS=10&hits=10&RESULTFORMAT=&fulltext=physician+supply+region&andorexactfulltext=and&searchid=1&FIRSTINDEX=0&resourcetype=HWCIT

Council on Graduate Medical Education. (2005). *Physician workforce policy guidelines for the United States: 2000–2020.* Retrieved from http://www.hrsa.gov/advisorycommittees/bhpradvisory/cogme/reports/sixteenthreport.pdf

Cunningham, P. J., & Hadley, J. (2008). Effects of changes in incomes and practice circumstances on physicians' decisions to treat charity and Medicaid patients. *The Milbank Quarterly, 86*, 1. Retrieved from http://www.ncbi.nlm.nih.gov/pmc/articles/PMC2690335/

Dill, M. J., & Salsberg, E. S. (2008). *The complexities of physician supply and demand: Projections through 2025*. Washington, DC: Association of American Medical Colleges. Retrieved from https://members.aamc.org/eweb/upload/The%20Complexities%20of%20Physician%20Supply.pdf

Enthoven, A. C., Crosson, F. J., Stephen, M., & Shortell, S. M. (2007). Redefining health care: Medical homes or archipelagos to navigate? *Health Affairs, 26*(5), 1366–1372.

Fadiman, A. (1997). *The spirit catches you and you fall down: Hmong child, her American doctors, and the collision of two cultures*. New York, NY: Farrar, Straus and Giroux.

Field, R. I. (2007). *Health care regulation in America: Complexity, confrontation and compromise*. New York, NY: Oxford University Press.

Fox, M. (2012, September 14). Lia Lee dies; life went on around her, redefining care. *The New York Times*. Retrieved from http://www.nytimes.com/2012/09/15/us/life-went-on-around-her-redefining-care-by-bridging-a-divide.html?_r=0

Freidson, E. (1970). *Profession of medicine: A study of the sociology of applied knowledge*. New York, NY: Dodd, Mead.

Gawande, A. (1999, February 1). When doctors make mistakes. *The New Yorker*, p. 40.

Gawande, A. (2005, November 14). The malpractice mess: Who pays the price when patients sue doctors. *The New Yorker*. Retrieved from http://www.newyorker.com/archive/2005/11/14/051114fa_fact_gawande

Goodman, D. C. (2004). Trends: Twenty-year trends in regional variations in the U.S. physician workforce. *Health Affairs* [Web exclusive]. Retrieved from http://content.healthaffairs.org/cgi/content/full/hlthaff.var.90/DC2?maxtoshow =&HITS=10&hits=10&RESULTFORMAT=&author1=Goodman&fulltext=trends&andorexactfulltext=and&searchid=1&FIRSTINDEX=0&resourcetype=HWCIT

Goodman, D., & Fisher E. S. (2008). Physician workforce crisis? Wrong diagnosis, wrong prescription. *New England Journal of Medicine, 358*, 16. Retrieved from http://www.nejm.org/doi/full/10.1056/NEJMp0800319

Groopman, J. (2007, March 19). The mistakes doctors make: Errors in thinking too often lead to wrong diagnosis. *Boston Globe*. Retrieved from http://www.boston.com/news/globe/health_science/articles/2007/03/19/the_mistakes_doctors_make/

Hart, L. G., Skillman, S. M., Fordyce, M., Thompson, M., Hagopian, A., & Konrad, T. R. (2007). International medical graduate physicians in the United States: Changes since 1981. *Health Affairs, 26*(4), 1159–1169.

Health Resources and Services Administration. (2008). *The physician workforce: Projections and research into current issues affecting supply and demand*. Retrieved from http://bhpr.hrsa.gov/healthworkforce/reports/physwfissues.pdf

Healthcare Association of New York State. (2009). *Expanding access, improving outcomes: The essential role of primary care*. New York, NY: Albany. Retrieved from http://www.hanys.org/communications/publications/2009/the_essential_role_of_primary_care.pdf

Heisler, E. J. (2013). *Physician supply and the Affordable Care Act*. Retrieved from http://op.bna.com/hl.nsf/id/myon-93zpre/$File/crsdoctor.pdf

Hillman, A. L., Pauly, M. V., & Kerstein, J. J. (1989). How do financial incentives affect physicians' clinical decisions and the financial performance of health maintenance organizations? *New England Journal of Medicine, 321*, 86–92.

Institute of Medicine, Committee on Quality of Health Care in America. (2000). *To err is human: Building a safer health system*. Washington, DC: National Academies Press.

Jones, J. T. (2013). A new, evidence-based estimate of patient harms associated with hospital care. *Journal of Patient Safety, 9*(3). Retrieved from http://www.ncbi.nlm.nih.gov /pubmed/23860193

Kane, C. K., & Emmons, D. W. (2013). *New data on physician practice arrangements: Private practice remains strong despite shifts toward hospital employment.* Retrieved from http://www .ama-assn.org/resources/doc/health-policy /prp-physician-practice-arrangements.pdf

Kao, A. (2003). Teaching and evaluating students' professionalism in US medical schools, 2002–2003. *Journal of the American Medical Association, 290*(9), 1151–1152.

Kassirer, J. P. (2005). *On the take: How medicine's complicity with big business can endanger your health.* New York, NY: Oxford University Press.

Knowles, J. H. (1970). *Higher education and the nation's health.* Berkeley, CA: Carnegie Commission on the Future of Higher Education.

Komaromy, M., Grumbach, K., Drake, M., Vranizan, K., Lurie, N., Keane, D., & Bindman, A. B. (1996). The role of black and Hispanic physicians in providing health care for underserved populations. *New England Journal of Medicine, 334*(20), 1305–1310.

Leapfrog Group. (2009). *How Leapfrog works.* Retrieved from http://www.leapfroggroup.org /about_us/how_leapfrog_works

Ludmerer, K. M. (1999). *Learning to heal: The development of American medical education.* New York, NY: Oxford University Press.

Marmor, T. (1973). *The politics of Medicare.* Chicago, IL: Aldine.

Mechanic, D. (1996). Changing medical organization and the erosion of trust. *The Milbank Quarterly, 74*(2), 171–189.

Mechanic, R. E., & Altman, S. H. (2009). Payment reform options: Episode payment is a good place to start. *Health Affairs, 28*(2), w262–w271.

Medscape. (2013). *Physician compensation report.* Retrieved from http://www.medscape.com/ features/slideshow/compensation/2013/public

Mello, M. M., Chandra, A., Gawande, A. A., & Studdert, D. M. (2010). National costs of the medical liability system. *Health Affairs, 29*(9), 1569–1577.

Mishler, E. G. (1981). Viewpoint: Critical perspectives on the biomedical model. In E. G. Mishler, L. R. AmaraSingham, S. T. Hauser, R. Liem, S. D. Osherson, & N. E. Waxler (Eds.), *Social contexts of health, illness, and patient care (pp. 1–23).* New York, NY: Cambridge University Press.

Mitchell, J. M. (2007). The prevalence of physician self-referral arrangements after Stark II: The evidence from advanced diagnostic imaging. *Health Affairs, 26*(3), w415–w424.

Mullan, F. (1997). The National Health Service Corps and inner-city hospitals. *New England Journal of Medicine, 336*(22), 1601–1603.

Nickitas, D. M. (2009). Moral courage or moral imperative: Which is it? *Nursing Economic$, 27*(6), 361–362.

O'Malley, A. S., Tynan, A., Cohen, G., Kemper, N. M., & Davis, M. M. (2009). *Coordination of care by primary care practices: Strategies, lessons and implications.* Retrieved from http://www.hschange. org/CONTENT/1058/?words

Pentecost, M. (2007). The future of employer-based health insurance. *Permanente Journal, 11*(2). Retrieved from http://www.thepermanente-journal.org/files/Spring2007/future.pdf

Pham, H. H., Ginsburg, P. B., McKenzie, K., & Milstein, A. (2007). Redesigning care delivery in response to a high-performance network: The Virginia Mason Medical Center. *Health Affairs, 26*(4), w532–w544. Retrieved from http://content.healthaffairs.org/cgi/content /full/26/4/w532

Price-Wise, G. (2008). *Language, culture, and medical tragedy: The case of Willie Ramirez.* Retrieved from http://healthaffairs.org /blog/2008/11/19/language-culture-and-medi-cal-tragedy-the-case-of-willie-ramirez/

RAND. (2013). *Payment reform and new models of care.* Retrieved from http://www.rand.org

/health/aca/payment_reform_care_delivery. html

Reid, R. J., Coleman, K., Johnson, E. A., Fishman, P. A., Hsu, C., Soman, M. P., . . . Larso, E. B. (2010). The group health medical home at year two: Cost savings, higher patient satisfaction, and less burnout for providers. *Health Affairs, 29*(5) 835–843.

Rosenbaum, S., Jones, E., Shin, P., & Ku, L. (2009). *National health reform: How will medically underserved communities fare.* Retrieved from http://www.gwumc.edu/sphhs/departments/healthpolicy/dhp_publications/pub_uploads/dhpPublication_5046C2DE-5056-9D20-3D2A570F2CF3F8B0.pdf

Rothman, D. T. (2000). Medical professionalism: Focusing on the real issues. *New England Journal of Medicine, 342,* 1284. Retrieved from http://content.nejm.org/cgi/content/full/342/17/1284

Sardell, A. (1988). *The U.S. experiment in social Medicine: The community health center program, 1965–1986.* Pittsburgh, PA: University of Pittsburgh Press.

Schoen, C., Radley, D., Piley, P., Lippa, J., Berenson, J., Dermody, C., & Shih, A. (2013). *Health care in the two Americas: Findings from the scorecard on state health system performance for low-income populations, 2013.* New York, NY: The Commonwealth Fund.

Schroeder, S. A. (1992). Physician supply and the U.S. medical marketplace. *Health Affairs, 11*(1), 235–243. Retrieved from http://content.healthaffairs.org/cgi/reprint/11/1/235?maxtoshow=&HITS=10&hits=10&RESULTFORMAT=&fulltext=generalist+and+specialist&andorexactfulltext=and&searchid=1&FIRSTINDEX=20&resourcetype=HWCIT

Schroeder, S. A., & Showstack, J. A. (1978). Financial incentives to perform medical procedures and laboratory tests: Illustrative models of office practice. *Medical Care, 16,* 289–298.

Starfield, B., Shi, L., Grover, A., & Macinko, J. (2005). The effects of specialist supply on populations' health: Assessing the evidence [Web exclusive].

Health Affairs. Retrieved from http://healthaff.highwire.org/cgi/reprint/hlthaff.w5.97v1.pdf

Starr, P. (1982). *The social transformation of American medicine.* New York, NY: Basic Books.

Stensland, J., & Winter, A. (2006). Do physician-owned cardiac hospitals increase utilization? Physician-ownership has primarily affected where people get cardiac surgery, not who gets the surgery. *Health Affairs, 25*(1), 119–129.

Stockburger, W. T. (2004). CT imaging, then and now: A 30-year review of the economics of computed tomography. *Radiology Management, 26*(6), 20–22, 24–30.

Studdert, D. M., Mello, M. M., Gawande, A. A., Gandhi, T. K., Kachalia, A., Yoon, C.,…Brennan, T. A. (2006). Claims, errors, and compensation payments in medical malpractice litigation. *New England Journal of Medicine, 354.* Retrieved from http://www.nejm.org/doi/pdf/10.1056/NEJMsa054479

Thomas, E. J., Studdert, D. M., Burstin, H. R., Orav, E. J., Zeena, T., Williams, E. J.,…Brennan, T. A. (2000). Incidence and types of adverse events and negligent care in Utah and Colorado. *Medical Care, 38*(3), 261–271.

Town, R., Wholey, D. R., Kralewski, J., & Dowd, B. (2004). Assessing the influence of incentives on physicians and medical groups. *Medical Care Research Review, 61*(Suppl. 3), 80S–118S.

Trinkoff, A. M., & Stor, C. L. (1998). Substance use among nurses: Differences between specialties. *American Journal of Public Health, 88*(4), 581–585.

Tu, H. T., & Ginsburg, P. B. (2006). *Losing ground: Physician income, 1995–2003.* Retrieved from http://www.hschange.com/CONTENT/851/#ib5

U.S. Bureau of Labor Statistics. (2013). *Occupational employment and wages.* Retrieved from http://www.bls.gov/news.release/ocwage.htm

Wachter, R. M., & Goldman, L. (2002). The hospitalist movement 5 years later. *Journal of the American Medical Association, 287*(4), 487–494.

Wazana, A. (2000). Physicians and the pharmaceutical industry: Is a gift ever just a gift? *Journal of the American Medical Association, 283*(3), 373–380.

Welch, P. W., Cuellar, A. E., Stearns, S. C., & Bindman, A. B. (2013). Proportion of physicians in large group practices continues to grow in 2009-2011. *Health Affairs, 32*(9). Retrieved from http://content.healthaffairs.org/content/32/9/1659.full.pdf+html

Wennberg, J. E., Goodman, D. C., Nease, R. F., & Keller, R. B. (1993). Finding equilibrium in US physician supply. *Health Affairs, 12*(2), 89–103.

Werner, R. M., & Dudley, R. A. (2009). Making the "pay" matter in pay-for-performance: Implications for payment strategies. *Health Affairs, 28*(5), 1498–1508.

Young, A., Chaudhry, H. J., Rhyne, J., & Dugan, M. (2013). A census of actively licensed physicians in the United States, 2012. *Journal of Medical Regulation, 99*(2). Retrieved from http://www.fsmb.org/pdf/census.pdf

CHAPTER 7

Healthcare Quality

Donna Middaugh

Overview

This chapter presents an overview of human error, error theory, quality improvement, and the application of these concepts to healthcare delivery. Error measurement tools and injury prevention models are applied to healthcare settings. Public reporting systems and regulatory agency requirements are analyzed in conjunction with nursing performance measures. New national initiatives and their impact on quality care are explored. In the United States, nearly one-fifth of all spending is devoted to health care. This will only accelerate with the aging of the population and its increased dependence on federal and state financing of health care. Yet despite our high national spending, health care in the United States is uneven in quality and is often wasteful, uncoordinated, and inefficient (Bipartisan Policy Center, 2013).

Objectives

- Explain relevant theories of error as they relate to patient care.
- Apply effective error management techniques from aviation and industry to healthcare delivery.
- Identify examples of quality care initiatives that are cost driven.
- Discuss the role of quality care mandates from regulatory agencies.
- Describe the impact of national initiatives on quality care.

Quality Care and Public Policy

Above all, do no harm.

—*Hippocratic oath*

Public belief and trust in the healthcare system was shaken in 1999 when the Institute of Medicine (IOM) reported that between 44,000 and 98,000 Americans die each year as a result of medical errors (Kohn, Corrigan, & Donaldson, 2000). The November 1999 report of the IOM, published in a book titled *To Err is Human: Building a Safer Health System*, alerted healthcare institutions and professionals to the true scope of the quality problem (Kohnet al., 2000). Errors occur in every healthcare delivery setting: clinics, physicians' offices, pharmacies, homes, nursing homes, and hospitals.

Every day, Americans expect to receive high-quality health care to maintain or restore their health and well-being. Unfortunately, every day, thousands of Americans do not receive quality health care and are injured or die in the course of treatment. For example, a hospital study conducted in New York state found that 3.7% of patients experienced adverse events: 12.6% of those events led to death, and 2.6% led to permanent disability. One-fourth of the events resulted from negligence (Agency for Healthcare Research and Quality [AHRQ], 2002). A Harvard study reported in 2003 that one-fourth of patients with health problems in five countries declare they have suffered from a medical or prescription error in the past 2 years. A minimum of 750 persons were surveyed in the United States, Canada, the United Kingdom, New Zealand, and Australia. Twenty-eight percent of those surveyed in the United States reported errors—the highest of all countries studied. The United Kingdom was the lowest, with 18%. This study suggests that the most significant risks to patients appear to occur when they are treated by multiple healthcare professionals. At least 25% of all those surveyed reported having duplicate tests performed but received conflicting information from different doctors (Dorschner, 2003).

The IOM released its staggering report on medical errors more than 13 years ago. It estimated that the United States loses more patient lives to safety incidents every 6 months than it did in the entire Vietnam War (Kohn et al., 2000). Statistics indicate that more deaths occur in the United States each year from medical errors than from motor vehicle accidents, breast cancer, or AIDS. Put in other terms, medical errors, if documented by the Centers for Disease Control and Prevention, would rank as the sixth leading cause of death in the United States (Healthgrades, 2005).

The IOM has estimated that more than 7,000 patients die each year in hospitals alone because of medication errors, and other reports have estimated that 100,000 hospital deaths occur each year because of adverse drug reactions (Kohn et al., 2000). These studies focused only on hospitalized patients. When one considers the billions of medications that are prescribed at clinics and physician offices and taken home, it is staggering to think of the possible scope of error. All medication mistakes may be preventable.

Since the IOM report, healthcare providers, the public, and federal and state governments have been seeking facts and answers as to why these errors are so prevalent. A report published in 2013, *American Hospital Quality Outcomes 2014: Healthgrades Report to the Nation*, focused on the performance of more than 4,500 U.S. hospitals and covered 31 of the most common inpatient procedures and conditions during 2010–2012. This report showed that hospitals, physicians, and patients each have a role to play, and each group must take specific actions to help improve quality outcomes at lower costs. The report identifies the following (Healthgrades, 2013):

- Quality disparities persist within hospitals among different procedures and conditions, as well as among hospitals within local service areas.
- Patient complications and mortality in hospitals increase direct costs.
- The use of minimally invasive surgical techniques may hold promise for reducing mortality and length of stay.

Hospitals must focus on quality and strive for continued improvement. The Healthgrades report demonstrates that there is significant variation in hospital outcomes, even after accounting for patients' severity of illness and population demographics. This translates into the fact that physicians should stay current on the latest approaches and techniques; perform procedures that have been shown to have lower complication and mortality rates; and use referral networks with surgeons who are trained in minimally invasive surgery options when appropriate. Patients should use quality performance data to make informed choices by finding out about the performance of hospitals based on complication and mortality rates. They should also be aware of the variation in direct costs incurred by hospitals, which are passed on to the consumer in the form of higher premiums, deductibles, and copays. The Healthgrades report highlights the connection between higher complication rates and increased costs.

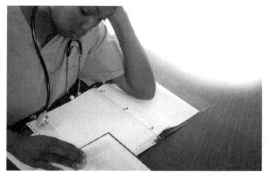

© Dewayne Flowers/ShutterStock, Inc.

Human Error

Errors can occur in all phases of healthcare delivery. Diagnostic errors can occur with improper testing, misread or misinterpreted laboratory results, or failure to act on the results. During patient treatment, technical errors can result in the inaccurate preparation or delivery of treatments. Treatment can be delayed, missed, or performed incorrectly. A medical error might mean the healthcare provider chose an inappropriate method of care, or the provider chose the right course of care but carried it out incorrectly (Nordenberg, 2000). Medical errors are not purposeful or reckless actions that are intended to harm a patient (Liang, 2001), and errors do not always result in harm. Adverse events, on the other hand, do imply harm to an individual.

Throughout the literature, the term *error* is used to denote a mistake, close call, near miss, or active or latent error. Active errors occur at the level of the frontline provider—for example, administering the wrong medication. Active errors are limited in time and space, so they are easier to measure. Latent errors involve system defects, such as faulty maintenance on equipment, poor design, or inadequate staffing. Latent errors are more difficult to measure because they occur over greater periods of time and space and because they may exist for a long time before they lead to an error or adverse event (Thomas & Petersen, 2003).

Error Settings

The use of outpatient settings, including physician offices, has risen dramatically in the past 2 decades, from 202 million visits in 1980 to 521 million visits in 2000 (Landro, 2002). Healthcare reform efforts have primarily focused on studies that have linked deadly errors to hospital settings; however, experts say that patients can face equal or greater risks in doctors' offices and outpatient settings (Landro, 2002). These errors can occur during routine visits or during outpatient surgery procedures. Very little data exist from malpractice insurers, medical societies, or federal researchers to document the scope of this problem.

The California Academy of Family Physicians identified key sources of errors in primary care and provided recommendations for family physicians to reduce the risk of errors and adverse outcomes in primary care practice settings (California Academy of Family Physicians, 2002). They note that errors are inevitable and expected, so healthcare delivery systems must be designed to prevent and absorb errors. They strongly believe that a culture must be created to support error reporting and that blame and punishment will not correct the problem.

The California Academy of Family Physicians has also reported a study that analyzed 330 errors made by 50 family physicians over the course of 1 year. These errors fell into the following categories (California Academy of Family Physicians, 2002):

- Communication problems (staff/patients): 24%
- Discontinuity of care: 20%
- Lab results: 19%
- Missing values or charting: 13%
- Clinical mistake with knowledge/skill: 8%
- Prescribing errors: 8%
- Other: 8%

Interestingly, this list conflicts with the common beliefs that medical errors are synonymous with prescriptions for medications and that errors are clinical errors made by bad practitioners. In this study, prescribing medications and clinical judgment errors accounted for only 16% of the total errors. The study found that errors were largely the result of latent conditions or system properties rather than active failure on a practitioner's part (California Academy of Family Physicians, 2002).

Nursing Errors

Woods and Doan-Johnson (2002) developed a taxonomy of nursing errors with prevention as the goal. To achieve this goal, they identified eight categories of errors, all of which include system, individual, and practice contributions. It is unclear whether the Practice Breakdown Research Advisory Panel studied subjects from all levels of nursing, including registered nurses and nurse practitioners; however, the following eight categories of nursing errors can be applied to all levels of nursing practice (Woods & Doan-Johnson, 2002):

- Lack of attentiveness
- Lack of agency/fiduciary concern
- Inappropriate judgment
- Medication errors
- Lack of intervention on the patient's behalf
- Lack of prevention
- Missed or mistaken patient orders
- Documentation errors

Lack of attentiveness can be caused by system-level problems, such as understaffing or fluctuations in patient acuity, and it often translates into lack of monitoring. Patient safety depends on attentiveness to both predictable and unpredictable conditions.

Agency concern is defined as the moral agency of the nurse or his or her trustworthiness in working for the patient's and family's best interest. Moral agency is lacking when nurses do not advocate for the best interests of their client. Failing to question an order, failing to call a physician for consultation, failing to heed a patient or family request for assistance, and breach of confidentiality are examples of lack of fiduciary concern. These can all contribute to causing harm to the patient.

The Practice Breakdown Research Advisory Panel identified various types of inappropriate judgment, including insufficient evaluation, faulty logic, flawed intervention, and inappropriate delegation. Interestingly, the panel also acknowledged a subclass of inadequate assessment, which occurred when nurses in the study did not understand or recognize the implications of the signs and symptoms they identified in their patient assessments (Woods & Doan-Johnson, 2002).

The advisory panel (Woods & Doan-Johnson, 2002) identified five types of medication errors in their study population:

- Missed doses of medications
- Wrong administration time
- Delivery of too much intravenous medications or delivery too fast
- Wrong route of medication delivery
- Medications delivered to wrong patient

Eight of the nine cases of medication errors found that the patient died as a direct result of the nurse's action. Because medication errors can encompass a wide range of causes and categories, the root cause and practice responsibility for the error must be analyzed on an individual basis.

Intriguingly, four of the panel's cases involved the death of a patient related to the nurse's lack of attentiveness or failure to intervene on the patient's behalf. These cases involved a combination of situations in which patient signs and symptoms of postoperative bleeding, pregnancy-induced hypertension, acute cardiovascular accident, high blood glucose levels, or dehydration were missed, or the nurse failed to obtain assistance in an acute situation (Woods & Doan-Johnson, 2002).

The prevention of patient complications, threats to patient safety, and errors is essential to good nursing care. Breaches of infection control, failure to prevent complications of immobility, and failure to prevent harm from environmental causes were all present in the panel's study sample (Woods & Doan-Johnson, 2002).

The category of missed or mistaken patient orders included all instances when nurses carried out orders that were inappropriate, or orders that were misread or misunderstood, resulting in patient harm. As with medication errors, this type of error necessitates in-depth investigation of each specific incident to categorize the root cause correctly.

Finally, documentation errors in this study included charting procedures before they were completed, or charting medications before they were administered to the patient, and failure to chart observations of the patient (Woods & Doan-Johnson, 2002). These resulted in serious harm to patients by masking a patient's true condition, causing a medication error, or generally failing to communicate vital information to other healthcare providers. Wood and Doan-Johnson's study attempted to develop a guide for statistically analyzing nursing errors.

Error Theory

Human error has been studied extensively by professor James Reason (2000), who identified two approaches to the problem of human error: the person approach and the system approach. A person approach concentrates on the unsafe acts of individuals, which usually result in blame for forgetfulness, inattention, or moral weakness. A systems approach focuses on the conditions under which the person works and assumes that humans are fallible and errors are to be expected. Errors are then viewed as consequences rather than causes.

The person approach has been the tradition in medicine, blaming someone for having made an unsafe choice of behavior (Reason, 2000). Shame and blame have been the method traditionally used by the medical profession to reduce medical errors. The person approach shames an individual into believing that his or her error denotes lack of professionalism and incompetence. It does not recognize the systems-based nature of successful error reduction (Liang, 2001).

The culture of blame seems to be reinforced throughout the education and training of physicians. Clinicians are led to believe that errors are caused by carelessness. This, combined with the public's and media's quick-to-blame mentality, results in fear of both making a mistake and being caught (Weinberg, 2002). There are experts who argue that in complex environments that undergo constant change, such as our healthcare environment, complete elimination of all error will never be possible (Ebright, Urder, Patterson, & Chalko, 2004).

Reason's theory of error has been used by airlines, railroads, nuclear power plants, financial management companies, and the military (Wachter & Shojania, 2004). Reason's research led him to develop a model of system accidents. High-technology systems, such as health care, have many defensive layers. These can include technological barriers (alarms, automatic shutdowns, etc.), people (surgeons, nurses, etc.), and procedures or administrative controls. The function of these layers is to protect victims and assets from hazards. In an ideal world, each defensive layer would be solid and intact.

Reason (2000) emphasizes that by nature, there are always weaknesses or holes in these layers, making them similar to Swiss cheese. He calls this a Swiss Cheese Model for latent errors. Each slice of cheese represents a safety defense or system, which can have either small holes or large holes. Each hole allows errors to penetrate—the larger the hole, the more errors get through.

Reason (2000) argues that when these holes in the cheese align, a number of slips can occur, so an error finally reaches the patient. The presence of holes in one layer does not normally cause an adverse event, but these holes are constantly opening and shutting. This allows mistakes or errors to slip through, hopefully to be caught by the next layer. Adverse events can happen only when the holes in many layers momentarily line up to permit a trajectory of accident opportunity, which brings the hazards into contact with victims (Reason, 2000). These holes arise because of active failures or latent conditions. This suggests the need for a systems perspective toward patient safety.

Byers and White (2004) discuss three major approaches to the causes of medical errors. The first is Reason's (2000) Swiss Cheese Model. The second is related to the visibility of the practitioner's actions. There are many visible and invisible factors involved in any single error. Usually, however, only the final action receives blame or attention, although a true systems analysis must look at all those involved in the process leading up to the error. Finally, Byers and White noted that too often, a simplified analysis is undertaken after an error occurs because of hindsight bias. It is easy to look back and determine that a different course of action should have been taken, but this is not easily accomplished during complex patient care situations.

Error Management

Reason (2000) believes that error management has two dimensions: limiting the occurrence of dangerous errors, and creating systems that are better able to tolerate errors and contain their damaging effects. He argues that there are high-reliability organizations that operate in hazardous conditions yet have few adverse events. He proposes that systems in health care should be modeled after these high-reliability organizations, such as U.S. Navy nuclear aircraft carriers, nuclear power plants, and air traffic control centers (Reason, 2000).

These organizations anticipate the worst and equip themselves to deal with the worst at all levels. This literally means asking individuals in these systems to remain chronically uneasy, yet the culture of these high-reliability organizations provides employees with reminders and tools to help them remember to be afraid. They have created a culture that makes their system as robust as practicable in the face of both human and operational hazards. Characteristics that allow high-reliability organizations to accomplish this include the following (Reason, 2000):

- Being internally dynamic, complex, and interactive

- Performing exacting tasks under time pressure
- Carrying out demanding activities with low incident rates
- Managing complex, demanding technologies to avoid major failures
- Maintaining the capacity to meet periods of peak demand

Medical Errors and Aviation

Research on the factors that cause human error has been in existence since the 1940s. Some of the early studies involved aviation. The IOM's 2000 report noted that the number of Americans who die each year as a result of medical errors is the equivalent of more than 230 full jumbo jets crashing each year (Kohn et al., 2000). The aviation and nuclear power industries learned long ago not to rely on human perfection to prevent accidents. These industries have implemented sound risk-management techniques, such as training, rules, and high standards to aid their systems (Spath, 1999). Experts have tried to assure the public that the United States healthcare system is safe despite the IOM statistics; however, compared to the complex aviation industry, the healthcare system is not safe. Nordenberg (2000) reports that a person would have to fly nonstop for 438 years before expecting to be involved in a deadly airplane crash. This places health care at least 10 years behind aviation in safeguarding consumers (Nordenberg, 2000).

Aircraft accidents are infrequent, but when they occur, they often involve a massive loss of life and therefore gain world attention. Aviation accidents immediately stimulate an enormous, exhaustive investigation into the causes and needed remedial action. Adverse events in health care, on the other hand, involve individual patients and seldom receive even local, let alone national, publicity. There is no standardized method of investigation or remedial action (Helmreich, 2000).

Errors can result from the following (Helmreich, 2000):

- Psychological limitations
- Physiological limitations
- Fatigue
- Heavy workload
- Cognitive overload
- Fear
- Poor interpersonal communications
- Imperfect information processing
- Flawed decision making

These factors are present among workers in both aviation and health care, but the aviation industry is doing something right to maintain the low incidence of disasters, whereas the healthcare industry continues to have a high accident rate.

Rivers, Swain, and Nixon (2003) looked at whether the safety techniques used in aviation could be applied to the healthcare delivery system. To test this idea, an aviation training team implemented 12 hours of error-reducing skills training for operating room personnel. The findings revealed a significant effect on the behaviors of operating room staff. Specific error-reducing behaviors resulted in more effective, efficient communication among team members, a 50% decrease in surgical count errors, early identification of potential red flags, standardized checklists and protocols, fewer delays in procedures, and savings in time and resources for the operating room as a whole (Rivers et al., 2003).

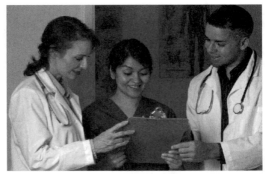

© JHDT Stock Images LLC/ShutterStock, Inc.

Error Management in Healthcare Settings

Preventable adverse events can occur in any healthcare setting despite the best intentions. The National Quality Forum and the Agency for Healthcare Research and Quality (AHRQ) together have identified 30 safe practices that evidence shows can work to reduce or even prevent adverse events (AHRQ, 2005). These 30 practices have been endorsed by the National Quality Forum, which includes 215 of the nation's leading healthcare providers, purchasers, and consumer organizations. All healthcare practitioners and organizations are strongly urged to adopt these practices to reduce the risk of harm to patients. The 30 practices are grouped under five major categories (AHRQ, 2005):

- Creating a culture of safety
- Matching healthcare needs with delivery capabilities
- Facilitating information transfer and clear communication
- Providing specific settings or processes of care
- Increasing safe medication use

All of the 30 recommended safe practices can be used by physicians and nurses. Of particular relevance to nurses are the safe practices that relate to communication with other healthcare providers and patients, and thorough regular evaluation and monitoring of clients for change in health status or risk of complications.

Strategies for Error Management

The American Society of Anesthesiologists was one of the first groups to adopt specific error-reduction strategies. Their clinical practice guidelines and system improvements have significantly reduced anesthesia-related mortality (Spath, 1999). The risk management and error-reduction strategies listed here have been successfully applied in numerous industries, and Spath suggests that these system and task redesigns could serve as the basis for improving quality in healthcare delivery as well:

- Improve information access: Information should be readily available to all who need it.

- Reduce reliance on memory: Checklists, computerized decision aids, and protocols can minimize the need for reliance on human memory.

- Error-proof processes: Critical tasks should be structured so that errors cannot be made.

- Standardize tasks: Tasks are to be done in a standardized process.

- Reduce the number of hand-offs: Processes and procedures should be restructured to minimize the number of people who are involved in transferring materials, information, people, instructions, or supplies.

The California Academy of Family Physicians proposes that a wide-ranging approach must be taken to reduce errors in health care. Their research has led them to suggest the following error-reduction methods (California Academy of Family Physicians, 2002):

- Pay more and hire great staff. Hire people who have a positive attitude and good communication and teamwork skills. Check references carefully and have a thorough orientation and training program.

- Invest in new technologies. Use technologies that will enhance communication, prescription writing, email, messaging, and electronic medical records.

- Simplify and standardize. Have an office-wide formulary with standardized prescription-writing standards. Spread authority and accountability in the office to enable checks and balances. Use office flow sheets and checklists. Reward staff for identifying an actual or potential mistake. Create processes for patient and lab follow-up, and follow principles of evidence-based medicine.

- Listen to the patients. Collect data on patient satisfaction. Ask patients what they need and design services to meet these needs.

- Create a culture of healthcare safety. Always look for weak links. Take ownership for safety and establish a clear chain of command. Empower and incentivize staff to report errors, and minimize the punishment of those who commit errors. Keep policies and procedures up to date. Provide in-service training to all staff regarding error identification.

Patient-Centered Care

One principle for transforming health care is patient-centered care. DuPree, Anderson, and Nash (2011) believe that health care should be designed around the interests and needs of patients and their families. The most crucial element is patient safety, where no deaths or injuries would occur due to preventable errors. Patients and their families have the best knowledge about their conditions, the evolution of symptoms, and response to treatments. In short, bring the patient and the family more deeply into care conversations.

Institute for Healthcare Improvement

Mathews (2013) states that today's healthcare system is still dominated by a fee-for-service system, which results in inefficiencies—namely, high service volume and unnecessary care. These are a detriment to quality. To address this, the Institute for Healthcare Improvement (IHI) developed a framework called Triple Aim. It describes an approach to optimizing health system performance through three aims (Institute for Healthcare Improvement, 2013):

- Improve the patients' experience of care.
- Improve the health of populations.
- Reduce the per capita cost of health care.

Organizations that attain the Triple Aim will have healthier populations, in part because of new designs that better identify problems and solutions further upstream and outside of acute health care. Patients can expect less complex and more coordinated care. Businesses will have the opportunity to be more competitive with stabilization or reduction of the per capita cost of care for populations.

Error Measurement Tools

The abundance of scientific articles and news accounts of medical errors and adverse events has stimulated great efforts and research geared toward identification, measurement, and management of errors and adverse events (Kohn et al., 2000). Thomas and Petersen

(2003) offer a conceptual model for measuring latent errors, active errors, and adverse events. They identify the following methods to measure errors and adverse events:

- Morbidity and mortality (M and M) conferences and autopsy
- Error reporting systems
- Administrative data analysis
- Chart review
- Electronic medical records
- Observation of patient care
- Clinical surveillance
- Malpractice claims analysis

Their research has documented that the ability of M and M conferences to improve care is unproved, although there is strong belief in the effectiveness of such conferences, especially when they are combined with autopsy; however, this method of detecting errors and adverse events is the weakest form of study design. Error reporting systems can provide details about latent errors that lead to active errors and adverse events, but used alone they are not a reliable measure because of the underreporting of errors. Administrative or billing data are sometimes used to measure errors and adverse events; however, these data may be incomplete and subject to bias.

Chart reviews have served as the foundation for research into errors and adverse events; however, Thomas and Petersen (2003) found this method to be fraught with limitations, including low reliability and incomplete documentation in medical records. The method may be strengthened if it is combined with provider reporting. Electronic medical record review uses computers to search electronic documentation for errors and adverse events that may not be detected by traditional chart reviews. Thomas and Petersen suggest that as hospital computerized systems become more sophisticated, this will become an accurate and precise method for measuring errors and adverse events.

Observation or videotaping of patient care has been effective in measuring active errors; however, this method is limited by the need to protect confidentiality. It is time intensive. Hindsight bias may be present, and the method focuses on the provider instead of the system of care delivery. Clinical surveillance is identified by Thomas and Petersen (2003) as the most precise and accurate method of measuring adverse events; however, this is an active and costly surveillance method that focuses on specific events in a specific time and place, and thus it may provide less information on latent errors.

Medical malpractice claims analysis is a strong method of identifying latent errors, and it has led to important patient safety standards; however, claims may be highly selected cases from which it is difficult to generalize. Thomas and Petersen (2003) suggest that a comprehensive monitoring system for patient safety should include combinations of all these measurement tools. They recommend using incident reporting, M and M conferences with autopsies, and malpractice claims analysis as the strongest tools for latent error identification. Direct observation is recommended for active error detection and clinical surveillance for adverse event recognition (Thomas & Petersen, 2003).

Agency for Healthcare Research and Quality

The AHRQ is the health services research division of the U.S. Department of Health and Human Services. It works in conjunction with the biomedical research mission of the National Institutes of Health. AHRQ research endeavors center on the following:

- Quality improvement and patient safety
- Outcomes and effectiveness of care
- Clinical practice and technology assessment
- Healthcare organization and delivery systems
- Primary care (including preventive services)
- Healthcare costs and sources of payment

This includes how people get access to health care, how much that care costs, and what happens to patients during that care. The ultimate goal is to improve patient safety. The AHRQ was established in 1989 to spearhead efforts to boost the quality of health care in the United States and to fund research on the comparative effectiveness of interventions. As a result of the 2009 American Recovery and Reinvestment Act, $473 million was invested in research supported by AHRQ (Kuehn, 2012). Comparative effectiveness research (CER) is a tool that generates and synthesizes evidence that compares benefits and harms of different interventions and strategies to prevent, diagnose, treat, and monitor health conditions and to improve the delivery of care (Largent, 2011). The goal is to determine which interventions are most effective for which patients and thereby enable consumers, practitioners, and policy makers to develop informed decisions to improve population health.

AHRQ developed the *Guide to Patient and Family Engagement in Hospital Quality and Safety*, which is an evidence-based resource to guide hospitals and families in order to improve quality and safety. The guide describes critical opportunities for hospitals to engage patients and families and to create partnerships between patients, families, and hospitals around the same goals. It also addresses real-world challenges and helps hospitals engage patients and families. This, in turn, helps hospitals improve quality and safety and helps them respond to healthcare reform and accreditation standards (AHRQ, 2013a).

Patient Safety Indicators

A key research area for AHRQ has been the nursing workforce and patient care environment, linking healthcare staffing and workflow design to medical errors (Clancy, Farquhar, & Collins Sharp, 2005). The AHRQ continues to develop patient safety indicators, which are tools to help healthcare agencies identify potential adverse events that occur during hospitalization. Failure to rescue is one of the AHRQ patient safety indicators that has garnered much attention and research. Failure to rescue is measured by comparing the number of patients who die after surgery when they develop a postoperative complication with the number of patients who survive these complications and are discharged (Simpson, 2004). These postoperative complications may include sepsis, acute renal failure, cardiac arrest, pneumonia, hemorrhage, or thrombosis/embolus. Although the concept of failure to rescue a patient is not new, AHRQ research suggests that it is a sensitive indicator of both the quality and quantity of nursing care (Simpson, 2004).

National Database of Nursing Quality Indicators

The National Database of Nursing Quality Indicators (NDNQI) is a repository for nursing-sensitive indicators developed by the American Nurses Association and managed by the University of Kansas School of Nursing. More than 1,200 hospitals across the United States participate, volunteering unit-level data on structure, process, and outcome measures quarterly (Kurtzman & Jennings, 2008). The NDNQI nursing-sensitive indicators are designed to be a sign of the structure, process, and outcomes of nursing care. Structure is indicated by the availability of nursing staff, skill level of nurses, and education and certification of nursing staff. Process indicators measure assessment, intervention of patient care, and registered nurse job satisfaction. Outcomes measured for nursing sensitivity are those that improve if there is a greater quantity or quality of nursing care. These might include patient falls, intravenous infiltrations, pressure ulcers, and so forth (American Nurses Association, 2009). Recently, the NDNQI has worked in conjunction with the National Quality Forum and The Joint Commission, using their nursing-sensitive indicators.

National Error Reduction Efforts

The Code of Silence

A serious question is why the statistics of the IOM 2000 report were such a shock to people. Part of the answer is that fear of being sued suppresses discussion of medical errors. If procedures are done with the best intentions and skill, yet something does not turn out the way it was supposed to, the doctor often has to compensate the patient with a huge settlement. The culture is that physicians are going to lose no matter what they do, so physicians remain closed among themselves (Nordenberg, 2000).

All professional codes of conduct require that breaches of professional behavior by colleagues be reported to the profession or appropriate licensing body. This is to ensure that there will be some form of investigation and discipline for conduct or service below standards. Williams (2004) notes that there is a deadly conspiracy of silence in health care today. This silent negligence is a marriage between a conspiracy to remain silent and negligence that is witnessed (Williams, 2004). Healthcare providers who witness negligent care share in the guilt if they refuse to speak out about it. Williams describes today's health environment as having no system of professional accountability, which reinforces physicians' suspicion that the need for a conspiracy of silence far outweighs the demand for ethical behavior. By definition, professionals self-regulate their practice, which requires a protective system for the society they serve. This concept is not unique to physicians. It is essential for all professionals, including advanced practice nurses. Self-regulation allows for mutual obligations shared between healthcare providers and society.

In 2002 a major newspaper in South Carolina reported that about 30 of the lawyers who specialized in suing doctors, nurses, and hospitals had won more than $57 million that year in settlements and verdicts for those killed or injured by medical negligence (Monk, 2002). In interviews, these malpractice lawyers stated that they turned down dozens of cases for each suit they accepted. They only accepted cases with strong evidence and expected doctors and their insurance companies to fight hard when sued. One factor causing patients to sue is that hospitals and doctors rarely volunteer information about errors. One attorney told the newspaper that it was easier to win malpractice cases if they went to trial because of the increasingly businesslike atmosphere in medical care. The attorney added that when relationships between medical providers and

patients are abrupt, questions are unanswered, and time is not spent, people were driven to sue (Monk, 2002).

The newspaper also reported that secrecy about medical errors is common, and facts about medical mistakes are often concealed (Monk, 2002). *The State* reported that doctors and hospitals regularly made secret payouts to victims of medical mistakes, and those hospitals did not always tell patients or families about mistakes that injured or killed their loved ones. Although courts are routinely open in South Carolina, hundreds of secret settlements are made in courthouses involving hospitals, doctors, and nurses (Monk, 2002). Other states, such as Florida, mandate that court settlements must be open and part of the public record. Some argue that confidentiality encourages quick resolution of lawsuits, whereas others argue that confidentiality conceals information that is essential to the public about healthcare providers.

Sorry Works! Coalition

The Sorry Works! coalition began in 2005 and is composed mostly of doctors, insurers, lawyers, and patient advocates (Sorry Works!, 2013). The organization advocates that full disclosure and apologies for medical errors are a "middle-ground solution" to the medical malpractice crisis (Sorry Works!, 2013, p.1). It is surmised that apologies for bad outcomes, adverse events, or medical errors, combined with upfront compensation, help to reduce the anger of patients and families. The healthcare providers apologize to the patient/family, admit fault, provide an explanation of what happened and how the hospital will fix the procedures so the error is not repeated, and make a fair offer of upfront compensation (Wojcieszak, Banja, & Houk, 2006). This approach is taken only after a root-cause analysis shows that the standard of care was not met. It is hoped that this, in turn, will lead to a reduction in medical malpractice lawsuits and associated defense litigation expenses.

If the standard of care was met or if there was no medical error or negligence, the providers still meet with the patient/family and their attorney to explain what happened, apologize, and offer empathy. They do not admit fault or provide compensation or offer to settle any claim. These protocols are based on a disclosure program developed at the Veterans Administration Hospital in Lexington, Kentucky (Wojcieszak et al., 2006). It is expected that this approach will spread to all healthcare organizations committed to creating a culture of safety and quality.

Safety Culture

The Institute for Safe Medical Practices reported that 40% of clinicians either keep quiet or remain passive after witnessing an improper patient care event to avoid possible reprisals (Nurse.com, 2012). In 2012, the National Association for Healthcare Quality (NAHQ) issued a Call to Action for Enhancing Health Care Quality and Patient Safety. This initiative is designed to enhance overall quality of care, strengthen patient safety protection, and minimize costly medical errors. The call to action asks healthcare provider organizations to expect all clinical staff to be accountable for achieving meaningful quality improvements and to report potential safety risks. This helps create a strong safety culture in healthcare organizations, which will enhance best practices, improve quality, improve safety reporting, and protect staff. The NAHQ joined with more than 10 national organizations to develop recommendations.

SPEAK UP Campaign

The Joint Commission initiated a new national SPEAK UP campaign in January 2005, and this program urges Americans to take an active role in avoiding medication errors at the doctor's office, pharmacy, hospital, and clinic. The acronym SPEAK UP stands for the following (Hill, 2005):

- Speak up if you have questions or do not understand.
- Pay attention to the care you are receiving.
- Educate yourself about your diagnosis and tests.
- Ask a trusted family member or friend to be your advocate.
- Know what medications you take and why.
- Use a hospital or clinic that has been evaluated for quality.
- Participate in all decisions about your treatment.

Brochures and posters titled "Things You Can Do to Prevent Medication Mistakes" were mailed to the nation's Fortune 1000 companies because The Joint Commission believes employers have a crucial role in developing informed healthcare consumers among their employees.

National Patient Safety Goals

Quite a few years ago, through the AHRQ, the federal government adopted the term *patient safety* (Kohn et al., 2000). Patient safety endeavors are crucial components of quality improvement and risk management activities in healthcare institutions. The Joint Commission has developed a set of national patient safety goals (NPSGs) to help organizations address explicit areas of patient safety. Beginning January 1, 2003, all healthcare organizations accredited by The Joint

Commission were required to demonstrate how they met the first six Joint Commission NPSGs (Joint Commission on Accreditation of Healthcare Organizations, 2003). The Joint Commission has revised and expanded the NPSGs, which have been identified for the following specific healthcare arenas (The Joint Commission, 2013a):

- Ambulatory health care
- Behavioral health care
- Critical access hospitals
- Disease-specific care
- Home care
- Hospital
- Laboratory

- Long-term care and Medicaid/Medicare certification-based long-term care
- Office-based surgery

In June 2013, The Joint Commission approved a new NPSG, 06.01.01, on clinical alarm safety for hospitals and critical access hospitals. All these goals focus on problems in healthcare safety in hospital settings and how to solve them. The 2014 hospital NPSGs are summarized in Table 7-1.

The NPSGs have become a critical method by which The Joint Commission promotes and enforces major changes in patient safety. The criteria used for determining the value of these goals are based on the merit of their impact, cost, and effectiveness (AHRQ, 2013b).

Table 7-1   2014 Hospital National Patient Safety Goals

1. Identify patients correctly.

—Use at least two ways to identify patients.

—Make sure the correct patient gets the correct blood when a blood transfusion is done.

2. Improve staff communication.

—Get important test results to the right staff person on time.

3. Use medicines safely.

—Before a procedure, label medicines that are not labeled.

—Take extra care with patients who take medicines to thin their blood.

—Record and pass along correct information about a patient's medicines.

4. Use alarms safely.

—Make improvements to ensure that alarms on medical equipment are heard and responded to on time.

5. Prevent infection.

—Use the hand cleaning guidelines from the Centers for Disease Control and Prevention or the World Health Organization. Set goals for improving hand cleaning. Use the goals to improve hand cleaning.

(continued)

Table 7-1   2014 Hospital National Patient Safety Goals (*continued*)

—Use proven guidelines to prevent infections that are difficult to treat.

—Use proven guidelines to prevent infection of the blood from central lines.

—Use proven guidelines to prevent infection after surgery.

—Use proven guidelines to prevent infections of the urinary tract that are caused by catheters.

6. Identify patient safety risks.

—Find out which patients are most likely to try to commit suicide.

7. Prevent mistakes in surgery.

—Make sure the correct surgery is done on the correct patient and at the correct place on the patient's body.

—Mark the correct place on the patient's body where the surgery is to be done.

—Pause before the surgery to make sure that a mistake is not being made.

Source: The Jcount Commision, 2014 Hospital National Patient Safety Goals, http://www.jointcommission.org/assets/1/6/2014_HAP_NPSG_E.pdf

Patient Safety in Critical Access Hospitals

The Critical Access Hospital Program was created by the 1997 federal Balanced Budget Act as a safety net to ensure that Medicare beneficiaries have access to healthcare services in rural areas. It was designed to allow more flexible staffing options relative to community need, simplify billing methods, and create incentives to develop local integrated health delivery systems, including acute, primary, emergency, and long-term care (Washington State Department of Health, 2009).

Casey, Moscovice, and Klingner (2004) conducted a national survey of 474 critical access hospitals (CAHs) to identify their top patient safety priorities and their familiarity with and implementation of The Joint Commission NPSGs, limitations and supports for implementation of safety interventions, and efforts directed at medication safety. The results indicated that medication safety and prevention of patient falls were the most frequent categories of CAH safety initiatives. Sixty-three percent were familiar with The Joint Commission NPSGs, and 55–88% had implemented strategies to achieve the goals. At least 50% of the CAHs reported limitations of financial, staff, and technological resources. Sixty-three percent had a pharmacist on site for less than 40 hours per week, and half used software to aid with medication dosing.

The authors concluded that CAHs are implementing some patient safety activities and are aware of national goals; however, more than half report severe limitations to full implementation, and pharmacy/medication safety efforts are still lacking (Casey et al., 2004). The Joint Commission began accrediting CAHs in 2001. As of December 2012, there were 1,330 CAHs in the United States (The Joint Commission, 2013c). The benefits of CAH accreditation are listed in Table 7-2.

Table 7-2   Benefits of Critical Access Hospital Accreditation

Organizes and strengthens patient safety efforts

Strengthens community confidence in the quality and safety of care, treatment, and services

Provides a competitive edge in the marketplace

Improves risk management and risk reduction

May reduce liability insurance costs

Provides education to improve business operations

Provides professional advice and counsel

Provides a customized, intensive review

Enhances staff recruitment and development

Provides deeming authority for Medicare certification

Recognized by insurers and other third parties

Provides a framework for organizational structure and management

May fulfill regulatory requirements in some states

Provides quality improvement tools for accredited organizations

Source: The Joint Commission, Facts about Critical Access Hospital Accreditation, http://www.joint-commission.org/assets/1/6/Facts_about_Critical_Access_Hospital_Accreditation.pdf

Public Quality Reporting Systems

Since the 2000 IOM report about medical errors, there have been considerable attempts to hold healthcare providers accountable for the quality of care. To accomplish this, an abundance of national policies, performance measurement tools, and public and private reporting mechanisms have been put into place. The effort to hold healthcare providers accountable has come in response to lagging performance, mounting healthcare costs, and misaligned reimbursement systems (Kurtzman & Jennings, 2008).

Hospital Consumer Assessment of Healthcare Providers and Systems

The Centers for Medicare and Medicaid Services (CMS) partnered with AHRQ to develop the Hospital Consumer Assessment of Healthcare Providers and Systems (HCAHPS). Data submitted to the HCAHPS data warehouse are analyzed by CMS, which then calculates the hospital HCAHPS scores and publically reports them on the Hospital Compare website (Medicare, 2014). In 2013, the HCAHPS scores were one of 13 measures used by CMS to calculate $850 million in payments from its Hospital Value-Based Purchasing Program. Inpatient hospitals will see a 1% reduction in their Medicare payments, which will be used to fund incentives that must be earned back by hospitals on the basis of their quality of care (Kennedy, Craig, Wetsel, Reimels, & Wright, 2013).

The HCAHPS survey is a standardized instrument and methodology that was developed in 2006 to measure patients' perspectives of hospital care. This provides a national standard for collecting and reporting information to the public that allows valid comparisons of hospitals to enhance consumer decision making. Table 7-3 lists the HCAHPS goals for the survey.

The HCAHPS survey contains 27 items and is available in five languages. It is designed to take respondents an average of 7 minutes to complete. The survey contains 18 patient

Table 7-3   HCAHPS Survey Goals

HCAHPS has three broad survey goals:

1. The survey will produce comparable data on patients' perspectives of care to allow objective comparisons among hospitals on topics that are important to consumers.

2. Public reporting of the survey results is designed to create incentives for hospitals to improve quality of care.

3. Public reporting serves to enhance public accountability in health care by increasing transparency.

perspectives on care in 8 key topics: communication with doctors; communication with nurses; responsiveness of hospital staff; pain management; communication about medicines; discharge information; cleanliness of the hospital environment; and quietness of the hospital environment. It also includes four screener questions and five demographic items.

Centers for Medicare and Medicaid Services

Hospital Compare

In 2005, Hospital Compare was started through a combined effort with CMS, the American Hospital Association, the American Association of Medical Colleges, and the Federation of American Hospitals. To date, it is one of the largest volunteer hospital public reporting systems for short-term acute-care hospitals. Hospital Compare is a consumer-based website that provides information about how well hospitals provide recommended care to patients who experienced congestive heart failure, heart attack, pneumonia, or surgery. In 2008, data from the HCAHPS survey was added to provide

a standardized method for measuring patient perspectives on their hospital care (Centers for Medicare and Medicaid Services, 2009). Approximately 90% of the facilities that report their scores are acute-care hospitals, and the remaining 10% are CAHs (Laschober, Maxfield, Felt-Lisk, & Miranda, 2007). All CAHPS surveys can be found online at the Agency for Healthcare Research and Quality (AHRQ, 2014). .

CMS Reporting Hospital Quality Data for Annual Payment Update

CMS collects 30 quality measures as part of its Reporting Hospital Quality Data for Annual Payment Update program. This program requires hospitals to submit data for specific quality measures for health conditions that are common among people with Medicare and that typically result in hospitalization. The initiative is designed to furnish consumers with quality of care information so they can make more informed decisions about their health care. It is also designed to encourage clinicians and hospitals to improve the quality of inpatient care provided to all patients. Hospitals that do not participate in the Reporting Hospital Quality Data for Annual Payment Update initiative or that do not meet the reporting requirements are subject to a 2% reduction in their Medicare Annual Payment Update for the upcoming fiscal year (U.S. Department of Health and Human Services & Centers for Medicare and Medicaid Services, 2008).

Preventable Complications

CMS is now withholding payment for preventable complications of care (Pronovost, Goeschel, & Wachter, 2008). The preventable complications include those that are nurse sensitive and hospital acquired, including pressure ulcers, falls with injuries, and nosocomial infections. For example, nursing homes will no longer receive insurance reimbursement from Medicare for treatment provided to patients with hospital-acquired (iatrogenic) stage 3 pressure ulcers. A community-acquired pressure ulcer that a patient comes into the hospital with, which is not documented on admission or within the time frame required by hospital policy, is considered iatrogenic. Nurses must assess the patient's skin with the same attention as the patient's respiratory and cardiac status. This new Medicare standard essentially mandates that registered nurses who admit patients conduct a thorough skin assessment and document it appropriately. After the initial skin assessment is completed by the registered nurse, it is incumbent on the physician to order appropriate treatments specific to the pressure ulcer stage and thus reduce the risk of advancement of a stage 1 pressure ulcer to stage 3. Although pressure ulcers are widely viewed as a result of poor nursing care, the collaborative effort of the multidisciplinary healthcare team, or lack thereof, is responsible for the patient.

The Joint Commission Quality Check

In 1996, The Joint Commission launched a directory of commission-accredited organizations and performance reports titled Quality Check. This all-inclusive guide includes performance results on measures for common treatment areas, accreditation decisions, compliance with NPSGs, and Magnet status. In 2007, Quality Check was expanded to include organizations that are not accredited by The Joint Commission (Kurtzman & Jennings, 2008).

Hospital Rating Systems

Healthgrades

Healthgrades, founded in 1999, is a private healthcare rating organization that is publically traded on NASDAQ. They provide profiles and independent ratings of hospitals and nursing homes to physicians, consumers, corporations, and insurance companies (Healthgrades, 2009a). In their annual reports, Healthgrades identifies the top 5% of hospitals in terms of mortality and complication rates across 26 procedures and diagnoses. These top hospitals receive the designation of Distinguished Hospitals for Clinical Excellence. In 2009, a study of Medicare patients found that 152,666 lives may have been saved and 11,772 major complications may have been avoided during the 3 years studied had the quality of care at all hospitals matched the level of those in the top 5% (Healthgrades, 2009b).

America's Best Hospitals

In 1990, *U.S. News & World Report* magazine initiated an annual appraisal of U.S. hospitals. Patients who truly need outstanding care are the target of the magazine's annual Best Hospitals rankings. Hospitals are judged not on routine procedures but on difficult cases across 16 specialties. Twelve of the 16 specialty rankings are driven largely by hard data; the other 4 rankings are based on 3 years of nominations by specialists. To be considered for the 12 data-driven specialties, a hospital had to meet at least one of three requirements: membership in the Council of Teaching Hospitals, affiliation with a medical school, or availability of at least 6 of 13 key technologies, such as robotic surgery. In 2008, nearly two-thirds of all hospitals failed the first test, and only 170 of 5,453 hospitals scored high enough to appear in any of the specialty rankings (Camarow, 2008).

Conclusion

This chapter has focused on the tremendous impact the seven primary IOM studies have had on quality efforts to reduce errors in health care. These studies include the following:

- *The Future of Nursing*
- *Preventing Medication Errors*
- *Patient Safety: Achieving a New Standard for Care*

Table 7-4   Red Flag Alerts for Patient Safety

Healthcare practitioners must be educated and alerted to red flags in their care of patients. When a red flag is identified, appropriate action should be taken to remedy the situation. Specific red flags include the following:

- Poor treatment results
- A lack of follow-up care
- Repetitious problems
- Equipment malfunctioning
- Dissatisfied patients or family members
- Poor staff–patient relations
- Intimidated patients
- Poorly maintained medical records
- A lack of policies or procedures
- Excessive volume of patients
- Acting outside the scope of practice
- Personality conflicts
- Performance of a procedure without needed supervision

Source: Data from Kavaler & Spiegel (2003).

- *Keeping Patients Safe: Transforming the Work Environment of Nurses*
- *Health Professions Education: A Bridge to Quality*
- *Crossing the Quality Chasm: A New Healthcare System for the 21st Century*
- *To Err Is Human: Building a Safer Health System*

Theories of error and error management were explored, along with numerous national healthcare initiatives and mandates. Healthcare providers must be committed to developing a culture of safety in which errors are accepted as inevitable, but members of the healthcare team are ever vigilant and committed to the prevention of error. This new culture of safety includes support and counseling for those who make mistakes, and open communication of errors and safety issues (Ttable 7-4).

Case Study

Patient Risk Assessment Tools
Helen Werner

Patient Falls: Morse Fall Scale

Fall incidence and subsequent injuries are of great importance as nursing quality indicators. The Morse Fall Scale is not always an accurate assessment of fall risk, according to the guidelines developed by Morse (2009); therefore, the predictive value is indeterminate. A study conducted in Australia by McFarlane-Kolb (2004) found that the Morse Fall Scale, in combination with other risk factors, more accurately reflected fall risk among older persons admitted to an acute surgical unit. Major tranquilizer use and male gender were the most significant predictors of fall risk in this population. The Morse Fall Scale can easily be modified to include additional risk factors that are more accurate predictors of fall risk for the indigenous population. This is important in terms of guidelines that are developed by the hospital, which may be formulated based on the calculated fall risk that may be inaccurate for the population being served. If a patient is identified to be at risk for falls, a more in-depth assessment is needed to determine the causative factors, especially those that are treatable.

Several fall-risk assessment tools were evaluated for validity by Ang, Mordiffi, Wong, Devi, and Evans (2007). The Morse Fall Scale, the St. Thomas Risk Assessment Tool in Falling Elderly Inpatients, and the Heindrich II Fall Risk Model were all validated for interrater reliability and validity studies; however, only the Heindrich II Fall Risk Model had a higher level of specificity (61.5%) than the Morse Fall Scale (48.3%). The Morse Fall Scale is the gold standard for fall-risk assessment in the United States; however, if nurses demonstrate difficulty scoring a patient's fall risk accurately, it may be necessary to consider piloting the use of another scale that may be more user friendly.

Patient Skin Assessment Tools

It is not uncommon for clinicians to shorten or modify risk assessments, like the Braden Scale, according to Braden and Maklebust (2005). This reduces the likelihood that a skin assessment will be predictive of pressure ulcer development during a hospitalization. The explanation is rather simple. The complete tool was tested for validity and reliability. Even minor changes can impact the accuracy of the scale. Research has been conducted by Bergquist (2001) testing modified Braden Scales and subsets to determine the extent of accuracy for predicting patients at greater risk of developing pressure ulcers. Bergquist found that the summative score, rather than any subset of the Braden Scale, was most predictive of pressure ulcer risk for older persons receiving home health care; however, researchers in China (Kwong et al., 2005) found a modified

Braden Scale more predictive for pressure ulcer development, with the addition of skin and body build for height and the exclusion of nutrition, which was a surprising finding. One explanation offered by the researchers was that the focus of oral intake and protein only does not accurately represent patients' nutritional status. It may also be necessary to explore modifications of the Braden Scale based on cultural differences.

Assessment tools such as the Braden Scale may not be as accurate as nurses' judgment. A study conducted by Lewicki, Mion, and Secic (2000) for cardiac surgery patients found that the sensitivity of the Braden Scale was 40% and its specificity was 70%, compared with nurses' judgment, which was found to have a sensitivity of 49% and a specificity of 73%. Additionally, the researchers suggested that the cutoff score, which has been 16 or less, is more applicable to long-term care than acute care and may need to vary for each postoperative day.

The NDNQI accepts data from hospitals that use other skin assessment scales. Data from the Norton Scale are also acceptable and, in fact, are noted on the data collection tool that the designated NDNQI site coordinator must use to enter data. Unfortunately, there is no way to determine whether the calculated score using the Braden Scale/Norton Scale published on the NDNQI website for the participating hospitals is based on use of the complete Braden Scale/Norton Scale or a modified version that had been previously tested for validity and reliability. The accuracy of these data is of great importance to the participating hospitals so individual units can compare themselves with similar types of participating NDNQI units across the country. The collection and entry of data for quality improvement as a participating hospital in NDNQI is deemed necessary to attain Magnet certification.

Discussion Questions

1. Identify a common error in healthcare delivery and work through Reason's Swiss Cheese Model, identifying how the holes can occur and what layers of protection should stop the error from getting to the patient.
2. How has the code of silence changed over the past few years? Is it more or less prevalent? Why?
3. What impact will the 2014 Hospital national patient safety goals have on hospital care? How will they affect reimbursement?
4. Discuss how public reporting of the HCAHPS survey will create incentives for hospitals to improve quality of care.

Case Study References

Ang, N. K. E., Mordiffi, S. Z., Wong, H. B., Devi, K., & Evans, D. (2007). Evaluation of three fall-risk assessment tools in an acute care setting. *Journal of Advanced Nursing, 60*(4), 427–435.

Bergquist, S. (2001). Subscales, subscores, or summative score: Evaluating the contribution of Braden Scale items for predicting pressure ulcer risk in older adults receiving home health care. *Journal of Wound, Ostomy and Continence Nurses Society, 28*, 279–289.

Braden, B., & Maklebust, J. (2005). Preventing pressure ulcers with the Braden Scale. *American Journal of Nursing*, 105(6), 70–72.

Kwong, E., Pang, S., Wong, T., Ho, J., Shao-ling, X., & Li-Jun, T. (2005). Predicting pressure ulcer risk with the modified Braden, Braden, and Norton Scales in acute care hospitals in mainland China. *Applied Nursing Research, 18*, 122–128.

Lewicki, L. J., Mion, L. C., & Secic, M. (2000). Sensitivity and specificity of the Braden Scale in the cardiac surgical population. *Journal of Wound, Ostomy and Continence Nurses Society, 27*, 36–41.

McFarlane-Kolb, H. (2004). Falls risk assessment, multitargeted interventions and the impact on hospital falls. *International Journal of Nursing Practice, 10*, 199–206.

Morse, J. M. (2009). *Preventing patient falls* (2nd ed.). New York, NY: Springer.

References

Agency for Healthcare Research and Quality. (2002). *Improving health care quality. Fact sheet* (Agency for Healthcare Research and Quality Publication Number 02-P032, September, 2002. ed., Vol. 2003). Rockville, MD: Author.

Agency for Healthcare Research and Quality. (2005). *30 safe practices for better health care* (Agency for Healthcare Research and Quality Publication No. 05-P007). Retrieved from http://www.ahrq.gov/research/findings/factsheets/errors-safety/30safe/index.html

Agency for Healthcare Research and Quality. (2013a). *Guide to patient and family engagement in hospital quality and safety*. Retrieved from http://www.ahrq.gov/professionals/systems/hospital/engagingfamilies/index.html

Agency for Healthcare Research and Quality. (2013b). *National patient safety goals*. Retrieved from http://psnet.ahrq.gov/resource.aspx?resourceID=2230 Agency for Healthcare Research and Quality. (2014). *CAHPS surveys and tools to advance patient-centered care*. Retrieved from https://cahps.ahrq.gov/

American Nurses Association. (2009). *Nursing sensitive indicators*. Retrieved from http://www.nursing-world.org/MainMenuCategories/ThePracticeof-ProfessionalNursing/PatientSafetyQuality

/Research-Measurement/The-National-Database /Nursing-Sensitive-Indicators_1

Bipartisan Policy Center. (2013). *A bipartisan Rx for patient-centered care and system-wide cost containment.* Retrieved from http://bipartisan-policy.org/library/report /health-care-cost-containment

Byers, J. F., & White, S. V. (2004). *Patient safety: Principles and practice.* New York, NY: Springer.

California Academy of Family Physicians. (2002). *Diagnosing and treating medical errors in family practice.* Retrieved from www.familydocs.org /positions.html

Camarow, A. (2008). A look inside the hospital rankings: How 170 out of 5,453 centers made the cut. *U.S. News & World Report.* Retrieved from http://health.usnews.com/articles/health /best-hospitals/2008/07/10/a-look-inside-the-hospital-rankings.html

Casey, M., Moscovice, I., & Klingner, J. (2004). *Quality improvement activities in critical access hospitals: Results of the 2004 National CAH survey* (Briefing Paper No. 2). Minneapolis, MN: Flex Monitoring Team. Retrieved from http://www.flexmonitoring.org/publications/bp2/

Centers for Medicare and Medicaid Services. (2009). *Hospital compare.* Retrieved from http://www.medicare.gov/hospitalcompare/About /What-Is-HOS.html

Clancy, C. M., Farquhar, M. B., & Collins Sharp, B. A. (2005). Patient safety in nursing practice. *Journal of Nursing Care Quality 20*(3), 193–197.

Dorschner, J. (2003, May 6). Study finds healthcare error prone. *The Miami Herald.* Retrieved from http://www.highbeam.com /doc/1G1-101283308.html

DuPree, E., Anderson, R., & Nash, I. S. (2011). Improving quality in healthcare: Start with the patient. *Mount Sinai Journal of Medicine, 78,* 813–819.

Ebright, P., Urder, L., Patterson, E., & Chalko, B. (2004). Themes surrounding novice nurse near-miss and adverse-event situations. *Journal of Nursing Administration, 34*(11), 531–538.

Healthgrades. (2005). *Healthgrades second annual patient safety in American hospitals report.*

Retrieved from http://hg-article-center.s3-web-site-us-east-1.amazonaws.com/a6/43 /b94f277e492d9a416af1d51b487d/PatientSafe-tyInAmericanHospitalsReport2005.pdf

Healthgrades. (2009a). *About us.* Retrieved from http://www.healthgrades.com/about-us

Healthgrades. (2009b). *Top hospitals have 27% lower mortality: Annual Healthgrades study.* Retrieved from http://health.usnews.com /health-news/managing-your-healthcare /treatment/articles/2009/01/27/americas-top-hospitals-cut-patient-death-rate-27

Healthgrades. (2013). *American hospital quality outcomes 2014: Healthgrades report to the nation: Executive summary.* Retrieved from https://d2dc-gio3q2u5fb.cloudfront.net/56/90/e07df9f64a5 fb741ab59924a9e0d/2013-american-hospital-quality-outcomes-2014-healthgrades-report-to-the-nation.pdf

Helmreich, R. L. (2000). On error management: Lessons from aviation. *British Medical Journal, 320,* 781–785.

Hill, C. D. (2005). *SPEAK UP: New national campaign offers Americans tips to prevent medication mistakes.* Retrieved from http://www.jcaho.org

Institute for Healthcare Improvement. (2013). *The IHI Triple Aim.* Retrieved from http://www.ihi.org/offerings/Initiatives/TripleAim/Pages /default.aspx

Joint Commission on Accreditation of Healthcare Organizations. (2003). Special report! 2003 JCAHO national patient safety goals: Practical strategies and helpful solutions for meeting these goals. *Joint Commission Perspectives on Patient Safety, 3*(1). Retrieved from http://www.teacherweb.com/ NY/StBarnabas/Law-PublicPolicy/JCAHO-2003.pdf

Kavaler, F., & Spiegel, A. D. (2003). *Risk management in health care institutions: A strategic approach* (2nd ed.). Sudbury, MA: Jones And Bartlett.

Kennedy, B., Craig, J. B., Wetsel, M., Reimels, E., & Wright, J. (2013). Three nursing interventions' impact on HCAHPS scores. *Journal of Nursing Care Quality, 28*(4), 327–334.

Kohn, L. T., Corrigan, J. M., & Donaldson, M. S. (Eds.). (2000). *To err is human: Building a safer health system*. Washington, DC: National Academy Press.

Kuehn, B. M. (2012). *A push for comparative effectiveness: US initiatives aim to empower patients, physicians*. Retrieved from http://jama.jamanetwork.com/data/Journals/JAMA/23306/jmn0418_1570_1571.pdf%3FresultClick%3D1&rct=j&frm=1&q=&esrc=s&sa=U&ei=PhyaU7fhDai68AHKjIFg&ved=0CCQQFjAE&sig2=8E3pcUHEs9FsgG16mNVx7A&usg=AFQjCNGozwDwR3bY8xv8qWImCPKtYGnHig

Kurtzman, E. T., & Jennings, B. M. (2008). Trends in transparency: Nursing performance measurement and reporting. *Journal of Nursing Administration*, *38*(7/8), 349–354.

Landro, L. (2002, August 29). Deadly errors dog procedures at doctors' offices and clinics. *The Wall Street Journal*, p. D3.

Largent, E. (2011). Comparative effectiveness research: What effects for nurses? *Dimensions of Critical Care Nursing*, *30*(1), 19–24.

Laschober, M., Maxfield, M., Felt-Lisk, S., & Miranda, D. J. (2007). Hospital response to public reporting of quality indicators. *Health Care Financing Review*, *28*(3), 61–76.

Liang, B. A. (2001). The adverse event of unaddressed medical error: Identifying and filling the holes in the health-care and legal systems. *Journal of Law and Medical Ethics*, *29*(3/4), 346–368.

Mathews, C. (2013, January). *Healthcare's triple aim: How technology is facilitating collaboration among members, providers and payers*. Retrieved from http://www.healthmgttech.com/articles/201301/healthcares-triple-aim.php

Medicare. (2014). *Hospital compare*. Retrieved from http://www.medicare.gov/hospitalcompare/search.html?AspxAutoDetectCookieSupport=1

Monk, J. (2002, June 16). Medical mistakes kept secret. *The State*, pp. A1, A6–A7.

Nordenberg, T. (2000, September/October). Make no mistake: Medical errors can be deadly serious. *FDA Consumer Magazine*. Retrieved from https://groups.yahoo.com/neo/groups/csen-anesthesia-mailing-list/conversations/messages/6087

Nurse.com (2012). *Statement urges accountability for patient safety*. Retrieved from http://news.nurse.com/article/20121017/NATIONAL02/110290006

Pronovost, P. J., Goeschel, C. A., & Wachter, R. M. (2008). The wisdom and justice of not paying for preventable complications. *The New England Journal of Medicine*, *299*(18), 2197–2199.

Reason, J. (2000). Human error: Models and management. *British Medical Journal*, *320*, 768–770.

Rivers, R. M., Swain, D., & Nixon, W. R. (2003). Using aviation safety measures to enhance patient outcomes. *Association of Operating Room Nurses Journal*, *77*, 158–162.

Simpson, K. R. (2004). Failure to rescue: Implications for evaluating quality of care during labor and birth. *Journal of Perinatal Neonatal Nursing*, *19*(1), 24–34.

Sorry Works! (2013). *Sorry Works! History*. Retrieved from http://sorryworkssite.bondwaresite.com/history-cms-29

Spath, P. L. (Ed.). (1999). *Error reduction in health care: A systems approach to improving patient safety*. San Francisco, CA: Jossey-Bass.

The Joint Commission. (2013a). *2012 national patient safety goals*. Retrieved from http://www.jointcommission.org/mobile/standards_information/national_patient_safety_goals

The Joint Commission. (2013b). *2014 hospital national patient safety goals*. Retrieved from http://www.jointcommission.org/assets/1/6/2014_HAP_NPSG_E.pdf

The Joint Commission. (2013c). *Facts about critical access hospital accreditation*. Retrieved from http://www.jointcommission.org/assets/1/6/Facts_about_Critical_Access_Hospital_Accreditation.pdf

Thomas, E. J., & Petersen, L. A. (2003). Measuring errors and adverse events in health care. *Journal of General Internal Medicine*, *18*(1), 61–67.

U.S. Department of Health and Human Services & Centers for Medicare and Medicaid Services. (2008). *Fact sheet: CMS updates the national hospital quality measure acute myocardial infarction set for discharges as of April 1, 2009.* Retrieved from https://www.cms.gov/Medicare/Quality-Initiatives-Patient-Assessment-Instruments/HospitalQualityInits/downloads/HospitalAMI-6FactSheet.pdf

Wachter, R. M., & Shojania, K. G. (2004). *Internal bleeding: The truth behind America's terrifying epidemic of medical mistakes* (1st ed.). New York, NY: Rugged Land.

Washington State Department of Health. (2009). *Rural health programs: What is a critical access hospital?* Retrieved from http://www.doh.wa.gov/ForPublicHealthandHealthcareProviders/RuralHealth/HealthcareFacilityResources/CriticalAccessHospitals.aspx

Weinberg, J. K. (2002). Medical error and patient safety: Understanding cultures in conflict. *Law & Policy, 24*(2), 93–113.

Williams, I. E. (2004). *First, do no harm: The cure for medical malpractice.* Mount Pleasant, SC: Corinthian Books.

Wojcieszak, D., Banja, J., & Houk, C. (2006). Forum: The Sorry Works! coalition: Making the case for full disclosure. *Joint Commission Journal on Quality and Patient Safety, 32*(6), 344–350.

Woods, A., & Doan-Johnson, S. (2002). Executive summary: Toward a taxonomy of nursing practice errors. *Nursing Management, 33*(10), 45–48.

Global Health: Past Progress, Future Directions

CHAPTER 8

Global Health: Policy, Politics, and Partners

Franklin Shaffer, Carol Tuttas, and Janice Phillips

Overview

Global health issues and priorities are increasingly being addressed by a number of entities and stakeholders worldwide. Stakeholders include, but are not limited to, the World Health Organization (WHO), the United Nations, governmental and nongovernmental agencies, private philanthropists, health professionals, and concerned citizens worldwide, to name a few. While progress has been made in alleviating the global burden of disease, much remains to be done. The authors of this chapter provide a beginning overview of a number of issues on the global health agenda and identify the critical role of policy, politics, and partners in addressing these issues and priorities. An interdisciplinary team approach, coupled with a working knowledge of the sociocultural, political, economic, and environmental factors influencing global health, is essential to effectively address a rapidly evolving global health agenda.

The WHO, the leading authority on global health issues, provides a comprehensive overview of the health profile of countries worldwide. It publishes *The World Health Statistics*, a comprehensive report on global public health in 194 countries. This information is derived from numerous databases from a number of entities, such as the World Bank, the United Nations, and the International Telecommunication Union (World Health Organization [WHO], 2013e). The following information provides a brief snapshot of the voluminous amount of data that is used to shape and evaluate the global health agenda:

- Approximately 800 women die each day secondary to complications of pregnancy and childbirth.

- When compared to children in high-income countries, children in low-income countries are 16 times more likely to die before age 5.

- China is now a front-runner in life expectancy at birth and enjoys a higher life expectancy than 7 out of 10 eastern European countries (WHO, 2013e).

Worldwide, a number of entities and stakeholders are advancing the global health agenda. A concerted, sustained, and interdisciplinary approach is critical to alleviating the well-documented global burden of disease. The authors of this chapter provide a beginning overview of this burden while highlighting the interconnectivity of policy, politics, and partners in achieving better health for all. The chapter concludes with discussion questions and a case study to illustrate the interconnectivity between health policy and potential health outcomes.

Objectives

- Articulate the urgent need to achieve the United Nations's 2013 Millennium Development Goals.
- Highlight three factors that influence the adequacy of a global nursing workforce.
- Describe potential barriers to the worldwide adoption of advanced technology.

Longevity and Leading Causes of Death Worldwide

Worldwide, chronic diseases and noncommunicable diseases (NCDs) have become the leading causes of death. These NCDs—including diabetes, cancer, and cardiovascular and chronic lung diseases—account for approximately two-thirds of all deaths worldwide. In 2000, NCDs were responsible for 60% of deaths worldwide (WHO, 2013c).

In 2011, the 10 leading causes of death in the world were as follows: (1) ischemic heart disease; (2) stroke; (3) lower respiratory infections; (4) chronic obstructive pulmonary disease (COPD); (5) diarrheal diseases; (6) HIV/AIDS; (7) tracheal, bronchial, and lung disease; (8) diabetes mellitus; (9) road injuries; and (10) prematurity. Notably, tuberculosis (TB) is no longer among the top 10 leading causes of death; it is now among the 15 leading causes of death, and it killed 1 million people in 2011 (WHO, 2013c). Cardiovascular diseases alone

killed approximately 17 million people worldwide (WHO, 2013e). Not surprisingly, the leading causes of death vary according to the socioeconomic status of the respective country, as does the average life span. High-income countries experienced the highest proportion of NCD deaths (87%), followed by upper-middle-income countries (81%), lower-middle-income countries (56%), and low-income countries (36%).

In high-income countries, 7 of every 10 deaths occur among people aged 70 years and older, and they typically die from chronic conditions. In low-income countries, 4 of every 10 deaths occur among children aged 15 years and younger, and only 2 in every 10 deaths occur among those aged 70 years and older. Infectious diseases, such as lower respiratory infections, HIV/AIDS, diarrheal diseases, malaria, and TB, account for one-third of deaths in low-income countries. Deaths among newborns and infants are widely attributed to prematurity, asphyxia, and birth trauma (WHO, 2013c).

Notably, in 2011, the overall global life expectancy at birth was 70 years. High-income countries experienced the highest life expectancy at birth, 80 years, and low-income countries experienced the lowest life expectancy at birth, 60 years (WHO, 2013b).

Whereas high-income countries have a better capability to record and measure the leading causes of death, other countries, particularly low-income countries, often lack this capability. The subsequent underreporting of the leading causes of death and other pertinent health information often provides an incomplete picture of the country's overall health and well-being. Nonetheless, measuring the cause of death in various countries is an essential tool for assessing the overall health and well-being of populations and evaluating the effectiveness of a country's healthcare delivery system.

Millennium Development Goals

Any discussions about global health would be incomplete without mention of the Millennium Development Goals (MDGs), which are the United Nations's eight development goals to achieve improvements in the health and well-being of all countries by 2015. These goals were established by 189 United Nations members following the Millennium Summit in 2000 and are included in the United Nations Millennium Declaration (United Nations, 2013). The goals are as follows:

1. Eradicate extreme poverty and hunger.
2. Achieve universal primary education.
3. Promote gender equality and empower women.
4. Reduce child mortality rates.
5. Improve maternal health.

6. Combat HIV/AIDS, malaria, and other diseases.
7. Ensure environmental sustainability.
8. Develop a global partnership for development.

While much has been done to alleviate malaria and tuberculosis and improve water sources and primary education, much more is needed to fully address this agenda. Indeed, progress toward achieving the goals has been substantial in some areas of the world and less than hoped for in other areas (Fehling, Nelson, & Venkatapuram, 2013; United Nations, 2013). Table 8-1 provides a brief synopsis of current progress in achieving the MDGs by 2015.

There is no doubt that a concerted and sustained action on all fronts by current and potential stakeholders is imperative for continued and sustainable progress if the MDGs are to be met by 2015. Intense and focused efforts are sorely needed in the areas of sanitation, hunger, maternal health, and environmental protection. United Nations Secretary-General Ban Ki-moon is hopeful that accelerated efforts and outcomes will provide the impetus and momentum for framing a 2015 postdevelopment agenda (United Nations, 2013).

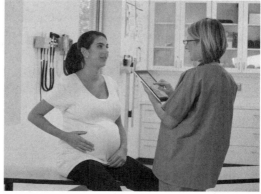

© Blend_Images/iStockphoto.com

Table 8-1   Progress toward Achieving the 2015 Millennium Development Goals

Target	Current Status	Future Directions
Eradicate extreme poverty and hunger.	• In developing areas, the poverty rate fell from 47% in 1990 to 22% in 2010. • Approximately 700 million fewer people lived in extreme poverty in 2010 than in 1990. • The % of global population using these sources is up from 76% in 1990 to 89% in 2010. • Hunger reduction is near target; decreased from 23.2% in 1990-1992 to 14.9% between 2010 and 2012.	• 1 in 8 people remain undernourished despite progress. • More than 100 million children remain undernourished; 1 in 4 show signs of stunted growth worldwide. • Poverty rates halved, but 1.2 billion still live in extreme poverty.
Achieve universal primary education.	• Progress in this area remains slow. • Between 2000 and 2011, the number of children out of school declined from 102 million to 57 million. • Worldwide, 123 million youth (15-25) lack basic reading and writing skills; majority young women.	• Poorest children remain more likely to be out of school. • Slow progress makes the goal of primary education unlikely by 2015.
Promote gender equality and empower women	• Women continually denied decision-making power. • Gender parity most likely to be achieved at the primary level; 2 out of 130 countries have achieved the educational targets. • 40 out of 1,000 wage earning jobs in non-agricultural sector are occupied by women.	• Steady progress regarding equal access to education, but more targeted approaches are needed in many regions.
Reduce child mortality rates by 2/3 between 1990 and 2015	• Global increases in child survival notable; 41 % reduction from 87 deaths per 1,000 live births in 1990 to 51 in 2011.	• Bolder action and redoubled efforts needed to reach targeted goal 2/3 reductions in child deaths and increased deaths during the first month of life in poor regions.
Improve maternal health	• Global reductions by 47%—400 maternal deaths/100, 00 live births to 201 between 1990 and 2010.	• Accelerated political backing needed to reach target of 3/4 reductions.

	• Only half of pregnant women receive the minimum number of 4 prenatal visits.	• Maternal deaths are preventable, and progress is limited.
Combat HIV/ AIDS, malaria, and other diseases	• Improved gains in eliminating malaria/ TB. • 25% reduction in malaria rates globally, averting 1.1 million deaths between 2000 and 2010. • Reductions in TB deaths likely to be halved by 2015 globally. • Successful treatment of 51 million patients with TB, saving 20 million lives. • In 2011, 230,000 fewer children under age 15 were infected with HIV than in 2001.	• Continued lack of knowledge about HIV transmission and prevention among young people. • Achieving universal access to antiretroviral drugs lags behind but may be reachable by 2015. • Universal access to antiretroviral treatment within reach, but sustained political action is critical.
Ensure environmental sustainability	• Environmental sustainability requires bolder action. • Global emissions of carbon dioxide increasing, with higher emissions up 46% compared with 1990 levels. • Birds, mammals, and many other species are rapidly approaching extinction. • More than 2.1 billion and 1.9 billion people have improved water and sanitation sources, respectively. • Decreased proportion of urban slum dwellers in cities and metropolises in developing world.	• Gains in sanitation are good but not good enough. • Rapid progress is needed to meet sanitation goals by 2015. • Deforestation remains a major threat to environmental sustainability. • The number of slum dwellers continues to grow, although the MDG slum target has been met. Stronger, more focused efforts are needed.
Develop a global partnership for development	• Development assistance at a standstill in 2012 at 126 billion = a 4% drop in real terms in 2011, affecting the least developed countries proportionately. • Aid is increasingly addressing gender issues, enhancing gender equality and women's empowerment. • 31% of the population in the developing world has internet access compared with 77% of the population in the developed world.	• Aid money continues to decline, especially for the poorest countries. • Continued efforts are needed to address the global financial issues and ensure official development assistance.

Source: Data from United Nations (2013). *The Millennium Development Goals.* New York, NY: Author.

Partners for Continued Progress

Advancements in global health have been facilitated by substantial contributions and support from a number of global health donors, organizations, institutions, and philanthropists. There are too many to mention, but Table 8-2 provides a short list of critical partners who are actively engaged in advancing global health. A new stream of financial resources, and even new partnerships, will be needed to meet the goals, especially in light of the recent declines in funding that disproportionately affect poorer countries.

Professionals across Borders

According to a recent report titled *The Universal Truth: No Health Without a Workforce*, "Acting on human resources for health is now in the hands of governments and all interested stakeholders. Political and technical leadership is critical to seize the opportunity to attain, sustain and accelerate progress on universal health coverage by transformative action on human

Table 8-2   Select Leaders/Partners in Advancing the Global Health Agenda and Related Priorities

The World Health Organization	http://www.who.int/en/
The United Nations Foundation	http://www.unfoundation.org/
UNICEF	http://www.unicef.org/
The World Bank	http://www.worldbank.org/
The US Government	http://www.globalhealth.gov/ global-programs-and-initiatives/ global-health-initiative/
The Centers for Disease Control and Prevention	http://www.cdc.gov/globalhealth/ghi/
United States Agency for International Development (USAID)	http://www.usaid.gov/
Bill and Melinda Gates Foundation	http://www.gatesfoundation.org/
The Clinton Foundation	http://www.clintonfoundation.org/
The Rockefeller Foundation	http://www.rockefellerfoundation.org/
Pfizer Pharmaceuticals	http://www.pfizer.com/responsibility/ global_health/global_health
Merck & Company	http://www.merck.com/index.html
International Council on Nursing	http://www.icn.ch
European Federation of Nurses Association	http://www.efn.be/
International Labour Organization	www.ilo.org
Global Workforce Alliance	www.who.int/workforcealliance/

resources for health" (Global Health Workforce Alliance [GHWA] & WHO, 2013). The report highlights the problems associated with some significant shortages of healthcare personnel:

- Eighty-three countries fall below the threshold of 22.8 skilled health professionals per 10,000 population.

- One hundred countries fall below the threshold of 34.5 skilled health professionals per 10,000 population.

- One hundred eighteen countries fall below the threshold of 59.4 skilled health professionals per 10,000 population.

- Only 68 countries exceed 59.4 skilled health professionals per 10,000 population.

Government political will to ensure the safety and well-being of national populations is evidenced in part through the promotion, development, and support of a well-educated healthcare workforce that can be mobilized within and across borders. Today's healthcare workforce requires preparation to meet acute needs and to implement preventive measures to promote optimal health among culturally diverse client populations that are characteristic of many countries. Policy that underpins such aims exemplifies responsible and cooperative action on the part of governments by protecting health interests of people worldwide.

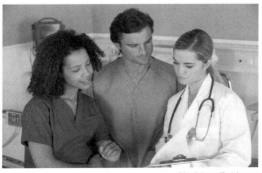

Global Competence of Healthcare Professionals

Since global travel has become a ubiquitous constituent of daily business and social activity, pathogens are not constrained by international borders to the extent that they once were. In recent years, swine flu episodes of epidemic proportions have served as ominous reminders that health and health care do not occur within the confines of national borders and that population health issues in one country boldly command the attention of all countries. It is imperative that the healthcare workforce stay abreast of newly released literature, knowledge, and statistics relative to global health to maintain currency and effectiveness in practice. World health information and statistical updates are made available on a frequent basis from reliable global sources. Some examples that reinforce this concept include the following:

- Two thousand people in the United States were diagnosed with and treated for malaria in 2011, nearly all of whom acquired the disease while abroad; among them were five fatalities (Centers for Disease Control and Prevention [CDC], 2013b).

- China, the country that boasts the world's largest population and was certified in 2000 by the World Health Assembly as a poliomyelitis-free region, experienced an outbreak of the disease in 2011 (Luo et al., 2013). With prompt action to institute robust symptom surveillance among the population and administration of 43 million doses of oral polio vaccine, the outbreak was brought under control within 90 days.

- A 45% drop in deaths from TB between 1990 and 2012 showed promising potential for the achievement of the MDGs to reverse the trend in the spread of TB by 2015. Nonetheless, 8.9 million people became ill with TB worldwide in 2012 (530,000 of them children), resulting in 1.3 million TB deaths (WHO, 2013d).

- The Centers for Disease Control and Prevention (CDC) reported that the global presence of dengue fever has been increasing over recent years due to a number of factors, including climate change (CDC, 2010). In September 2012, one person was diagnosed with dengue fever in Kosrae, one of the Federated States of Micronesia, and by March 2013, 3.7% of those residing in Kosrae had been hospitalized with symptoms of infection with the vector-transmitted virus (CDC, 2013a).

Global Mobility of Healthcare Professionals

Natural disasters—such as earthquakes, typhoons, tsunamis, volcanic eruptions, hurricanes, flooding, mudslides, and tornadoes—in countries across the globe call for a mobile healthcare workforce outfitted with current scientific knowledge combined with corresponding cultural sensitivity to effectively administer care to diverse populations of affected countries. In the most recent report published jointly by the Global Health Workforce Alliance (GHWA) and the WHO, known distribution-related shortages within countries are acknowledged, as is the probability of even more severe distribution challenges among countries (GHWA & WHO, 2013). This misdistribution calls for a competent healthcare workforce that is flexible and motivated to migrate to where they are most needed. From this perspective, it is fitting to collectively refer to professional healthcare workers

from countries around the world as the global healthcare workforce.

Healthcare workers need not leave their native country to be considered part of the global healthcare workforce, due to the progressive increase in migration among the general population worldwide and the corresponding increase in diversity among populations of all countries. Hence, it is essential for today's global healthcare workforce to maintain current knowledge, skills, and mobility to reach, educate, and treat diverse composites of populations worldwide while aiming to prevent outbreaks of diseases once thought to be controlled or eradicated.

Diversity among Global Healthcare Professionals

As general populations in countries around the world evolve toward broader mixes in terms of ethnic and cultural diversity, there is a need for a corresponding increase in diversity among the healthcare workforce in primary, secondary, and tertiary care settings. For decades, countries worldwide have capitalized on the willingness and motivation of healthcare workers to migrate to alleviate shortages. This phenomenon has been well documented, primarily in nurse migration to destination countries such as the United Kingdom, Australia, the United States, and Canada (Alexis, Vydelingum, & Robbins, 2007; Allan, Cowie, & Smith, 2009; Deegan & Simkin, 2010; Smith, Allan, Henry, Larsen, & Mackintosh, 2006).

Although the purpose of recruiting internationally has been to fill vacant nursing positions for which domestic supply was lacking, hiring migrant healthcare workers has yielded other benefits, such as diversifying the workforce, which dovetails with the increasing cultural diversity of the patient population. Promotion of diversity among healthcare workers of all disciplines in countries across the globe facilitates increased sensitivity to patients' cultural needs and practices, enhances communication and innovation in health teaching, and supports conditions that lead to a harmonized workforce and better outcomes (Shaffer, 2014; Spetz, Gates, & Jones, 2014).

Ethical Recruitment of Global Healthcare Professionals

Much has been published about the ethical implications associated with the global migration of healthcare workers (Mackey & Liang, 2012; Pittman, Herrera, Spetz, & Davis, 2012; Plotnikova, 2012). Nonetheless, much remains to be instituted in terms of policies, practice, and surveillance.

The Alliance for Ethical International Recruitment Practices (AEIRP) revised its original voluntary code of ethical conduct document that was published in 2008 to expand beyond a foreign-educated nurse-centered aim to include other foreign-educated healthcare professionals who are being recruited to the United States (Alliance for Ethical International Recruitment Practices, 2011; Chen, Auerbach, Muench, Curry, & Bradley, 2013). Whether the recruiting entity is a third party (i.e., recruitment or staffing agencies) or an employer (i.e., hospital, long-term care organization, etc.), the AEIRP established a number of standards that comprise the ethical implications associated with recruitment behavior. Compliance with laws, such as fair labor standards, civil rights and other anti-discrimination laws, and immigration laws, are examples of legal parameters impacting recruitment behaviors that call for sufficient monitoring. Open and transparent communication

pertaining to the nature of the job and venue of employment are essential to the practice of ethical recruitment. The code provides transitional provisions for recruited foreign healthcare workers and requires that recruiters abstain from seeking healthcare workers from countries in crisis. While subscription to and compliance with the standards documented in the code are voluntary, it is a step in the right direction toward calling out unethical recruitment practices and establishing a monitoring system to hold recruiting entities accountable.

The WHO's Global Code of Practice on the International Recruitment of Health Personnel (WHO, 2010) is another voluntary code reflecting global concern about the ethical implications of international healthcare worker recruitment activity. Subscribing members are states (countries) rather than individual recruitment entities. Concerns forming the basis for the development of the WHO code included threats to healthcare worker supplies in countries already facing shortages and for which the potential to achieve MDGs would be undermined as a result of losing the human clinical and intellectual capital necessary to improve health systems and outcomes.

Both of these voluntary codes emphasize the need to respect the rights and responsibilities of migrant healthcare workers as well as the source and destination countries. To advance the scope and effectiveness of these efforts to protect vulnerable stakeholders associated with international recruitment of healthcare workers, the next logical step may be to evaluate the effectiveness of voluntary subscription to these standards and consider moving toward international policy mandating compliance, in combination with auditing activities, to enforce the ethical recruitment of healthcare workers worldwide.

Interprofessional Education of Global Healthcare Professionals

At a 2008 global conference held in Ethiopia, the concept of task shifting was introduced and promoted as an effective means to achieve population health goals despite the apparent shortage of healthcare professionals in a country or region (WHO, 2013a). Task shifting refers to the appropriate delegation of tasks to a less intensely prepared healthcare worker, which frees up a more specialized healthcare worker to be better utilized. As a result, access to health care expands substantially simply by using existing resources efficiently. Findings of recent studies reflect that task shifting is associated with favorable clinical outcomes in practice settings including, but not limited to, HIV treatment (Fairall et al., 2012), midwifery (Colvin et al., 2013), mental health care (Petersen, Lund, Bhana, Flisher, & Mental Health and Poverty Research Programme Consortium, 2012), tuberculosis control (Mafigiri, McGrath, & Whalen, 2012), and anesthesiology (Tromp Meesters, Hettinga, Brink, Postma, & Scheffer, 2013). This notion suggests that traditional barriers among healthcare specialties may pose a barrier to optimal population health outcomes.

A growing number of countries are subscribing to the concept of interprofessional education. This term describes a rather nontraditional education concept where those who are studying to practice in one health discipline learn shoulder to shoulder with students of other health disciplines (Reeves, Perrier, Goldman, Freeth & Zwarenstein, 2013). In 2007, the Canadian Interprofessional Health Collaborative (CIHC) published core competencies for interprofessional education (2007). Interprofessional exposure during prelicensure enhances the potential to eliminate traditional silos that serve as barriers to interprofessional practice. A meta-analysis of 15 studies showed interprofessional education to be associated with positive patient and process outcomes (Reeves et al., 2013).

The Policy and Politics of Global Nursing

Diverse treaties, politically inspired policies, educational preparation, and the laws of various countries profoundly affect the migration of nurses. Nonetheless, there are common factors that influence all professionals who are considering migrating to another country. The push factors, which motivate nurses to depart from their countries of origin (commonly described as source countries in the global migration context), include low-paying jobs, lack of career advancement, and limited professional growth. The pull factors, which draw them to specific destinations, include better quality of life, higher wages, and better working conditions (Davis & Richardson, 2009). It seems that destination countries also have a common new set of requirements that impact their willingness to pull various professionals to their borders—such as the country's need for certain expertise; the applicant's educational preparation, skill set, and current income; and salary potential—and have been deciding factors in some cases.

Impact of Economic Factors

In some cases, the deciding factors include the destination country's economic status and internal politics. Retrogression in the United States is one example. Retrogression refers to the delay in obtaining an immigrant visa when there are more people applying for immigrant visas in a given year than the total number of available visas.

In October 2005, the U.S. Department of State significantly retrogressed the employment-based immigrant visa (also known as employment green cards) in many categories. As the U.S. Department of Labor and the U.S. Citizenship and Immigration Services began to adjudicate applications more expediently, the demand for employment-based green cards started to exceed the annual allocated supply. Therefore, the Department of State was forced to establish priority date cutoffs in many employment-based immigrant visa categories. Thus, many international registered nurses, physical therapists, and other skilled professionals have already waited 3 or 4 years for U.S. Permanent Residency visas (green cards). With the prospect of having to wait perhaps another 3–5 years, they are actively looking to immigrate to other countries where permanent residency visas are more readily accessible.

Impact of Educational Factors

Nursing education, which occurs on a postsecondary level in the United States, forms the foundation for evaluating eligibility for entry to practice. In some, but not all, countries, educational requirements for entry in nursing programs emulate those of the United States. Modeled to an extent after the bachelor of science in nursing (BSN) degree in the United States, Philippine nursing programs lead to a baccalaureate degree; however, some courses are incorporated into the secondary school education. India offers both diploma and baccalaureate programs, and the entrance requirement is the completion of 12 years of primary and secondary education. China offers three types of nursing programs: midassociate's degree, associate's degree, and bachelor's degree. In Mexico, many practicing nurses received their nursing education during the first 12 years of their education, although recent changes now place nursing programs on the postsecondary level. In the United Kingdom (before 1990) and other former British colonies, nurses are educated through a specialist pathway (Shaffer & Yuen-Heung To Dutka, 2012).

Competitive Sustainability

As described in Chapter 1.2 of the *Global Competitiveness Report 2013–2014*, competitive sustainability is built on specified pillars that are categorized under two major headings: the social sustainability pillar and the environmental sustainability pillar. The social sustainability pillar measures the set of institutions, policies, and factors that enable all members of society to experience the best possible health, participation, and security and to maximize their potential to contribute to and benefit from the economic prosperity of the country in which they live. The environmental sustainability pillar measures the institutions, policies, and factors that ensure an efficient management of resources to enable prosperity for present and future generations (Bilbao-Osorio et al., 2013).

Legislation and Regulation

Legislation and regulation of professionals affects their dissemination and use. It is fundamental to their identity and the types of services a professional provides. The way a profession is regulated either facilitates or impedes its ability to remain relevant and its capacity to offer needed services. Meaningful legislation and regulation of healthcare professionals depends on an examination and analysis of the content and approaches that various countries take in their education. Nursing is one case in point. Despite a shared purpose in preparing nurses to provide direct patient care, nursing education differs markedly from country to country.

Although not all countries require nursing registration, many do, chief among which is the United States. To determine educational comparability, credentialing organizations use one or both of two types of assessment for migration purposes: determinative assessment and advisory assessment. In a determinative assessment, credentials are evaluated against a set of standards. The evaluator determines, on the basis of evidence, whether an applicant has met the requirements. A certificate is awarded when an applicant is deemed to have met all program requirements. The VisaScreen: Visa Credentials Assessment Service and the Certification Program offered by CGFNS International are examples of determinative assessment.

In an advisory assessment, a detailed report is compiled based on a critical analysis of the education and professional credentials of the applicant. The standards upon which the applicants are evaluated are provided either by a specific state board of nursing that will receive the reports or by a standards committee composed of professionals drawn from academic and practice sectors of the nursing profession. "Credential evaluation will continue to gravitate toward measuring comparability of education as the basis for assessing the portability of education and professional qualifications required in determining

occupational mobility . . . Regulatory authorities and credential evaluation organizations need to work closely to continually refine assessment processes and tools to achieve this shared goal" (Shaffer & Yuen-Heung To Dutka, 2012).

Given the variations in nursing education among countries, the search for equivalence with U.S. standards can be a contrived exercise. CGFNS International and many state U.S. boards of nursing use the concept of comparability to drive their evaluation. In examining the evidence in verified documents provided directly by primary sources, the evaluator renders a judgment on the comparability of the education using prevailing standards in the United States.

Impact of Trade Agreements

Trade Agreements and Mutual Recognition Agreements have enormous impacts on the migration of healthcare professionals. Such agreements facilitate the movement of goods, services, or people across national borders. Among them are the following: General Agreement on Trade in Services (GATS); European Union (EU); North American Free Trade Agreement (NAFTA); and Central America Free Trade Agreement (CAFTA). The aim of trade agreements is to reduce barriers and liberalize international trade. The World Trade Organization (WTO) deals with the rules of trade between nations globally. While recognizing a national authority's right to regulate professions, WTO's GATS aims to ensure that licensing requirements and procedures do not constitute unnecessary barriers to trade.

Mutual Recognition Agreements (MRAs) are agreements between national entities that allow respective licensing authorities to accept, in whole or in part, the credentials obtained in the jurisdiction of the other party. MRAs include

East, Central and South African College of Nursing (ECSACON); Trans-Tasman Mutual Recognition Agreement (TTMRA); and Caribbean Community and Common Market (CARICOM). MRAs are bilateral or multilateral agreements that establish and promote fair and objective criteria for licensing foreign-educated professionals. MRAs encourage international mobility of professions by extending the right to practice to qualified foreign-educated individuals.

Global Health Technology

The rapid growth and interoperability in the development, certification, and dissemination of medical apps enables all healthcare workers, not necessarily just professionals, to bring health information, monitoring, diagnostic testing, and even intervention to the most remote regions. According to O'Connor (2012), there are about 40,000 medical apps available for download on smartphones and tablets; however, these apps are of varying quality and accuracy. Unfortunately, evidence-based research has not kept up with technological innovation, so their efficacy has yet to be demonstrated. Moreover, in some countries, there is physician opposition and a lack of infrastructure to support the new technologies. However, the biggest obstacle to effective research, development, and use of medical apps may be the regulation, licensure, and control issues that governments are grappling with in different ways. The challenge now faced by regulators and lawmakers of every country is how to come up with solutions that balance public interest with innovation.

Implications for Nursing

Worldwide, nurses are well positioned to help advance the global health agenda by nature of the work they do as nurse clinicians, researchers,

educators, and policy advocates. Beck, Dosey, and Rushton (2013) emphasized the need for such engagement when they issued a clarion call for greater nursing involvement in the global health arena. These authors encourage nurses to lend their voices to promote an awareness of global health issues. In doing so, nurses must utilize the advancements in social media and global networking opportunities as tools to advance worldwide nursing activism and advocacy. The need for nurses to display their worldwide contributions to care cannot be overemphasized (Beck et al., 2013).

As authors of this chapter, we offer some additional implications for nursing that support the need to act locally and think globally:

- Advocate for policies that eradicate the sociodeterminants of health, a major contributing factor to the global burden of disease worldwide.

- Incorporate substantive global health content into interdisciplinary health professions curricula.

- Advance the international nursing agenda by generating and disseminating research in alignment with the WHO health priorities.

Conclusion

This chapter has provided an overview on the global health environment in terms of politics, policies, and partners, which are germane to advancing a global health agenda. There is no doubt that consistent and concerted efforts on a number of fronts are sorely needed to improve global health and development. Because they represent the largest number of healthcare professionals worldwide, nurses are well positioned to expand their contributions to global health as they engage in interprofessional education, conduct global health research, and advocate for better health and health care worldwide. As global health issues and initiatives continue to transcend borders, nurses, in collaboration with other stakeholders, will be called upon to utilize a broader set of core competencies to effectively address a plethora of complex and growing global health concerns. Issues such as the unprecedented growth in global migration, the increased emphasis on achieving the 2015 MGDs, and the ongoing priority of reducing the global burden of health care will require that stakeholders demonstrate a working knowledge of the sociocultural, political, economic, and environmental factors that influence health worldwide. Nurses and other healthcare professionals need to be directly involved in the development of global health policy, drawing from a combined interdisciplinary body of scientific and experiential knowledge. This interdisciplinary approach is an essential component of the effective management of a rapidly evolving global healthcare milieu.

Case Study

When Policy Dictates Treatment Options for HIV-Positive Women in Resource-Constrained Settings

Kathleen M. Nokes

According to the AIDSinfo Drug Database from the National Institutes of Health, efavirenz (Sustiva) is a type of anti-HIV medicine called a non-nucleoside reverse transcriptase inhibitor. There is a warning in the database that says, "Women should not become pregnant while taking efavirenz and for 12 weeks after stopping the drug. Serious birth defects have been seen in the babies of animals and women treated with efavirenz during pregnancy. Whether efavirenz caused the birth defects is unknown" (AIDSinfo Drug Database, 2014).

The AIDSinfo Drug Database also says that Atripla is a combination medication containing efavirenz and two other anti-HIV medications, and the same pregnancy warning is shown (AIDSinfo Drug Database, 2014).

A March 2, 2014, memo from the deputy director general of the South African Department of Health, titled *Urgent FDC Roll Out*, advised that all HIV-positive patients who are eligible for anti-HIV medications—including all pregnant women, regardless of CD4 count, and all HIV-positive pregnant women and breast-feeding mothers who are currently stable on other drugs—should be switched to the fixed dose combination that includes efavirenz (Pillay, 2014). These South African recommendations are consistent with the 2013 WHO guidelines that state, "A once-daily fixed-dose combination of TDF + 3TC (or FTC) + EFV is recommended as first-line ART in pregnant and breastfeeding women and adults with TB and HBV coinfection" (WHO, 2013, section 7.2.2). The WHO says the recommendation was made after balancing the benefits of starting anti-HIV medications in pregnant and breastfeeding women with the possible risks of drug toxicity to the mother and fetus or infant during pregnancy and breastfeeding. The toxicity associated with efavirenz is neural tube defects, which are birth defects of the brain, spine, or spinal cord that happen in the first month of pregnancy; the two most common neural tube defects are spina bifida and anencephaly. Although the WHO Guidelines Development Group emphasized that better data on birth defects were needed, it felt confident that this potential low risk should be balanced against the programmatic advantages and the clinical benefit of efavirenz in preventing HIV infection in infants and for the mother's health.

Treatment costs have declined, mainly due to the sustained efforts of organizations such as the

President's Emergency Plan for AIDS Relief (PEP-FAR) (2013) and the Global Fund (2014). According to the 2013 PEPFAR report, there has been a striking decline in treatment costs over time, from more than $1,100 to approximately $338 per patient per year. The three-drug combination regimen is economic and simple because it requires dosing only once per day. The choice to continue women on other treatments has been eliminated since the policy is to switch all HIV-positive patients to the three-drug combination.

The paradox is that HIV-positive women in the United States would probably be counseled about the potential neural tube defect in the fetus and given a choice about the type of HIV treatment, while an HIV-positive woman in a resource-constrained country would probably not be given the choice because policy dictates treatment supplies and options. How does a healthcare provider in a resource-constrained setting ensure that HIV-positive women are making an informed consent about treatment when the choice is no treatment or taking a medication that has a very slight chance of causing neural defects in the fetus during the first trimester? Not treating HIV infection results in about a 25% chance that the baby will be HIV infected, which is associated with higher infant mortality rates and lifelong chronic illness. Is there a choice? The health literacy levels of many of the women being treated are limited because poverty has constrained educational and healthcare setting options. Healthcare providers can be on heightened awareness for the incidence of neural tube

defects and know how to report these occurrences to international bodies monitoring the incidence of medication toxic effects, such as the U.S. Food and Drug Administration. Healthcare providers can acknowledge that they are forced once again into a difficult situation for which there are limited solutions and try to take the course of least harm.

Case Study References

AIDSinfo Drug Database. (2013). *Efavirenz.* Retrieved from http://aidsinfo.nih.gov /drugs/269/efavirenz/0/patient

AIDSinfo Drug Database. (2014). *Efavirenz/emtricitabine/tenofovir disoproxil fumarate.* Retrieved from http://aidsinfo.nih.gov/drugs/424 /atripla/0/patient

Global Fund. (2014). *The Global Fund to fight AIDS, tuberculosis, and malaria.* Retrieved from http://www.theglobalfund.org/en/

President's Emergency Plan for AIDS Relief. (2013). *Report on costs of treatment in the President's Emergency Plan for AIDS Relief (PEPFAR).* Retrieved from http://www.pepfar.gov/docu-ments/organization/212059.pdf

Pillay, T. (2014). *Urgent FDC roll out.* Retrieved from http://www.sahivsoc.org/upload/documents /FDC%20ROLLOUT_URGENT%20CIRCULAR%20 NDOH-1.pdf

World Health Organization. (2013). *Consolidated guidelines on the use of antiretroviral drugs for treating and preventing HIV infection: Recommendations for a public health approach.* Retrieved from http://apps.who.int/iris/bitstr eam/10665/85321/1/9789241505727_eng.pdf

Discussion Questions

1. Within your area of influence, what initiatives are devoted to advancing global health?
2. How might nursing assume leadership in addressing the United Nations 2013 MDGs?
3. What are some opportunities to employ an interdisciplinary approach to advance a WHO global health agenda?

References

Alexis, O., Vydelingum, V., & Robbins, I. (2007). Engaging with new reality: Experiences of overseas minority ethnic nurses in the NHS. *Journal of Clinical Nursing, 16*, 2221–2228. doi:10.1111/j.1365-2702.2007.02080.x

Allan, H., Cowie, H., & Smith, P. (2009). Overseas nurses' experiences of discrimination: A case of racist bullying? *Journal of Nursing Management, 17*, 906–906. doi:10.1111/j.1365-2834.2009.00983.x

Alliance for Ethical International Recruitment Practices. (2011). *Voluntary code of ethical conduct for the recruitment of foreign-educated health professionals to the United States.* Retrieved from http://www.fairinternationalrecruitment .org/index.php/the_code/

Beck, D., Dosey, B., & Rushton, C. H. (2013). Building on the Nightingale Initiative for Global Health–NIGH: Can we engage and empower the public voices for nurses worldwide? *Nursing Science Quarterly, 26*(4), 366–371.

Bilbao-Osorio, B., Blanke, J., Campanella, E., Crotti, R., Drzeniek-Hanouz, M., & Serin, C. (2013). Assessing the sustainable competitiveness of nations. In K. Schwab (Ed.), *The global competitiveness report 2013–2014: Full data edition* (pp. 54–82). World Economic Forum, Geneva, Switzerland. Retrieved from http://www.weforum.org/reports /global-competitiveness-report-2013-2014

Canadian Interprofessional Health Collaborative. (2007). *Interprofessional education and core competencies.* Retrieved from http://www.cihc.ca/ files/publications/CIHC_IPE-LitReview_May07. pdf

Centers for Disease Control and Prevention. (2010). *Dengue and climate.* Retrieved from http: //www.cdc.gov/dengue/entomologyEcology /climate.html

Centers for Disease Control and Prevention. (2013a). Dengue outbreak—Federated States of Micronesia, 2012–2013. *Morbidity and Mortality Weekly Report, 19*(62), 570–573.

Centers for Disease Control and Prevention. (2013b). *Malaria cases in U.S. hit 40-year high.* Retrieved from http://www.cdc.gov/features /malaria/

Chen, C., Auerbach, D., Muench, U., Curry, L., & Bradley, E. (2013). Policy solutions to address the foreign-educated and foreign born health care workforce in the United States. *Health Affairs, 32*(11), 1906–1913. doi:10.1377/hlthaff.2013.0576

Colvin, C., de Heer, J., Winterton, L., Mellenkamp, M. G., Glenton, C., Noyes, J., . . . Rashidian, A. (2013). A systematic review of qualitative evidence on barriers and facilitators to the implementation of task-shifting in midwifery services. *Midwifery, 29*(10), 1211–1221.

Davis, C. D., & Richardson, D. R. (2009). Preparing to leave your home country. In B. L. Nichols & C. D. Davis (Eds.), *The official guide for foreign-educated nurses: What you need to know about nursing and health care in the United States* (pp. 20–42). New York, NY: Springer.

Deegan, J., & Simkin, K. (2010). Expert to novice: Experiences of professional adaptation reported by non-English speaking nurses in Australia. *Australian Journal of Advanced Nursing, 27*(3), 31–37.

Fairall, L. B., Bachman, M., Lombard, C., Timmerman, V., Uebel, K., Zwarenstein, M., . . . Bateman, E. (2012). Task shifting of antiretroviral treatment from doctors to primary-care nurses in South Africa (STRETCH): A pragmatic, parallel, cluster-randomised trial. *Lancet, 380*(9845), 889–898. doi:10.1016/S0140-6736(12)60730-2

Fehling, M., Nelson, B. D., & Venkatapuram, S. (2013). Limitations of the Millennium Development Goals; A literature review. *Global Public Health, 8*(10) 1109-22 doi:10.1080/17441692.2013.845676.

Global Health Workforce Alliance and World Health Organization. (2013). *A universal truth: No health without a workforce.* Retrieved from http: //www.who.int/workforcealliance/knowledge /resources/hrhreport_summary_En_web.pdf

Luo, H., Zhang, Y., Wang, X., Yu, W., Wen, N., Yan, D. M....& Yang, W. Z. (2013). Identification and control of a poliomyelitis outbreak in Xinjiang, China. *New England Journal of Medicine, 369*(21), 1981–1990. doi:10.1056/NEJMoa1303368

Mackey, T. K., & Liang, B. A. (2012). Rebalancing brain drain: Exploring resource reallocation to address health worker migration and promote global health. *Health Policy, 107,* 66–73.

Mafigiri, D., McGrath, J., & Whalen, C. (2012). Task shifting for tuberculosis control: A qualitative study of community-based directly observed therapy in urban Uganda. *Global Public Health, 7*(3), 270–284. doi:10.1080/17441692.2011.552067

O'Connor, M. (2012). *mHealth: Barriers to global implementation.* Retrieved from http://healthworkscollective.com/marie-ennis-ocon-nor/34718/mhealth-barriers-and-solutions-global-implementation

Petersen, I., Lund, C., Bhana, A., Flisher, A., & Mental Health and Poverty Research Programme Consortium. (2012). A task shifting approach to primary mental health care for adults in South Africa: Human resource requirements and costs for rural settings. *Health Policy & Planning, 27,* 42–51. doi:10.1093/heapol/czr012

Pittman, P., Herrera, C., Spetz, J., & Davis, C. D. (2012). Immigration and contract problems experienced by foreign-educated nurses. *Medical Care Research and Review, 69*(3), 351–365. doi:10.1177/1077558711432890

Plotnikova, E. (2012). Cross-border mobility of health professionals: Contesting patients' right to health. *Social Science & Medicine, 74,* 20–27.

Reeves, S., Perrier, L., Goldman, J., Freeth, D., & Zwarenstein, M. (2013). Interprofessional education: Effects on professional practice and healthcare outcomes (update) (review). *The Cochrane Library, 3,* 1–47.

Shaffer, F. (2014). Ensuring a global workforce: A challenge and opportunity. *Nursing Outlook 62*(1), 1–4.

Shaffer, F., & Yuen-Heung To Dutka, J. (2012). Perspectives on credential evaluation: Future trends and regulatory implications. *Journal of Nursing Regulation, 3*(1), 27–31.

Smith, P., Allan, H., Henry, L., Larsen, J., & Mackintosh, M. (2006). *Researching equal opportunities for internationally recruited nurses and other health professionals: Valuing and recognising the talents of a diverse health workforce.* Retrieved from www.rcn.org.uk/publications/pdf/survey-2002-p1-45.pdf

Spetz, J., Gates, M., & Jones, C. B. (2014). Internationally educated nurses in the United States: Their origins and roles. *Nursing Outlook, 62*(1), 8–15.

Tromp Meesters, R. C., Hettinga, A. M., Brink, G., Postma, C. T., & Scheffer, G. J. (2013). Task shifting and quality of care in practice: Physician assistants compared with anaesthesiology residents in the preoperative anaesthesiology outpatient clinic. *Nederlands Tijdschrift Voor Geneeskunde, 157*(19), A5518.

United Nations. (2013). *The millennium development goals report—2013.* Retrieved from http://www.un.org/millenniumgoals/pdf/report-2013/mdg-report-2013-english.pdf

World Health Organization. (2010). *WHO global code of practice on the international recruitment of health personnel.* Retrieved from http://www.who.int/hrh/migration/code/code_en.pdf

World Health Organization. (2013a). *First global conference on task shifting.* Retrieved from http://www.who.int/healthsystems/task_shifting/en/

World Health Organization. (2013b). *Life expectancy.* Retrieved from http://www.who.int/gho/mortality_burden_disease/life_tables/situation_trends_text/en/#

World Health Organization. (2013c). *The top 10 causes of death: Fact sheet no. 310.* Retrieved from http://www.who.int/mediacentre/factsheets/fs310/en/index1.html#)

World Health Organization. (2013d). *Tuberculosis fact sheet no. 104.* Retrieved from http://www.who.int/mediacentre/factsheets/fs104/en/

World Health Organization. (2013e). *World health statistics—2013.* Retrieved from http://www.who.int/gho/publications/world_health_statistics/EN_WHS2013_Full.pdf

CHAPTER 9

Population Health: Vulnerable Populations' Access to Care

Marie Truglio-Londrigan and Sandra B. Lewenson

Overview

Vulnerability and living in a state of vulnerability have been experienced by individuals, families, communities, and populations over time. The strategies developed to improve the health of vulnerable populations, such as political advocacy and legislation, have evolved. To illustrate this unfolding evolution, this chapter has been developed from a historical to a contemporary perspective. The historical perspective highlights the work of nurses with vulnerable populations as these nurses engaged in political advocacy. It shows the work of one local rural community in upstate New York during the late 19th and early 20th century that joined forces to provide healthcare access, specifically nursing care, to those who typically lacked services. The more contemporary aspect of this chapter introduces vulnerability and its complexity as it is understood today and continues to highlight nursing's work with vulnerable populations. These sections of the chapter explore vulnerable populations today, what factors may facilitate and sustain these vulnerabilities, and what potential positions and actions may be taken in advocacy for vulnerable people. To do so, it uses an interview with a contemporary public health nurse to illustrate how public policy initiatives influence care delivered at the local level. This interview demonstrates how politics and policy play a role in how programs are developed, negotiated, and delivered, and, in turn, it addresses the health needs of vulnerable populations.

Objectives

- Understand nursing's historical role in primary health care and care of vulnerable populations.
- Discuss factors that have the potential to facilitate vulnerability in an individual or population.
- Examine the relationship between vulnerability and disparity.
- Explore the relationships among ethical norms, ideas, values, and beliefs related to the public policy agenda.
- Examine how nursing ideas, values, and beliefs play a role in setting the policy agenda.
- Consider the role that politics, policy, and law have in protecting the rights of vulnerable populations.

Lessons from Nursing History on Political Advocacy

In 1922, noted nursing leaders and public health nursing activists Lavinia Dock and Fannie Clement described how a pioneer rural nursing association was started by a Johns Hopkins nursing school graduate, Ellen M. Wood, in the northern region of Westchester County, just north of New York City. This new service that began in 1898 provided families living in the northern reaches of the county, which is now considered a suburb but then was a rural setting, access to much-needed healthcare services. These services were not readily available because of geographic isolation and economic circumstances. The founding of the District Nursing Association of Northern Westchester County (DNA) predated the start of the American Red Cross Rural Nursing Service, which began in 1912 and would later bring public health nursing to the far reaches of American life, where access to care was at a minimum and vulnerability was at a premium.

This was not an entirely new concept, but it is a good example for understanding the relationship between the lack of access and the politics of health. Noted public health leader Lillian Wald had already established primary healthcare services in 1893 on New York's Lower East Side at the Henry Street Settlement, bringing vital nursing services to immigrant populations who came to New York seeking a better way of life (Keeling & Lewenson, 2013). It was Wald who recognized that all citizens, whether in the crowded urban environment or in isolated rural areas, required healthcare services. She started the visionary American Red Cross Rural Nursing Service in 1912 and called for additional educational training for public health nurses, in both urban and rural communities (Keeling & Lewenson, 2013). Wald also was a leader in advocating for healthcare reforms in New York City, effecting local laws to include placing school nurses in public schools, establishing playgrounds where children in crowded urban settings could play, and supporting tenement laws to protect the health of people who lived in unhealthy conditions.

In addition, Wald and many of her colleagues at Henry Street Settlement, including Lavinia Dock, advocated for women's suffrage to protect the health of the public (Lewenson, 1996). Dock called for nursing professionals "to look at social and political problems and include social reform among their professional obligations" (Lewenson, 1996, p. 144). For many nurses during this period of social activism, "nurses' concerns with injustices in the world rendered their political involvement unavoidable" (Lewenson, 1996, p. 150). The late 19th and early 20th century was a time of professional advancement, political advocacy, and local commitment to bettering health care for populations. The women in northern Westchester were part of this progressive movement and led healthcare reform efforts in their community.

Ellen Wood and the Use of Political Advocacy

The Wood family had a long history of caring for their rural neighbors prior to Ellen Wood's entrance into nurses' training at Johns Hopkins Training School for Nurses. Her brother, Hollingsworth Wood, wrote about his sister: "she decided to experience the training then given to nurses in order to take the best possible care of her neighbors" (District Nursing Association of Northern Westchester County [DNA], 1948, p. 13). When Ellen Wood graduated in 1896* she returned home and brought the nursing skills she learned at Johns Hopkins to her neighbors. Her brother wrote, "At first her daily rounds were made on foot, but soon her circle widened as cases of sickness in the remoter county districts came

*In an email dated February 28, 2013, archivist Marjorie Kehoe at Johns Hopkins University wrote that Ellen Wood graduated in 1895 and received postgraduate training in obstetrical nursing in 1896.

to her knowledge, until presently a horse and buggy were needed to take her to her patients" (DNA, 1948, p. 14). In these early years, Ellen Wood provided skilled nursing care and taught families how to care for themselves in her absence. Her work was considered "instructive, preventive, and social service work" (DNA, 1948, p. 14).

When the Spanish-American War broke out in 1898, Wood volunteered to serve and was assigned as superintendent of nurses at the Fort Hamilton Army base located in Brooklyn, New York. The Spanish-American War lasted less than a year, starting on April 25, 1898, and ending with the signing of Treaty of Paris on December 10, 1898. Wood's work in the American Red Cross continued following the war. She served on a committee to establish an Army Nurse Corps, something that professional nursing leaders also advocated. Wood worked alongside nursing leaders like Mary Adelaide Nutting, Anna Maxwell, Irene H. Sutliffe, and Isabel Hampton Robb in their efforts to have nursing recognized in the military. These leaders found support from several social-minded women who supported nursing's efforts in this area, including Mrs. Winthrop Cowdin, who later helped Wood establish the rural nursing service in their upstate community (Dock & Clement, 1922).

With the support of her family and friends, Wood went on to begin the DNA following the war. The women began the DNA with $250, which were the funds that remained after their short-lived Red Cross Auxiliary that they started to support the local boys who fought in the Spanish-American War. Four committees gathered the needed equipment either through loans or purchases to support this new endeavor. They collected items such as hot water bags, rubber sheets, sheets, towels, diapers, ice caps, thermometers, soap, Vaseline, bandages, and other items that were needed for care in the home. They provided instruction for home care to practical nurses and arranged for a "special nurse" from New York City to come to their community when needed (DNA, 1948, p. 15). The organizers of the DNA also asked community members to join by paying a $1 annual membership fee. These dues, along with other fund-raising activities, donations, and fees charged for nurses' visits, financed the growth of the organization. In addition, money from two insurance companies—Metropolitan Life Insurance Company and John Hancock Insurance Company—paid for nursing services for their policy holders. For those who could not pay, the DNA provided services free of charge.

The DNA organizers believed that trained nurses needed to bring health care to their rural communities and spoke highly of their pioneering effort. They acknowledged the challenges they faced when starting the association and recognized that although district nursing existed already in cities like Boston, New York, Buffalo, and Baltimore, none yet existed in rural communities. These women believed, like other reformers of that period, that health care must be learned and that nurses in the community could implement the ideas of sanitary reform by teaching the women in the community. Convincing the community of the need for public health nurses also meant winning the support of local physicians. Stories about the need to gain support from physicians include the following from one of the early pioneers, Miss Luquer:

> I remember sending the nurse to a patient who lived near me. I begged the doctor for his permission. He finally consented. I got the nurse and took her to the neighbor. She made the patient so comfortable that when the doctor called, she thanked him again and again for sending the nurse. He never said a word, but neither did he ever call the nurse again. (DNA, 1948, pp. 20–21)

Although it was not always successful in the beginning, the writers of the DNA's history noted that physicians ultimately became the organization's "mainstay" (DNA, 1948, p. 21).

Without calling the rural communities *vulnerable*, the late 19th and early 20th century community activists, mostly women, joined forces with early public health nurses to provide care to those in need and to those living in rural northern Westchester. Like in other rural settings, the lack of adequate roadways, hospitals, health departments, and healthcare facilities contributed to the vulnerability of the families in this community. The women who joined forces with Wood advocated for the start of the visiting nurses services that Wood and other nurses could provide. These women believed that joining people together was key to meeting the needs of those who required care. People must just "go ahead and do it" (DNA, 1948, p. 47). They were used to working together, as demonstrated in their earlier work in establishing a Red Cross Auxiliary during the Spanish-American War in 1899, and then again when they lobbied in Washington, DC, for the establishment of an Army nurses' corps. They were accustomed to working toward providing access to care, whether on the battlefield or in the civilian community, and sought support from organized nursing, local boards of health, other healthcare professionals, and insurance companies.

The history of the DNA shows how nurses in the past responded to primary healthcare needs, collaborated intra- and interprofessionally, and recognized the value of political advocacy for that care. This narrative about the 1920s era captures how nurses have responded to the needs of vulnerable populations on a local level and perhaps can help us shape how we consider the advocacy role that nurses continue to have in the 21st century. It also shows the collaborative nature of nurse advocates as they joined the work of rural and urban efforts (DNA and Henry Street Settlement, respectively).

> Late one summer evening a call came from Henry Street Settlement asking if it were possible to send a nurse to their camp at Secor's Lake where a boy had been taken very ill. There was no nurse, the camp doctor had gone to New York, and there was no night train. The need was urgent and Katonah was the only point of contact because there was a visiting nurse there. It took some time to locate the camp, but at last the livery man was awakened and the willing nurse set off with the livery team in a violent thunder storm. The picture she found was a gloomy one. The boy had been removed to a vacant barn for fear of contagion. The nurse stayed for hours doing all she could for his comfort, but the next day he was removed to a New York hospital where he died. Miss Wald's letter received later spoke with appreciation of the "link of co-operation" which brought help to the boy, and relief to the Henry Street Settlement from the Nursing Association of Northern Westchester. (DNA, 1948, p. 52)

Vulnerability can happen to any population living in urban or rural settings, and it is often compounded by race, class, and gender. As this historical example shows, nursing attempted to provide care to vulnerable populations in rural settings and urban settings. The DNA, the American Red Cross Rural Nursing Service, and the Henry Street Settlement on the Lower East Side of New York are just a few exemplars of how nurses cared for the populations living in the community. Nurses in each of these community-based organizations offered primary healthcare services, such as well-baby classes for new mothers, bedside care in the home for those in need, coordination of care with other healthcare providers, and collaboration with local governmental agencies like health departments, school boards, and local chambers of commerce to provide such care. The ability of the activists and the families in the northern Westchester community during the late 19th and early 20th century to work together and address the needs of the community offers insight into today's need for strong community partnerships, political advocacy for those who need healthcare services, and the recognition of nursing's role in providing primary health care in rural settings.

Vulnerability Today: A Continuum from History

Vulnerability and Disparity

Grabovschi, Loignon, and Fortin examined the relationship between healthcare disparities and vulnerability and found a direct correlation: "The people with the greatest health care needs receive the least health care services" (2013, p. 2). Furthermore, their findings suggest that "people who accumulate more vulnerability factors are more likely to face health care disparities" (p. 7). A conversation that focuses on vulnerability frequently incudes a discussion about the concept of disparity and begs the question, Is there a relationship between the two concepts? Healthcare disparity is addressed in the U.S. Department of Health and Human Services, Agency for Healthcare Research and Quality (AHRQ) *National Healthcare Disparities Report* (2011). Highlights of this report suggest that Americans who experience disparities have the following characteristics:

- They do not receive care they need, and/or
- The care they received causes harm, and/or
    - The care was delivered without consideration of the patient's preferences
    - The care was distributed in a way that was inefficient and uneven across populations

Furthermore, this report notes how these disparities may be due to "differences in access to care, provider biases, poor provider-patient communication, or poor health literacy" (U.S. Department of Health and Human Services, AHRQ, 2011, p. 1).

As a result of these differences, disparity will be noted to a greater or lesser extent in the health outcomes of various populations (U.S. Department of Health and Human Services [USDHHS], 2010a). Considering the preceding information, one may explore how vulnerable people may experience disparities in health. For example, as we will see later in this chapter, Rose lacks access to care due to a physical disability that prohibits her from driving, as well as geographical distances that prohibit easy access by alternative (and costly) means of transportation. These factors make her vulnerable and leave her open to greater disparities. Her inability to access much-need physical

therapy means she is more likely to continue having speech and motor deficits. This also might mean that she will be unemployed longer or may never be able to return to work and enjoy her former economic status. In another example, Jane faces increasing vulnerability due to aging. This increased vulnerability leads to greater healthcare disparities because fewer opportunities to socialize with friends makes her increasingly isolated and contributes to the potential for adverse health outcomes.

Vulnerable populations, the factors that facilitate and sustain these vulnerabilities, and what potential positions and actions may be taken to advocate for them are discussed and further highlight the complexities of vulnerability in our contemporary world. These questions and the interrelationship between vulnerability and disparity are explored.

Who Is Vulnerable?

Public health initiatives throughout the 20th century made great strides in addressing poverty and vulnerability. Yet, despite these great strides, there are still "vulnerable populations left behind" (Institute for Alternative Futures, n.d., p. 8). Some of these identified populations are as follows: high-risk mothers and infants; people who are chronically malnourished, homeless, ill, or disabled; people who are living with HIV/AIDS (including pediatric AIDS cases); people who abuse alcohol and drugs (including fetal alcohol syndrome and crack babies); people with health problems caused by chemical exposures; people who are mentally ill; veterans who suffer from posttraumatic stress disorder (PTSD); abusive families and relationships; gays and lesbians who suffer from discrimination; foster youth who are aging out of the foster care system; prisoners; and American Indians (Institute for Alternative Futures, n.d. pp. 8–9).

Discussions pertaining to vulnerability tend to focus on a population perspective. It is important to recognize, however, that individuals make up populations. An individual who is a member of a vulnerable population may not experience vulnerability; conversely, an individual who is a member of a nonvulnerable population may be vulnerable due to personal life events (de Chesnay, 2011). Changes in social, economic, and political contexts may create a state of vulnerability for an individual, such as an illness, a loss of a job, a move to an unfamiliar environment, or the loss of a loved one (Benatar, 2013; de Chesnay, 2011; Rogers, 1997). This notion introduces the fact that vulnerability is complex and that understanding the vagaries of life can help avoid stereotyping individuals and populations, and it allows for a more culturally competent practice.

Conversations about who vulnerable people are and the factors that precipitate the openness or exposure leading to vulnerability is crucial yet difficult. The tendency is to speak of each factor in isolation—such as age, economic status, lack of education, loss of a job, and so forth—but they coexist and thus highlight the multifactorial nature of vulnerability and demonstrate its complexity (Shi, Stevens, Faed, & Tsai, 2008). This is further noted by Stevens, Shi, and Faed, who explain this phenomenon as being "vulnerable in more than one way" (2008, p. 902). Flaskerud and Winslow (2010) illustrate this complexity by portraying and explaining the interrelationship and interplay among risk, resource availability, and health status. Aday (2003) furthered this conversation by illustrating how vulnerability may be considered from community and individual perspectives and examines the relationships among concepts such as ethical norms and values and policy (social and economic policy,

community-oriented health policy, and medical care and public health policy). We suggest that Aday's use of the term *medical care* (2003) does not represent the expansiveness of the needs of any population, and we propose that a broader term, such as *health care and public policy*, would be more useful. An example of this complexity is noted in the case study about Rose later in this chapter.

An interconnected relationship among the various causes of vulnerability exists and affects the advocacy required in addressing vulnerability and health care. The following case study highlights this complexity.

Case Study

Rose is a 42-year-old Hispanic female who is educated at the master's level and employed as an office worker. She had a stroke that left her with left-sided hemiplegia. She finds herself socially and physically isolated from family and friends as a result of living in a rural setting. Rose loses custody of her two children to her ex-husband and finds that her new live-in fiancé of less than 1 year (and her sole caretaker following the stroke) no longer wants to marry her. The economic vulnerability affecting her physical and mental recovery is compounded when she learns that the remaining disability payments from her job, which she can no longer perform, will be gone within a year. Being ineligible to enroll in Medicaid creates long-term economic concerns that add to her stress and ability to recover.

Rose's inability to drive, lack of funds, emotional and physical loss, geographic isolation, and lack of local physical therapy compound her increasing vulnerability and thus her health outcomes. As we will see later in this chapter, Healthy People 2020 considers health services to be one of the determinants of health; it supports the increasingly untoward experience of Rose and the need to advocate for better health services to achieve the desired health outcomes and is concerned with the other factors that compound her increasingly vulnerable state (USDHHS, 2010b).

Factors and Precipitators Leading to Potential Vulnerability

According to Mechanic and Tanner, vulnerability results from "developmental problems, personal incapacities, disadvantaged social status, inadequacy of interpersonal networks and supports, degraded neighborhoods and environments, and the complex interactions of these factors over the life course" (2007, p. 1200) and may arise from challenges evidenced not only in populations but in individuals and communities (de Chesnay, 2011; Mechanic & Tanner, 2007). The following case study depicts how an older adult, experiencing aging changes and the vagaries of life, creates a situation that precipitates vulnerability and potential adverse health outcomes. It is interesting to note that this individual is representative of other older adults and raises the real possibility that the *population* of older adults may be at risk for these same health outcomes.

Case Study

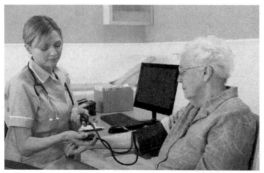
© iStockphoto/Thinkstock

A 75-year-old active woman named Jane has been living independently in her chosen community. She has been experiencing normal aging changes, and as a result, her family notes a difference in her ability to engage in activities of daily living and instrumental activities of daily living. In particular, Jane has not been able to go to follow-up appointments with her primary healthcare provider, attend lunch outings with her friends, or make needed trips to the pharmacy and grocery store. In addition, she has experienced several minor car accidents during her outings that frightened her and caused her to abandon these once enjoyable trips. These aging changes have introduced vulnerability into Jane's life. This new vulnerability places Jane at risk for negative health outcomes. Furthermore, Jane's family has been negotiating the health and social networks of Jane's community to look for social support for Jane, and they have noted that there is a limited network of support that would permit her to age successfully and safely in place; thus, Jane is vulnerable and at risk.

As you read this fictitious account, can you identify other possible factors or precipitators that may increase the vulnerability of Jane or other older adults living in this community, affecting their health outcomes?

There is a danger when making a list of vulnerable populations. Such a list gives the impression that the list is complete. The list presented earlier in this chapter is not complete and is provided as a demonstration of the breadth of this issue. Rather than discuss different populations, we have chosen to present and discuss some determinants or factors and precipitators that have the potential to facilitate vulnerability.

The interrelationship and interaction among these determinants of health may be considered factors or precipitators that can place individuals and populations at risk for being vulnerable and thus determine their health. These categories, as identified in Healthy People 2020, include social factors, health services, individual behavior, biology and genetics, and policy making (USDHHS, 2010c). Social factors, as determinants of health, are subdivided into social determinants and physical determinants. Some examples of social determinants include the following: availability of resources; social norms and attitudes, such as discrimination; crime and violence; social support; social networks and social interactions; socioeconomic conditions; transportation; and safety. Examples of physical determinants include the following: the built environment; housing; and environmental exposure to toxic substances (USDHHS, 2010d).

Social Factors Social factors are not all-inclusive but offer some evidence as to the strong influence of social determinants on vulnerability. Shi and colleagues state that the healthcare professions are now understanding the impact that "social position and social class, racism and discrimination, social networks, and other more relational community factors have on population health" (2008, p. 43). Furthermore, factors that have the potential to facilitate vulnerability—such as education, income, occupation, social networks, and social support—correlate with health outcomes. These social determinants of health have been positively associated with employment and higher paying jobs with benefits that result in favorable health outcomes (Moscou, 2013). This has been seen over time. One example can be found in the work of Carthon (2011) in which the author presented a historical study of the physical and social environments of blacks in early-20th-century Philadelphia. In what would fit under the description of today's Healthy People 2020 social determinants of health, the black community was faced

with economic hardships, housing shortages, insufficient toileting, lack of clean water, lack of educational opportunities, and limited social relief. This community banded together to address these issues through community activism. They organized the Little Mother Club, which offered health education to childbearing women as a means to reduce infant mortality in the city.

Health Services Health services, as a determinant of health, refers to both access to and quality of healthcare services. Vulnerable populations include those who are "not well integrated into the health care system because of ethnic, cultural, economic, geographic, or health characteristics" (Urban Institute, 2010, para. 1). Because of this lack of integration, they are put at further risk. This lack of *access* may mean that the population, and the individuals who are part of that population, may not be *aware* of needed resources or how to navigate the complex healthcare system. As a result, they are not able to *avail* themselves of services, further facilitating their vulnerability (Gallagher, & Truglio-Londrigan, 2004 Krout, 1986, 1994; Williams, Ebrite, & Redford, 1991; USDHHS, 2010e). As a result, they never were integrated into the system and thus were left behind. An individual who does not have access to needed healthcare services due to barriers such as cost, lack of availability, geographic location, or language may be at risk for being vulnerable and present with negative health outcomes (USDHHS, 2010e).

Individual Behavior Individual behavior, as a determinant of health, refers to personal choices regarding diet, physical activity, or the use of substances. The choices a person makes may have a direct implication on health (USDHHS, 2010f).

Biology and Genetics   Biology and genetics, as a determinant of health, refer to factors such as age, gender, and genetic predisposition (USDHHS, 2010g), which are not under an individual's control. There may be situations when these specific factors place an individual or population at risk, thus facilitating vulnerability with potential negative health outcomes. Age, for example, may have an impact on whether an individual is vulnerable, as evidenced in the case study about Jane and her increasing vulnerability and potential for adverse health outcomes. Yet the case study of Rose, who is only 42 years of age and is not typically part of a vulnerable population for the kind of illness she experienced, age plays a factor because she is a mother of two young children and is no longer able to care for them due to her disability. As a result, she faces a change in custody. According to Aday, "People are more or less vulnerable at different states of their lives" (2003, p. 54). For example, older adults experience normal aging changes (Smith & Cotta, 2012) and an increase in the incidence of chronic illness (Federal Interagency Forum on Aging-Related Statistics, 2012). These alterations in health may precipitate vulnerability along with the potential for negative health outcomes.

Policy Making   Finally, policy making, as a determinant of health, may have an impact on health outcomes. For example, increasing taxes on tobacco sales may correlate with decreased sales of cigarettes, or laws may facilitate greater safety and a decrease in injury rates (USDHHS, 2010h). The importance of health determinants as factors or precipitators of vulnerability in individuals or populations cannot be underestimated as nurses and other healthcare providers seek to address disparities with the goal of improving health outcomes.

Contemporary Political Advocacy toward Health Equity

Nurses engage in reflection individually and collectively as a professional group. They ask questions such as: Where do we stand, and where does the nation stand? It is important to ask these questions to clarify and answer them. Courtwright says, "If we take the social determinants of health seriously, we need to look beyond asking whether the conditions that create them are just or unjust and start with the more fundamental questions of whether it is *right* that some people have worse health care than others" (2008, p. 17). Over the decades, there has been a progressive movement in the work of Healthy People to address this issue, as noted in the evolution of its overall goals, where there has been a shift of emphasis concerning disparities. Initially, the focus was on the reduction of health disparities, then the focus shifted to the elimination of health disparities. More recently, Healthy People 2020 introduced the concept of health equity, which is defined as "attainment of the highest level of health for all people. Achieving health equity requires valuing everyone equally with focused and ongoing societal efforts to address avoidable inequalities, historical and contemporary injustices, and the elimination of health and healthcare disparities" (National Partnership for Action, 2011, para. 1).

Social Justice and Responsibility

Flaskerud and Winslow invite readers to reflect on and answer the following question: "Who has the ultimate responsibility for the well-being of the most vulnerable among us?" (2010 p. 298). Given the issues we face as a nation with regard to economics and the never-ending debate regarding the health of our people, it is a question that warrants a courageous and crucial conversation (Patterson, Grenny, McMillan, & Switzler, 2012). Fairman and D'Antonio (2013) speak about this national conversation throughout U.S. history, as seen in debates triggered by Social Security legislation in the 1930s, Medicaid and Medicare in the 1960s, and now the Affordable Care Act (ACA).

Rogers (1997) discussed how certain factors that lead to vulnerability are nonmodifiable, such as age and gender, and how others, such as poverty, education, and social support, are modifiable. Nurses, for example, with their knowledge base, are in a prime position to develop strategies to address these modifiable and nonmodifiable factors that may lead to vulnerability and disparity. According to Benatar (2013), the common response in terms of protecting the health and rights of vulnerable people is through the law. There is, however, conflicting discourse about this very notion of responsibility and accountability. Some say the responsibility rests solely with the individual, and others say it is a collective responsibility. This directly impacts politics and the policy agenda.

Even if there were agreement that health is a collective responsibility, as argued by Benatar (2013), and if responsibility were carried out through law, the laws themselves do not guarantee social justices. This is further explicated by Mechanic and Tanner:

> Federal and state government are more likely to provide assistance to those who are not seen as responsible for their vulnerability, such as children, the blind, disabled veterans, and the elderly. When people are seen as responsible for their life circumstance, such as in the case

> of substance abusers . . . There is less public compassion and often stigma. (2007, p. 1222)

Do we, as a nation, a profession, and a people, recognize and see a problem? Do we see and understand the issues experienced by vulnerable people as a priority, or do we neglect, ignore, or become bogged down in the dogma that reflects the diverse and wide variety of ideas pertaining to social and moral values (Mechanic & Tanner, 2007)? To talk about the policy necessary to address the needs of vulnerable people in this way implies an approach that is paternalistic without regard to the strengths of the vulnerable population in question. Purdy (2004) conducted a concept analysis of the term *vulnerable* and identified several positive consequences. One had to do with the term *open and exposed*. Purdy indicated that being open and exposed, with regard to vulnerability, may lead to positive opportunities. Dorsen (2010) took this a step further in a concept analysis of vulnerability in homeless adolescents and noted positive consequences of vulnerability as the homeless adolescents demonstrated increased resilience, self-reliance, resourcefulness, and innovation. In addition, the providers demonstrated a decrease in negative judgmental behavior and also illustrated a greater understanding of the struggles of this specific population.

The possibility exists, therefore, to view vulnerability in a different way, where healthcare providers and policy makers see those who are vulnerable as valuable partners working together to address the determinants that facilitate vulnerability and disparities. This new way emulates practice from a primary healthcare perspective. Truglio-Londrigan, Singleton, Lewenson, and Lopez (2013) view primary health care as a philosophical belief about social justice and health equity that nurses and the profession must consider in their work. They base their beliefs on the 1978 saying "Health for All" that was coined by the World Health Organization (WHO) and led to the idea of primary health care as the means of achieving this goal. So strong was this belief that at the International Conference on Primary Health Care, the Declaration of Alma-Ata was developed and expressed a call to action by all governments and world communities to promote and protect all people (World Health Organization [WHO], 1978). This declaration contains 10 points. The fifth point speaks specifically to the idea of primary health care. The declaration formally defined primary health care as follows:

> Essential health care based on practical, scientifically sound and socially acceptable methods and technology made universally accessible to individuals and families in the community through their full participation and at a cost that the community and country can afford to maintain at every stage of their development in the spirit of self-reliance and self-determination. It forms an integral part both of the country's health system, of which it is the central function and main focus, and of the overall social and economic development of the community. It is the first level of contact of individuals, the family and community with the national health system bringing health care as close as possible to where people live and work, and constitutes the first element of a continuing health care process. (WHO, 1978, para. 6)

The notion of full participation in this definition is further defined in the following statement:

> Requires and promotes maximum community and individual self-reliance and participation in the planning, organization, operation and control of primary health care, making fullest use of local, national and other available resources; and to this end develops through appropriate education the ability of communities to participate. (WHO, 1978, point 6, section 5)

Could this engagement for full participation by vulnerable people be another way of working with our elected officials in the policy arena? As individuals and populations who are living in vulnerable states partner with organizations in the development of strategies to address factors, precipitators, or determinants of health that facilitate these vulnerabilities, which may lead to negative health outcomes, is it possible to apply the insights of those considered vulnerable in the identification of priority policy agenda items and how these policies are implemented at local levels? The ability to fully operationalize partnering with all other parties in a community, while perhaps the goal, is difficult to achieve but not impossible. Using an example from the recent past allows us to view the way a public health nurse operationalized the idea of engaging vulnerable people in political advocacy for better healthcare outcomes by establishing beginning connections necessary for partnership development with the population being served. The following case study is from an interview with a public health nurse and illustrates the intersection of nursing social responsibility, laws to protect vulnerable people, and concern for the population in general, and how standards of care were executed with policies and procedures.

Case Study

A Public Health Nurse's Story: Responding to Local Need

This case study is based on the work of a public health nurse, Amanda, who served in the role of director of public health nursing in a county department of health services during the 1990s and early 2000s. While public health nursing focuses on populations, it also works with individuals, families, and communities. By virtue of their practice, public health nurses are connected with governments at local, county, state, and federal levels. This case illustrates how public health nursing practice is often based on legislation that must be enacted at the local level. "It is because federal, state, and local laws require enforcement, that public health nursing can be described as a combination of nursing practice and public health science, including the enforcement of all applicable, local health laws" (anonymous personal communication, August, 7, 2013). Amanda further explained that the U.S. Department of Health and Human Services (HHS) and the Centers for Disease Control and Prevention (CDC) guide public health practice, whereas the state commissioner of health and each state's legislated Standards of Performance for Local Boards of Health guide practice at a local level. The delivery of care at a local level to a vulnerable population of adults who are diagnosed with tuberculosis (TB) highlights the core functions of public health: assessment, policy development, and assurance.

Population at Risk

The population at risk is any resident within the county who had been diagnosed with TB

or was at risk for TB. Physicians at the County TB Chest Clinic and the public health nurses related to this specific County Department of Health Services (CDHS) were the main providers of TB care in the community.

The Problem

For a long time, Amanda reported, Chest Clinic physicians and the involved public health nurses were able to deliver the required care and meet standards of practice. Over time, however, there was a change in the population served; this was not recognized by the public health nurses and other professionals, resulting in diminished treatment compliance, reduced numbers of optimal outcomes, and increased risk of multi-drug-resistant tuberculosis (MDR-TB).

Demographic trends showed the county was changing due to increased migration from Korea, China, South America, and Central America. This created a shift from a mostly white, English-speaking population to a more culturally diverse population, with English as a second language or no English at all. This was compounded by the fact that these diverse populations often had a different cultural understanding of TB and its treatment. In addition, if a particular person was undocumented, he or she saw the public health nurse as a government person and wanted to avoid contact.

Although the population had changed, Amanda reported, the available public health nurses were still primarily white and English speaking. They sensed these shifts in demographics, but it had happened gradually, so its significance was not apparent. They were not culturally aware of what these shifts meant in terms of how TB care delivery needed to be changed. Strategies for the delivery of culturally competent and congruent care would be needed if positive health outcomes were going to be sustained. Instead, the nurses recognized only how increasingly difficult it was to meet client needs, obtain compliance, achieve standards of care, and reach positive outcomes.

Simultaneously, additional standards of care had been developed by the State Department of Health—Standards of Care for Tuberculosis Disease and Latent TB Infection—that stressed the use of Directly Observed Therapy (DOT) (standard 6) for all pulmonary and laryngeal TB cases. DOT means that a public health nurse, or a delegate, would meet with each TB patient to observe the self-administration of prescribed medications. As this standard was incorporated, each TB program throughout the state did its best to meet the DOT standard; however, it became apparent that provider agencies with a significant number of TB cases needed additional CDC funding or additional staff to meet the DOT standard, particularly in this county, where there was a significant shift in demographics.

This issue spurred an internal assessment to find out what was happening. Conducting the assessment was difficult because the CDHS system was not fully supported by technology, and data mining was impossible. What ensued was a massive chart audit that helped everyone see the changing demographics and created the context for collective reflection. Based on this audit, policies and staffing needed to change, as did the competencies of the staff and the involvement of key individuals living in the communities that were reflected in the vulnerable population being served.

Solution

Amanda, in concert with the CDHS health officer, applied for a grant that the CDC made available to state departments with demonstrated need. The previous audit outcomes allowed her to be successful in demonstrating need; the grant was awarded, and monies to enhance the department's abilities were received.

This financial resource permitted the CDHS to hire additional staff, purchase necessary equipment, and provide the public health nurses with culturally accurate educational materials for the target population of TB cases and their contacts. Amanda reported that these grant monies allowed the CDHS Office of Public Health Nursing to add bilingual nursing or outreach staff to meet the language needs of the population, have a designated car for DOT home visits, provide annual updated and culturally sensitive TB Standards of Care education to all involved public health personnel, and enhance involvement of the communities and populations being served.

Outcome

As a result of these interventions, the treatment policies changed. DOT was provided daily by culturally sensitive staff, community understanding and involvement increased, TB treatment compliance increased, and the incidence of MDR-TB conversions decreased. These positive outcomes resulted in continued grant funding from the state, thus ensuring continuance of care. The cycle of public health assessment, policy development, and assurance had come full circle.

Conclusion

Vulnerability can be assigned to populations, and it can occur in individuals. There is a relationship among factors that lead to vulnerabilities. Using various examples from history and contemporary times, we see an evolving overarching framework in which we can explore the ideas surrounding vulnerability, disparity, advocacy, and policy. Nurses have responsibly acted upon the needs of vulnerable people over the past 100 years. From Wald's leadership in both urban and rural settings to nurses' responses today as they meet the needs of vulnerable people, this commitment continues. This chapter illustrates how nurses have and continue to execute political advocacy to bring vulnerable populations to the collective table as a way to mitigate the potential for adverse outcomes. In this way, it is hoped that the Declaration of Alma-Ata phrase "Health for All," can be realized.

Discussion Questions

1. As a group, discuss political advocacy. After the group develops a common understanding, delve into nursing databases, such as CINHAL or nursing history databases. Identify an article from the past that depicts the work of nurses as they engaged in the role of advocacy.
   a. Identify the time in history and describe what the presiding issue of the time was and what the population was experiencing with regard to the issue.
   b. How did the nurses of that time exemplify the role of advocate for the population?
   c. How did the nurses of the time engage in political advocacy?
2. As a group, discuss the various vulnerable populations that you have encountered in your practice.
   a. Identify the population and the presiding issue you are concerned about.
   b. Gather information about the issue and population.
   c. How can you advocate for this particular population with regard to the issue?
   d. How can you engage in political advocacy? Provide specific exemplars.
   e. How might you partner with the identified population to work together?

References

Aday, L. A. (2003). *At risk in America: The health and health care needs of vulnerable populations in the United States* (2nd ed.). San Francisco, CA: Jossey-Bass.

Benatar, S. R. (2013). Global health, vulnerable populations, and law. *Journal of Law, Medicine & Ethics, 41*(1), 42–47.

Carthon, J. M. B. (2011). Bridging the gaps: Collaborative health work in the city of brotherly love, 1900–1920. In P. D'Antonio & S. B. Lewenson (Eds.), *Nursing interventions through time: History as evidence* (pp. 75–87). New York, NY: Springer.

Courtwright, A. (2008). The social determinants of health: Moving beyond justice. *The American Journal of Bioethics, 8*(10), 16–17.

de Chesnay, M. (2011). Vulnerable populations: Vulnerable people. In M. de Chesnay & B. A. Anderson (Eds.), *Caring for the vulnerable: Perspectives in nursing theory, practice and research* (3rd ed., pp. 3–15). Sudbury, MA: Jones & Bartlett Learning.

District Nursing Association of Northern Westchester County. (1948). *The District Nursing Association Northern Westchester County, 1898–1948, Mount Kisco, NY.* Found in the Pace University Lienhard School of Historical Nursing Archives of Westchester /Rockland Counties, Birnbaum Library, Pleasantville, New York, HNAWRC, RT 97, .D61.

Dock, L. L., & Clement, F. (1922). From rural nursing to the public health nursing service. In L. L. Dock, C. D. Noyes, F. F. Clement, E.G. Fox, & A. R. VanMeter (Eds.), *History of the American Red*

Cross nursing (pp. 1211–1292). New York, NY: Macmillan.

Dorsen, C. (2010). Vulnerability in homeless adolescents: Concept analysis. *Journal of Advanced Nursing, 66*(12), 2819–2827.

Fairman, J., & D'Antonio, P. (2013). History counts: How history can shape our understanding of health policy. *Nursing Outlook, 61*(5), 346–352.

Federal Interagency Forum on Aging-Related Statistics. (2012). *Older Americans 2012: Key indicators of well-being.* Washington, DC: Author.

Flaskerud, J., & Winslow, B. W. (2010). Vulnerable populations and ultimate responsibility. *Issues in Mental Health Nursing, 31,* 298–299.

Gallagher, L. P., & Truglio-Londrigan, M. (2004). Using the "Seven A's" assessment tool for developing competency in case management. *Journal of the New York State Nurses Association, 35*(1), 26–32.

Grabovschi, C., Loignon, C., & Fortin, M. (2013). Mapping the concept of vulnerability related to health care disparities: A scoping review. *BMC Health Services Research, 13*(1), 1–11.

Institute for Alternative Futures. (n.d.). *The history of vulnerability in the United States.* Retrieved from http://altfutures.org/pubs/vuln2030/history.pdf

Keeling, A., & Lewenson, S. B. (2013). A nursing historical perspective on the medical home: Impact on health care policy. *Nursing Outlook, 61*(5), 360–366.

Krout, J. A. (1986). *The aged in rural America.* Westport, CT: Greenwood.

Krout, J. A. (Ed.). (1994). *Providing community-based services to the rural elderly.* Thousand Oaks, CA: Sage.

Lewenson, S. B. (1996). *Taking charge: Nursing, suffrage, and feminism, 1873–1930.* New York, NY: NLN Press.

Mechanic, D., & Tanner, J. (2007). Vulnerable people, groups, and populations: Societal view. *Health Affairs, 26*(5), 1220–1230.

Moscou, S. (2013). Fundamentals of epidemiology and social epidemiology. In M. Truglio-Londrigan

& S. B. Lewenson (Eds.), *Public health nursing: Practicing population-based care* (2nd ed., pp. 103–129). Burlington, MA: Jones &Bartlett Learning.

National Partnership for Action. (2011). *Health equity and disparities.* Retrieved from http://www.minorityhealth.hhs.gov/npa/templates/browse.aspx?lvl=1&lvlid=34

Patterson, K., Grenny, J., McMillan, R., & Switzler, Al. (2012). *Crucial conversations: Tools for talking when stakes are high.* New York, NY: McGraw-Hill.

Purdy, I. B. (2004). Vulnerable: A concept analysis. *Nursing Forum, 39*(4), 25–33.

Rogers, A. C. (1997). Vulnerability, health and health care. *Journal of Advanced Nursing, 26,* 65–72.

Shi, L., Stevens, G., Faed, P., & Tsai, J. (2008). Rethinking vulnerable populations in the US. *Harvard Health Policy Review, 9*(1), 43–48.

Smith, C. M., & Cotta, V. T. (2012). Normal aging changes: Nursing standard of practice protocol: Age related changes in health. In M. Boltz, E. Capezuti, T. Fulmer, & D. Zwicker (Eds.), *Evidence based geriatric nursing protocols for best practice* (4th ed., pp. 23–47). New York, NY: Springer.

Stevens, G., Shi, L., & Faed, P. (2008). Vulnerable in more than one way. *Health Affairs, 27*(3), 894–902.

Truglio-Londrigan, M., Singleton, J., Lewenson, S. B., & Lopez, L. (2013). Conversation about primary health care. In M. Truglio Londrigan & S. B. Lewenson (Eds.), *Public health nursing: Practicing population-based care* (2nd ed., pp. 399–413). Burlington, MA: Jones & Bartlett Learning.

Urban Institute. (2010). *Health policy center: Vulnerable populations.* Retrieved from http://www.urban.org/health_policy/vulnerable_populations/

U.S. Department of Health and Human Services, Agency for Healthcare Research and Quality. (2011). *National healthcare disparities report 2011.* Rockville, MD: Author.

U.S. Department of Health and Human Services, Office of Minority Health. National Partnership for Action to End Health Disparities. The

National Plan for Action. (2011). *Health equity and disparities*. Retrieved from http://www.minorityhealth.hhs.gov/npa/templates/browse.aspx?lvl=1&lvlid=34

U.S. Department of Health and Human Services/Healthy People 2020. (2010a). *Disparities*. Retrieved from http://www.healthypeople.gov/2020/about/DisparitiesAbout.aspx

U.S. Department of Health and Human Services/Healthy People 2020. (2010b) *Health services*. Retrieved from http://www.healthypeople.gov/2020/about/DOHAbout.aspx#healthservices

U.S. Department of Health and Human Services/Healthy People 2020. (2010c). *Determinants of health*. Retrieved from http://www.healthypeople.gov/2020/about/DOHAbout.aspx

U.S. Department of Health and Human Services/Healthy People 2020. (2010d). *Social*. Retrieved from http://www.healthypeople.gov/2020/about/DOHAbout.aspx#socialfactors

U.S. Department of Health and Human Services/Healthy People 2020. (2010e). *Access to health care*. Retrieved from http://www.healthypeople.gov/2020/topicsobjectives2020/overview.aspx?topicid=1

U.S. Department of Health and Human Services/Healthy People 2020. (2010f). *Individual behavior*. Retrieved from http://www.healthypeople.gov/2020/about/DOHAbout.aspx#individual

U.S. Department of Health and Human Services/Healthy People 2020. (2010g). *Biology and genetics*. Retrieved from http://www.healthypeople.gov/2020/about/DOHAbout.aspx#biology

U.S. Department of Health and Human Services/Healthy People 2020. (2010h). *Policymaking*. Retrieved from http://www.healthypeople.gov/2020/about/DOHAbout.aspx#policymaking

Williams, M., Ebrite, F., & Redford, L. (1991). *In-home services for the elders in rural America*. Kansas City, MO: National Resource Center for Rural Elderly.

World Health Organization. (1978). *Declaration of Alma-Ata*. Retrieved from http://www.who.int/publications/almaata_declaration_en.pdf

Healthcare Providers: Understanding How Power, Markets, and Government Impact Organization and Delivery of Care

CHAPTER 10

Hospitals: Consolidation and Compression

Nancy Aries and Barbara Caress

Overview

This chapter discusses the critical role of hospitals in the delivery of health care. Hospitals have historically been viewed as the hub of the healthcare system, accounting for more than one-third of personal healthcare expenditures. They have functioned independently given their history, the context of the communities in which they are located, and the financing system that supports them. The role of hospitals in the delivery system is slowly changing as a result of the evolving nature of healthcare delivery. While they are still dominant as the provider of tertiary care, they are slowly being integrated into a model of care that is population based and seeks to provide comprehensive and integrated care. This integration of services can be seen in the changes taking place in the relations between other institutional providers, such as nursing homes.

Objectives

- Understand the transformation of hospitals from social welfare providers, to acute care facilities, to providers within integrated systems of care.
- Identify how hospitals became the hub of the healthcare delivery system and the competing pressures for change.
- Explain how external pressures are changing the nature of hospital services.
- Delineate the strategies being used by hospitals to ensure their centrality to the provision of services and their quality of care.
- Assess the impact of the Affordable Care Act on the role of hospitals.

The Role of Hospitals within the Delivery System

Hospitals, as currently organized, provide an excellent example of the limits of using competitive markets to provide healthcare services. Superficially, hospitals look like the competitive suppliers of salable services that economics textbooks hail as the necessary condition for market-driven efficiency. The term *market* means a situation in which the sellers and buyers of a product come together voluntarily to exchange money for goods at a price that is set by the competition among all the sellers to attract willing and able buyers of the service in question. According to the theory, the pressure of competition will drive sellers to provide the best possible care at the lowest possible price.

Because U.S. hospitals are not part of a singular healthcare system, like the hospitals in Canada or other industrial nations, it would seem that they can operate as efficient textbook competitors in search of paying customers. The difficulty with this idealized market-based and regulation-free approach to hospital-based care is that hospitals acting in their own best interests in a situation where few customers can cover the costs will not always act in the best interests of the entire population in need of medical care. The dilemma is most obvious for hospitals that are intended to serve financially vulnerable populations, who cannot afford to pay the full costs of the care and do not have insurance to cover the difference. Such hospitals become financially vulnerable because they must rely on nonmarket sources of funding. Not surprisingly, in an era of government cutbacks, this has resulted in a large number of hospital closures since the 1990s (Cutler, 2009).

Consequently, there has been growing pressure to rationalize the delivery of healthcare services by moving away from competition and toward integration and cooperation to improve health system effectiveness and efficiency. With the passage of the Affordable Care Act (ACA), there is now an enhanced emphasis on improving the complementarity among currently independent facilities. By reorienting the entire healthcare system away from its emphasis on competition for paying patients to one that creates incentives for improving the quality of care and controlling costs across specific populations, it is believed that there is a potential for hospitals to become more fully integrated into organized systems of care and not stand-alone competitors that inefficiently duplicate services to attract individual paying customers. In this chapter, the development of the hospital sector will be explained, as will the impact of healthcare reform on hospitals and the industry's response.

Hospitals in a Historic Context

The origin of hospitals is more tied to the provision of social services than medical services. Before the Civil War, there were just a handful of hospitals, including Philadelphia General, Massachusetts General, and New York Hospital. These were often founded at the urging of doctors as workshops in which to study and train physicians. They were endowed by city elites and supported by the public because they cared for persons who had no family to care for them (Starr, 1982). As cities grew in number and size after the Civil War, the number of hospitals increased dramatically (Rosner, 1982). Given the social stresses due to immigration, industrialization, and urbanization, hospitals were critical to urban stability, and there was a new wave of hospitals built to respond to the defined needs of specific communities. These hospitals were a principal tool whereby community elites organized assistance to the poor and dislocated. The names of the hospitals told of their affiliations: Mount Sinai, Lutheran, St. Luke's, Methodist, and St. Vincent's. The goal was not just medical; the goal was to provide assistance in whatever form it was needed (Starr, 1982).

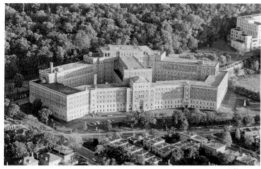

© Photos.com

The modern U.S. hospital industry was born between the 1860s and the 1920s as hospitals transformed from social welfare institutions to institutions that provided acute medical care. Rather than serving the generic needs of the community, the mission of the hospital became one of curing the acute problems of the sick. The change in purpose was related to the rise of biomedical sciences and medical technology. Scientific advances enabled physicians to provide services that could positively impact patient health, but many medical services could not be safely and efficiently provided in a patient's home. They required a centralized location where sterile conditions could be ensured and where equipment such as X-ray machines and pathology laboratories could be located. As a result, patients who would

benefit from medical intervention began to be treated in hospitals, whereas chronic or social problems, such as alcoholism or old age, that were not responsive to medical intervention were redefined as social services. By 1920, the transformation of the hospital was achieved in Philadelphia when Philadelphia General Hospital was reorganized as three distinct institutions: an acute care hospital, an asylum, and an almshouse (Rosenberg, 1982).

Beyond the growth of the hospital, two other transformations occurred. First, the hospital changed from an institution operated as charity into one run as a business. Hospitals were becoming costlier to operate because of changes resulting from scientific advances. Their business model that had relied on philanthropy was no longer tenable. Hospitals needed new sources of revenue. They began charging for services and opening their doors to private practitioners who had access to potentially paying middle-class patients. Once hospitals became dependent on private physicians to fill their beds, the second transformation occurred. Control passed from boards of trustees, drawn from among elite members of the community, to physicians who controlled admissions (the most important source of revenue) and ultimately the mission (Rosner, 1982). As hospitals grew in number and size, the role and influence of physicians also grew. One organized agent of the physician community, the American College of Surgeons, even sought to standardize hospital services. The college surveyed all hospitals to determine whether (1) physicians were licensed, (2) the medical staff met monthly, (3) there were accurate patient records, and (4) there were diagnostic and therapeutic facilities under competent supervision (Stevens, 1989).

By the late 1930s, hospitals had become the hub of the healthcare delivery system. It was the locus of both patient care and medical training. Centralizing care in increasingly complex institutions was the most important manifestation of the transformation of U.S. health care in the 20th century. Hospital care defined medical care as the treatment of injury and disease, not prevention and comfort, and physicians were its heart and soul (Rosenberg, 1982). Since that time, hospitals have fought to maintain their hegemony in this tremendously complex system and its disease-based focus on the provision of care.

Starting in the 1990s, the centrality of the hospital and its role in the organization of healthcare delivery became an important focus of health policy discussions. In part this was due to technological changes that meant care previously provided in hospitals could now be provided in ambulatory care settings. Changing surgical practices, for example, that enabled patients to be operated on and discharged the same day meant surgical suites could be disconnected from hospitals (Kalra, Fisher, & Axelrod, 2010). Second, managed care was becoming the dominant organization form for private health insurance, and its financial arrangements negatively impacted hospital utilization and costs (Baicker, Chenew, & Robbins, 2013). Taken together, these changes led the Clinton administration to advance integrated models of care in its national health insurance proposal. The common understanding was that the most complex patient care could be provided in a variety of settings. Therefore, the integration of services was critical so that patients did not become lost between care providers, and there was better management of healthcare costs.

Hospitals understood this need and looked for ways to integrate services under their roofs. Many hospitals, for example, purchased physician practices as a way to control the cost and

delivery of services. The movement toward integrated models of care, however, floundered with the move away from tightly controlled managed care and the possibility of healthcare reform. While it was an idea to which most policy analysts subscribed, reform was not formally on the public agenda until the passage of the Affordable Care Act (ACA) in 2010. The ACA makes the need for change more imminent. Medicare payments to hospitals will soon incorporate both physicians and posthospital care, meaning that independent providers must cooperate if they are to succeed financially. In addition, the incentives to organize Accountable Care Organizations (ACOs) for distinctive groups of patients will facilitate the development of integrated models of healthcare delivery that ultimately can be brought to scale.

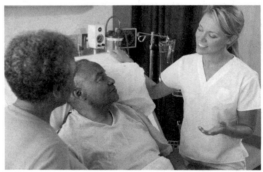

© Monkey Business Images/ShutterStock, Inc.

Baseline Information

In 1920, the second Hospital Census identified 5,700 institutions, practically the same number as today (Starr, 1982.) The number of hospitals peaked at approximately 6,500, and there are now 5,724 hospitals (American Hospital Association [AHA], 2013). Of these, 4,973 are community hospitals. A community hospital is broadly defined as a nonfederal, short-term, general, and other hospital whose services are available to the public (AHA, 2013). This definition excludes hospital units in institutions that are not available to the public, such as prisons. The average length of stay (LOS) in a community hospital must be less than 30 days. Discussions about hospitals typically refer to community hospitals. There are 751 noncommunity hospitals. Noncommunity hospitals include federal and long-term institutions (AHA, 2013). Federal hospitals refer to Veterans Health Administration hospitals, U.S. Public Health Service hospitals, and Marine hospitals. Long-term general hospitals refer to psychiatric hospitals, hospitals for tuberculosis and other respiratory diseases, institutions for the mentally disabled, alcohol and chemical dependency hospitals, and units in short-term institutions. The defining characteristic is a LOS that is greater than 30 days.

Tables 10-1 and 10-2 provide more detailed information about community hospitals. The number of community hospitals is declining. The hospitals that are currently closing include rural hospitals and urban hospitals that are financially at risk because they serve a patient population with limited ability to pay. The decreased number of beds results from the decreased average LOS despite the overall increase in admissions. With a growing and aging population, the number of surgical operations is increasing, as is the number of births—two of the primary services that filled the beds in midcentury U.S. hospitals; thus, one might expect increased demand for inpatient admissions. Nevertheless, as can be seen in Table 10-1, the number of hospital beds fell by more than 200,000 between 1982 and 2011, as have the number of admissions,

Table 10-1   Community Hospitals: 1980, 1990, 2000, 2010, and 2011

	1980	1990	2000	2011
Community hospitals	5,830	5,384	4,915	4,973
Beds	988,000	926,436	823,560	797,403
Beds/hospital	169	182	169	160
Admissions	36,143,000	31,181,046	33,089,467	34,843,085
Daily census	747,000	619,000	526,000	512,944
LOS	7.6	7.2	5.8	5.4
Inpatient days	2,784,060,002	225,971,653	192,420,368	187,072,013
Surgical operations	19,236,000	21,914,868	26,612,710	29,907,712
Inpatient surgeries	N/A	10,844,916	9,729,336	9,638,467
Outpatient surgeries	N/A	11,069,952	16,383,374	17,269,245
Bassinets	77,522	68,412	60,839	56,290
Births	3,408,482	3,958,263	3,880,166	3,730,342
Occupancy rate (%)	75.6	66.8	63.9	64.3
Outpatient visits	202,231,000	300,514,516	521,404,976	656,078,942

Source: Data from the American Hospital Association (2002, 2013).

despite the increase in the U.S. population and the increased number of births. During the same 25-year period, the number of outpatient encounters, however, has increased by more than 300%. When looking at surgical operations, for example, there is a steady increase in the number of outpatient surgeries and a slight decrease in the number of inpatients surgeries.

Table 10-2, which displays the U.S. hospital complement based on the average number of beds, is important because it shows that the typical community hospital is quite small—averaging between 50 and 200 beds. These are not large institutions endowed with facilities to provide the complexity of services required for many of the surgeries indicated in Table 10-1. It also stands in sharp contrast to a city like New York, where practically every hospital has more than 200 beds (New York State Department of Health, 2009). The larger hospitals tend to be academic medical centers that train physicians and care for people with complex medical and social problems. These hospitals find themselves in competition with smaller community hospitals. One dominates

in terms of numbers, and the other dominates in terms of prestige.

Hospital costs comprise the largest single portion of spending in the healthcare sector. More is spent on hospitals than on Social Security or defense (Kocher & Emanuel, 2012). In 2011, hospital spending was $850 billion, or 37%, of personal healthcare spending. As Table 10-3 indicates, the relative percentage of healthcare spending on hospitals rose dramatically between 1960 and 1980, to almost 50% of personal health care. Cost-control efforts on the part of the government and private health insurance companies have helped bring these costs down, and hospital spending is just slightly lower as a percentage of all healthcare spending than it was in 1960. Hospitals have been a prime driver of increasing healthcare costs since the passage of Medicare. As the average annual growth in healthcare spending has slowed, so has the growth in hospital spending. Since 2008, the rate of increase in hospital spending has been steadily declining. The source of payment has also changed considerably over the last 50 years.

Table 10-2 Number of Community Hospitals by Number of Beds: 1980, 1990, 2000, 2010, and 2011

Beds	1980	1990	2000	2010	2011
6–24	259	226	288	424	445
25–49	1,029	935	910	1,167	1,177
50–99	1,462	1,263	1,055	970	955
100–199	1,370	1,306	1,236	1,029	1,005
200–299	715	739	656	585	582
300–399	412	408	341	352	353
400–499	266	222	182	185	184
500+	317	285	247	273	272

Source: Data from Health, United States, 2013, Table 107.

Table 10-3   National Health Expenditures by Hospitals and Physicians and by Source of Funds: 1960, 1970, 1980, 1990, 2000, and 2011

Levels in $ millions	1960	1970	1980	1990	2000	2011
National health expenditures	27,487	74,857	253,389	714,148	1,352,855	2,700,700
Population	186	210	230	254	283	311
Personal health care	23,320	62,943	214,784	607,542	1,139,192	2,279,300
Hospital care	9,179	27,589	101,008	251,570	416,864	850,600
Private funds	5,301	12,357	47,444	119,607	179,669	378,000
Consumer payments	5,189	11,462	42,366	109,181	157,769	335,003
Out-of-pocket payments	1,904	2,491	5,406	11,319	13,651	28,113
Private health insurance	3,284	8,971	36,960	97,862	144,118	306,890
Other private funds	113	895	5,078	10,426	21,900	42,997
Public funds	3,878	15,233	53,564	131,963	237,196	464,388
Federal funds	1,552	9,961	40,537	101,690	191,866	385,548
State and local funds	2,326	5,272	13,027	30,273	45,330	78,840
Physician and clinical services	5,353	13,981	47,074	157,548	288,621	541.4
Hospital care as percentage of personal health care (%)	39.4	43.8	47.0	41.4	36.6	37.3
Contribution of source						
Private funds (%)	57.8	44.8	47.0	47.5	43.1	44.4
Consumer payments (%)	56.5	41.5	41.9	43.4	37.8	39.3
Out-of-pocket payments (%)	20.7	9.0	5.4	4.5	3.3	3.3
Private health insurance (%)	35.8	32.5	36.6	38.9	34.6	36.1
Other private funds (%)	1.2	3.2	5.0	4.1	5.3	3.3
Public funds (%)	42.2	55.2	53	52.5	56.9	54.6
Federal funds (%)	16.9	36.1	40.1	40.4	46	45.3
State and local funds %)	25.3	19.1	12.9	12.0	10.9	9.3

Source: Data from Centers for Medicare and Medicaid Services (2013b).

The government is the largest single payer of hospital costs. This is a direct result of the passage of Medicare and Medicaid in 1965. In 2011, public funds accounted for almost 55% of hospital costs. The federal share of hospital expenditures increased from 17% in 1960 to 45% in 2011. It is anticipated that the federal spending on health care will increase with the implementation of the ACA in 2014 as more persons have access to health insurance (Congressional Budget Office, 2013). The second largest source of funds is private. As government funding increased, there was a decline in consumer payments from 56% to almost 40%. This decline was also marked by the dramatic decline in out-of-pocket payments to hospitals. Between 1960 and 2011, these payments decreased from 20% to just over 3% of hospital expenditures, but they are rising as costs are shifted from private health insurers to patients.

There are three types of community hospitals, based on ownership. Nonprofit hospitals include both community-based hospitals and academic health centers. Public hospitals are state and locally owned hospitals. Last are privately owned or for-profit hospitals (Starr, 1982). Ownership creates different financial and legal constraints on the institutions that impact both the population served and the underlying financing of the institution. Two major shifts can be seen in the distribution of hospitals and hospital beds by ownership type, as seen in Table 10-4. The first is the steady decline in the number of nonprofit community hospitals. The hospitals that have been lost were the most financially vulnerable. They typically served low-income populations that were either uninsured or did not have adequate insurance coverage. In addition, they had fewer beds and decreased operating margins (Daugherty & Escobedo, 2013). Alternatively, there has been growth in the for-profit sector that can be attributed to the purchase of failing nonprofit hospitals (Ault, Childs, Wainright, Young, & Williams, 2011). These changes are

Table 10-4   Community Hospitals by Ownership Type

Year	1980	1990	2000	2010	2011
Nonprofit hospitals	3,339	3,191	3,003	2,904	2,903
Number of beds	692,459	657,000	583000	556,000	547,804
% of beds	70%	70.9%	71%	69%	69%
Public state/local hospitals	1,835	1,444	1,163	1,068	1,045
Number of beds	208,895	169,000	131,000	125,000	121,228
% of beds	21%	18.2%	15.9%	15.5%	15.2%
For-profit hospitals	730	749	749	1,013	1,025
Number of beds	87,033	101,000	110,000	125,000	128,371
% of beds	9%	10.9%	13.3%	15.5%	16.1%
Total number of hospitals	5,904	5,384	4,915	4,985	4,973
Total number of hospital beds	988,000	927,000	824,000	804,093	797,403

Source: Data from American Hospital Association (2002, 2009, 2013).

attributed to the increasingly market-based organization of health care. The concern is that the loss of community hospitals will result in low-income patients having even fewer options available for hospital care (Bazzoli, Lee, Hsieh, & Mobley, 2012).

Challenges Facing Community Hospitals

The pressures experienced by hospitals since the 1980s are related, in part, to the rapidly changing knowledge about the management and treatment of disease and in part to increased efforts to control costs that were

becoming an ever-larger share of domestic spending. Hospitals find themselves contending with excess capacity despite the closure of many hospitals and an increasing competitive market for hospital services that make survival dependent on them generating adequate revenues to cover costs.

Excess Capacity

Hospitals have been forced to deal with surplus inpatient capacity because of declining admissions and decreased LOS. There are almost 1.5 million fewer admissions today than there were in 1980 despite the fact that the population has increased by more than

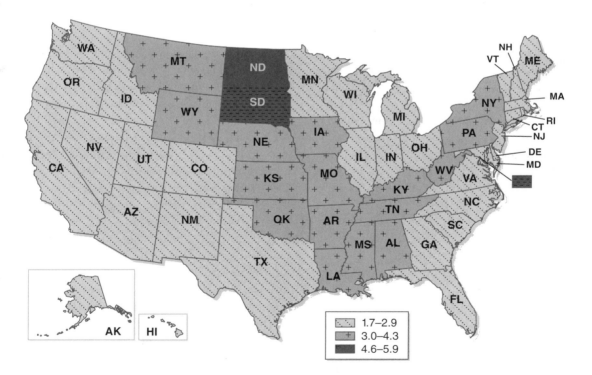

FIGURE 10-1 Hospital beds per 1,000 population, 2007

Data from: Kaiser Family Foundation. (2013). *Hospital beds per 1,000 population, 2011.* Retrieved from http://kff.org/other/state-indicator/beds/#

80 million persons. In addition to the declining rate of admissions, between 1980 and 2011, there has been a steady decline in the average LOS in the United States. In 1980, the average LOS was 7.6 days, and in 2011, the average LOS was 5.4 days, a decrease of 29%. (Table 10-1). As a result, the occupancy rate of U.S. hospitals is about 65% (Litvak & Bisognano, 2011).

While the number of inpatient beds has remained relatively flat, the number of beds per 1,000 population has decreased, as has the number of inpatient days per 100,000 persons. Despite lower ratios of beds and inpatient days to population, there remains a problem of excess capacity, but it is not equally distributed across all hospitals. There is little correlation between excess capacity and the number of inpatient beds. In areas where there are fewer beds and fewer inpatient days, there is excess hospital capacity. There may also be less excess capacity in areas where there are more beds and inpatient days per 1000,000 population. There is also variation in the number of of inpatient days per 100,000 persons and hospital occupancy rates across the country (DeLia & Wood, 2008). Long-standing variation in medical practice patterns contributes to this problem (Mechanic, 2011).

The decline in admissions and LOS is a result of many factors. First, there has been an improvement in the nation's health. The incidence of breast cancer in women younger than age 65 years, for example, is declining. The same is true for coronary disease, cardiovascular disease, and pneumonia. In addition, there are growing alternatives to hospitalization. The management of diseases and conditions that required hospitalization has changed dramatically. Scientific advances have minimized the invasive nature of many procedures and changed our understanding of how best to care

for patients (Kalra et al., 2010). Myriad surgeries and diagnostic and other procedures can be done in ambulatory settings, and ambulatory surgery centers, diagnostic imaging, and radiological centers are being opened throughout the country (Mitchell, 2007). The problem of excess capacity has also been attributed to the management of patient admissions for elective procedures (Litvak & Bisognano, 2011). During peak periods, hospitals operate at full capacity, and patients are boarded in the hallways of emergency departments. During periods of low demand, the hospitals and staff are underused.

Reductions in admissions and LOS have also been impacted by payment methodologies. The first studies of health maintenance organizations found that hospital admissions decreased by as much as 40% (Luft, 1981). The declining LOS picked up steam with the implementation of hospital payment based on Diagnosis-Related Groups (DRGs) in 1983.* DRGs reinforced the incentive to discharge patients more quickly because hospitals bore the cost for patients with extended hospital stays. The growth of managed care further impacted hospitals as physicians were incentivized through risk-sharing contracts to treat patients in less costly settings and better manage the length of hospital stays (Draper, Hurley, Lesser, & Strunk, 2002). The issue of hospital capacity will be further complicated by implementation of the Medicaid expansion and the health insurance exchanges because they are expected to increase demand for services. Given the cost of opening new beds, it is expected that

---

*Diagnosis-Related Group is a system of payment for hospital inpatient services based on predetermined rates per discharge for approximately 500 groupings. It was developed for Medicare and has been in use since 1983. A Medicare recipient is assigned to a payment group depending on the principal diagnosis. Other criteria include the patient's age, sex, secondary diagnoses, procedures performed, discharge status, complications, and comorbidities.

hospitals will be pressured to better manage patient flows (Litvak & Bisognano, 2011).

Increasingly Competitive Financial Environment

Hospital financing has gone through three distinct phases. Initially hospitals were financed by philanthropic giving. Hospital matrons would sit with wealthy trustees to negotiate a budget that they would fund through annual donations (Rosner, 1982). These donations became the means by which the hospital's small administration staff was expected to operate the facility. By the early decades of the 20th century, hospitals needed more income than their benefactors could regularly provide. They became increasingly dependent on patient payments for service. With the stock market crash of 1929 and ensuing financial calamity, hospital revenues fell dramatically. One response was the organization of Blue Cross as a way to guarantee patient payment for hospital services. The idea originated in Dallas, where Baylor Hospital contracted with the teachers' union to provide 21 days of care for $6 per year. Blue Cross, which began as a wholly owned subsidiary of the hospital trade group, the American Hospital Association brought this financing model to scale nationally (Law, 1976). Blue Cross and other retrospective payers covered the costs associated with a specific segment of the hospital's patients. Retrospective payment in simple terms meant there was an annual reckoning. At the end of the year, Blue Cross would pay its share of hospital costs. If 50% of the patient days were attributed to Blue Cross subscribers, Blue Cross would pay half of the hospitals' annual expenses. Medicare was established in 1965 with a similar reimbursement scheme.

This inherently inflationary payment mechanism was replaced in the 1980s with prospective payment. In this third phase of hospital financing, led by the introduction of Medicare's Prospective Payment System in 1983, hospitals were paid a fixed amount based on the type of illness and type of patient—known as DRGs. The theory underlying this reimbursement system was that hospitals would increase efficiency to cover their costs. There is some evidence that this happened (Lee, Berenson, Mayes, & Gauthier, 2003). On the other hand, critics charged that hospitals were discharging patients "sicker and quicker" to achieve the same ends (Qian, Russell, Valiyeva, & Miller, 2011, p. 1). Private insurers adopted similar reimbursement schemes. By the early 1990s, virtually all hospital reimbursement systems contained some element of the prospective payment, case-based system.

It is now the case that many payers are not paying hospitals for their full costs. With the growth of managed care and the power of private insurers to direct where patients receive care, hospitals have had to provide steep discounts in exchange for a guaranteed share of patients. Medicare and Medicaid, the public payers, accounted for 57% of all hospital care in 2010, but they reimbursed hospitals at less than full cost (AHA, 2012). Medicare paid only 92 cents for every dollar of care for a Medicare patient, and Medicaid paid only 93 cents on the dollar. The combined funding shortfall for hospital care was almost $28 billion. Whether hospitals discount rates to private insurers is more dependent on the market. When hospitals are part of systems, they can dictate prices to insurers. Where there is an insurance concentration, the payers can negotiate lower prices (Frakt, 2010).

The other area where financial stress can be seen is in access to capital (Robinson, 2002). Without adequate capital, hospitals cannot replace or modernize outdated facilities, respond to changing demands, such as the growth of outpatient surgery, or add new technology or equipment. Hospitals are encouraged to finance debt because all interest and depreciation expenses are treated as allowable costs and can be built into their hospital payments from public and private insurance companies. For-profit hospitals have greater access to capital because they can sell stocks and bonds in public markets. Nonprofit and public hospitals finance most capital needs through tax-exempt revenue bonds. Multihospital systems with substantial assets and cash flow have an easier time gaining access to capital markets than freestanding hospitals. Those in the worst position are inner-city hospitals. Competition for scarce resources reinforces the situation in which the strongest and best-financed hospitals get stronger, and the weak get weaker.

Vulnerable Hospitals Serve Vulnerable Populations

Financial shortfalls are not evenly spread across all hospitals. Hospitals with the highest proportion of paying patients are the most economically viable. Hospitals that disproportionately serve the working poor, unemployed, those with inadequate insurance, undocumented immigrants, and Medicaid patients are most vulnerable due to low reimbursement rates that do not cover costs (Tompkins, Altman, & Eilat, 2006). These might be public or nonprofit hospitals.

The financial well-being of public hospitals is further complicated by their provision of unprofitable services that are highly labor intensive (Horwitz, 2005). These are typically inpatient and outpatient services that combine medical and social services that many nonprofit hospitals find too costly to offer. In the 10 largest cities, public hospitals account for 12% of acute care hospitals, but they provide 24% of emergency visits and 33% of outpatient visits. These hospitals represent 37% of Level I trauma providers and 57% of the beds for burn patients (National Association of Public Hospitals and Health Systems, 2012). Their debt is picked up by local governments, but the tax base is not adequate in poorer communities to ensure their survival. Local tax revenues have risen less quickly than hospital costs.

Hospitals in rural areas were largely built as a result of the Hill-Burton legislation (Dowell, 1987). To distribute funds equitably across the 50 states, money went into the construction of hospitals in communities of less than 10,000 persons. There are currently 2,000 rural hospitals, which is 40% of all nonfederal hospitals. Rural hospitals are even more financially vulnerable than many inner-city community hospitals because they tend to be smaller, have fewer than 50 beds, and cannot offer highly complex care. As a result, many medical procedures that might have been done in such a facility can now be done on an outpatient basis. The result is occupancy rates of less than 40%. In addition, rural hospitals receive a lower DRG rate than urban hospitals, and they have increased debt from the uncollected bills of very poor patients (Chul-Young & Moon, 2005). Recognizing the need for hospitals in rural communities, Medicare has created a category of rural hospital called Critical Access Hospitals (CAHs). CAHs have an average LOS of 96 hours and no more than 25 beds, and they are reimbursed based on costs, as opposed to fixed reimbursement rates (Centers for Medicare and Medicaid Services, 2013a).

Hospital Strategies in a Competitive Market

With their survival dependent on generating adequate revenues to cover costs, hospitals have invested in two strategies to ensure their financial viability and control the market for healthcare services. The first is the creation of formalized networks so hospitals strengthen their competitive position vis-à-vis health insurers. The second is to affiliate with physicians so that hospitals do not compete with local doctors who can increasingly provide a wide range of services in ambulatory settings.

Networks and Systems

Hospitals have sought to control the healthcare market through consolidations and mergers (Kocher & Emanuel, 2012). Physicians and patients prefer the arrangement, and it has proved financially beneficial to hospitals. Because they control the supply of services, hospitals are in a position to dictate prices. As a result, prices for hospital care are reported to be 13–25% higher where there is market consolidation (Kendall, 2012).

Starting in 1999, the American Hospital Association began reporting statistics on the number of hospitals that were identified as part of hospital systems, which were defined as "a corporate body that may own and/or manage health provider facilities or health-related subsidiaries as well as non-health-related facilities including freestanding and/or subsidiary corporations" (AHA, 2013, Chart 2-4). The number of mergers per year has been increasing since 2000. Over the last 10 years, there have been more than 590 hospital takeovers. The number is once again on the rise following the recession; there were 51 mergers and acquisitions in 2009

(during the recession), 75 mergers and acquisitions in 2010, and 86 mergers and acquisitions in 2011 (Irving Levin Associates, 2012). In 2011, a total of 3,007, or 60%, of all community hospitals identified themselves as being part of a system (AHA, 2013).

Hospital–Physician Alignment

Hospitals have also sought to control patient admissions through their relationship to physicians who direct patient care. Affiliations with primary care physicians ensure referrals into hospitals from specialty practices whose services are highly lucrative, such as cardiothoracic surgery. Many younger physicians and physicians in primary care who face reimbursement rates that have been relatively constant and who want more balanced lifestyles also seek employment in hospitals. It is a way for them to have greater leverage when negotiating rates with insurers and have steadier hours (O'Malley, Bond, & Berenson, 2011).

Hospitals began purchasing physician practices in the 1990s. They initially lost money on these arrangements because compensation was based on salary, not productivity (Kocher & Sahni, 2011). Poorly developed contracts guaranteed physicians almost 100% of their previous year's salary, but physicians continued to provide lucrative services in settings not affiliated with the hospitals (O'Malley et al., 2011). Once again, hospitals are looking to employ physicians. In part this is driven by fear that physicians will become competitors by aggregating into larger integrated groups that direct referrals and utilization to their own advantage. Hospitals with robust employment strategies believe they will be positioned to compete under a variety of reimbursement scenarios because hospital-employed primary care physicians generally direct patients to their own hospitals and the specialists affiliated with them (Kocher & Emanuel, 2012). If the fee-for-service system persists, large physician networks will provide hospitals with greater negotiating power when contracting with health plans. Conversely, if the payment system moves toward risk-based reimbursement, large outpatient networks will allow a system to shift patients away from higher cost hospital-based care and capture revenue that otherwise would have been lost.

The ACA and the Rationalization of Hospital Care

The ACA will also impact the ways in which hospitals operate. Built into the legislation are provisions that address both the organizational fragmentation of the healthcare system and the financial incentives that have led to rapidly increasing costs. The provisions related to the organization of ACOs create a mechanism whereby providers who previously operated independently within a community develop mechanisms that assure patients of receiving comprehensive and continuous care. In addition, the ACA uses the reimbursement system to support the alignment of these providers. While ACOs and pay-for-performance are still in their infancy, they create legislative incentives to improve quality and control costs.

ACOs and the Alignment of Services

The concept of integrated care is not new. It originated with the development of health maintenance organizations in the 1930s. These organizations bore the risk of ensuring that patients received all-inclusive services. With the growth of managed care in the late 1980s,

there was pressure for hospitals to integrate services both vertically and horizontally. The rationale for integration was twofold. By creating a continuum of care, quality could be improved, and by reorganizing payment using global capitation and risk contracting, there could be greater efficiency. The assumptions that drove the growth of managed care were incorrect. The projected economies of scale did not follow the development of these first integrated systems. The synergies did not occur between the partners because integration became a financial strategy to protect hospital position (Burns & Pauly, 2001).

The term *Accountable Care Organization* was first used in 2006 as a new way to explain efforts to advance integration by making care providers responsible for both the quality and the costs of care. This would be achieved through payments linked to quality improvement. Demonstration programs funded by the Centers for Medicare and Medicaid Services (CMS) led to the inclusion of language pertaining to ACOs in the ACA. The ACA created the Medicare Shared Savings Program (MSSP) that encourages voluntary groups of physicians, hospitals, and other healthcare providers to become identified as ACOs. According to the legislation, over a 3-year period, the ACOs will accept responsibility for the overall quality, cost, and care of a defined group of at least 5,000 Medicare beneficiaries. By including the MSSP into the ACO, it becomes a permanent option under Medicare.

Achieving the goals stipulated by the MSSP requires better care coordination. Hospitals have already recognized the need for better internal coordination of services because poor coordination can result in longer lengths of stays as patients wait for needed services, or poor quality of care because services are not provided in a timely way. In addition, patients often experience avoidable readmissions. Better care coordination among providers can result in fewer hospitalizations, reduced hospital and nursing home stays, and lower monthly medical costs (Bielaszka-DuVernay, 2011). This is particularly true of an aging population, who has the highest rate of hospitalizations (Bynum, Andrews, Sharp, McCollough, & Wennberg, 2011). There are even studies documenting the success of multistate programs to address barriers to better coordination among providers (Boutwell et al., 2011). At this time, there is no one model to achieve this end, and multiple innovations have been tried. A shared feature of many programs is the use of nurses as care leaders (Naylor, Aiken, Kurtzman, Olds, & Hirschman, 2011). What is important is the growing evidence that a mix of providers is needed to provide continuous and comprehensive care for quality improvement.

There is also growing evidence that better care coordination will not be simple to achieve and that creating ACOs can be costly. They rely heavily on shared information systems that will enable providers in different practice settings to work from the same database and avoid unnecessary duplication of services or suffer from lack of information about prior medical care. The implementation of electronic health records, however, is expensive and raises complex problems related to data compatibility and data sharing (Friedman, Parrish, & Ross, 2013). At this time, 94% of hospitals have installed electronic health records, and 59% are sophisticated enough to receive certification for their electronic health record systems (Charles, Gabriel, & Furukawa, 2014). Small nonteaching hospitals and rural hospitals have been slow adopters, as have smaller physician practices (DesRoches, Worzala, Joshi, Kralovec, & Jha, 2012).

There are also mixed results as to whether care coordination reduces overall healthcare costs. In one Medicare demonstration that involved 15 programs in a randomized controlled trial, the cost of intensive support was comparable with the costs of the hospitalizations. Although hospitalizations were reduced and patients received what was deemed to be better care, lower costs were dependent on the ability to control the costs of the care coordination (Brown, Peikes, Peterson, Schore, & Razafindrakoto, 2012).

Payment Reform to Improve Quality

Payment methodologies can also influence how medicine is practiced. Policy makers attempt to design reimbursement systems that incentivize practitioners to coordinate care and control costs. Starting in 1983, when Medicare implemented prospective payment, LOS began to decline. The impact of DRGs on overall costs was clear as hospitals shifted costs to other payers and shifted services to more profitable areas (Altman, 2012). In 2011, Medicare extended the concept of DRGs and bundled physician services and postoperative care into the prospective payment system. By bundling payment, payment systems reinforce care coordination by aligning the interests of physicians, hospitals, and postoperative care providers. However, like the DRG system, if only one payer (Medicare) changes the way that payment is structured, hospitals will find alternative ways to minimize the potential impact of the change. To be effective, it is critical that all payers become part of the system.

Pay-for-performance is another strategy to control costs and improve quality by better aligning hospitals and doctors. Pay-for-performance adjusts the fee-for-service payment system by making higher payments for higher quality care. The concept is intuitively appealing, but pay-for-performance programs have had mixed results (Werner & Dudley, 2012). Whether the problem lies with the size of the incentive, the involvement of the hospital in related quality improvement efforts, or the availability of resources to support improvement efforts is unknown. CMS supported a demonstration that compared 260 hospitals that participated in the pilot program and 780 hospitals that participated in a control group. The hospitals that participated showed performance gains, but over 5 years, the control group caught up. In addition, hospitals that were well financed or in less competitive markets performed better. The Medicare pay-for-performance program that was included in the ACA is modeled on the CMS pilot program. As of October 2012, a pool of $850 million has been divided among more than 3,000 eligible hospitals. The program will impact current hospital payment because the pool was created by reducing DRG payments. However, the actual impact of the program on hospital quality is unknown because the change of payment is relatively small given the size of the pool. It is estimated that for two-thirds of the hospitals, the change might be only 1%, thus limiting the incentive for hospitals to change existing practices if no other initiatives are under way (Werner & Dudley, 2012).

Healthcare Policy, Health Reform, and the Role of Hospitals

Hospitals remain at the center of the U.S. healthcare delivery system. Although many hospitals have formed alliances with physicians and other providers and many have merged into multihospital systems, the hospital sector remains as it was at the beginning of the 20th century: roughly 5,000 separate institutions that function independently.

Since the 1970s, health policy experts have documented the need for greater integration. There is an emerging consensus among policy makers about the need to foster the growth of integrated systems and development of payment reform systems that support greater integration. The ACA has taken the first steps to incorporate the integration of healthcare providers into systems that serve population-based need and to restructure the payment system to incentivize providers who provide coordinated and continuous care. These are just the first steps to healthcare reform. Hospitals account for more than one-third of the $2.3 trillion spent in the U.S. health system in 2011 (Table 10-3). With such gigantic sums comes an enormous capacity to influence public policy. Although hospitals operate independently, they have banded together into a potent political force to defend that autonomy. According to the Center for Responsive Politics (2014), hospitals and nursing homes employed 875 lobbyists who spent $91 million to influence healthcare reform during 2013.

This is clearly a case where rational common interests and rational individual interests are in conflict. Our inability to transcend the conflict produces what Garret Hardin described more than four decades ago as a "tragedy of commons" (1968, p. 1244). The solution is simple to state but difficult to achieve. It is not enough to charge the stakeholders with acting irresponsibly and demand better behavior, but it is important to change what is in their best interest. Nurses can play a large role in making this happen because they are proving to be central players in the provision of efficient and effective care.

Discussion Questions

1. How do you explain the independence of any particular hospital and its centrality to the healthcare system?
2. Why have hospitals experienced declining LOS and admissions over time?
3. How have hospitals sought to ensure their position within the communities they serve?
4. To what extent are hospitals' quests for integration different from, and the same as, the drive for better care coordination under the ACA?

References

Altman, S. (2012). Lessons from Medicare's prospective payment for hospital bundled payment. *Health Affairs, 31*(9), 1923–1929.

American Hospital Association. (2002). *Hospital statistics*. Chicago, IL: Health Forum.

American Hospital Association. (2009). *AHA hospital statistics*. Chicago, IL: Health Forum.

American Hospital Association. (2012). *Underpayment by Medicare and Medicaid fact sheet, 2012 update*. Chicago, IL: Health Forum.

American Hospital Association. (2013). *AHA hospital statistics*. Chicago, IL: Health Forum.

Ault, K., Childs, B., Wainright, C., Young, M., & Williams, M. D. (2011). Relevant factors to consider prior to an investor-owned acquisition of a nonprofit healthcare entity. *Journal of Healthcare Management,56*(4), 269–281.

Baicker, K., Chernew, M., & Robbins, J. (2013). *The spillover effects of Medicare managed care: Medicare advantage and hospital utilization* (NBER Working Paper No. 19070. JEL No. I1,I13,I18). Retrieved from http://www.nber.org/papers/w19070.pdf

Bazzoli, G. J., Lee, W., Hsieh, H., & Mobley, L. R. (2012). The effects of safety net hospital closures and conversions on patient travel distance to hospital services. *Health Services Research, 47*(11), 129–150.

Bielaszka-DuVernay, C. (2011). Improving the coordination of care for Medicaid beneficiaries in Pennsylvania. *Health Affairs, 30*(3), 431–438.

Boutwell, A. E., Johnson, M. B., Rutherford, P., Watson, S. R., Vecchioni, N., Auerback, B. S., . . . Wagner, C. (2011). An early look at a four-state initiative to reduce avoidable hospital readmissions. *Health Affairs, 30*(7), 1272–1280.

Brown, R. S., Peikes, D., Peterson, G., Schore, J., & Razafindrakoto, C. M. (2012). Six features of Medicare coordinated care demonstration programs that cut hospital admissions of high-risk patients. *Health Affairs, 31*(6), 1156–1165.

Burns, L., & Pauly, M. (2001). Integrated delivery networks: A detour on the road to integrated health care? *Health Affairs, 20*(6), 128–143.

Bynum, J. P. W., Andrews, A., Sharp, S., McCollough, D., & Wennberg, J. E. (2011). Fewer hospitalizations result when primary care is highly integrated in to a continuing care retirement community. *Health Affairs, 30*(5), 975–983.

Center for Responsive Politics. (2014). *OpenSecrets.org*. Retrieved from https://www.opensecrets.org/lobby/indusclient.php?id=H02&year=2013

Centers for Medicare and Medicaid Services. (2013a). *Critical access hospital: Rural health fact sheet series*. Retrieved from https://www.cms.gov/Outreach-and-Education/Medicare-Learning-Network-MLN/MLNProducts/downloads/CritAccessHospfctsht.pdf

Centers for Medicare and Medicaid Services. (2013b). *The National Health Expenditure Accounts (NHEA)*. Retrieved from http://www.cms.gov/Research-Statistics-Data-and-Systems/Statistics-Trends-and-Reports/NationalHealthExpendData/index.html?redirect=/nationalhealthexpenddata/

Charles, D., Gabriel, M., & Furukawa, M. F. (2014). *Adoption of electronic health record systems among U.S. non-federal acute care hospitals: 2008-2013.* Office of the National Coordinator for Health Information Technology, ONC Data Brief, No. 16. Retrieved from http://www.healthit.gov/sites/default/files/oncdatabrief16.pdf

Chul-Young, R., & Moon, M. J. (2005). Nearby, but not wanted? The bypassing of rural hospitals and policy implications for rural health care systems. *Policy Studies Journal, 33*(3), 377–394.

Congressional Budget Office. (2013). *Updated budget projections: Fiscal years 2013 to 2023.* Retrieved from http://www.cbo.gov/sites/default/files/cbofiles/attachments/44172-Baseline2.pdf

Cutler, D. (2009). The next wave of corporate medicine—how we all might benefit. *New England Journal of Medicine, 361,* 549–551. Retrieved from http://dx.doi.org/10.1056/NEJMp0904259

Daugherty, D. A., & Escobedo, E. (2013). An empirical study of the determinants of safety-net hospital failures. *Global Conference on Business & Finance Proceedings, 8.2,* 79–88. Hilo, HI: Institute for Business and Finance Research.

DeLia, D., & Wood, E. (2008). TRENDS: The dwindling supply of empty beds: Implications for hospital surge capacity. *Health Affairs, 27*(6), 1688–1694.

DesRoches, C. M., Worzala, C., Joshi, M. S., Kralovec, P. D., & Jha, A. K. (2012). Small, nonteaching, and rural hospitals continue to be slow in adopting electronic health record systems. *Health Affairs, 31*(5), 1092–1099.

Dowell, M. (1987). Hill-Burton: The unfulfilled promise. *The Journal of Health Politics, Policy and Law, 12*(1), 153–176.

Draper, D. A., Hurley, R. E., Lesser, C. S., & Strunk, B. C. (2002). The changing face of managed care. *Health Affairs, 21*(1), 11–23.

Frakt, A. (2010). *Expert voices: The future of health care costs: Hospital-insurer balance of power.* Retrieved from http://www.nihcm.org/pdf/EV_Frakt_FINAL.pdf

Friedman, D. J., Parrish, R. G., & Ross, D. A. (2013). Electronic health records and US public health: Current realities and future promise. *American Journal of Public Health, 103*(9), 1560–1567.

Hardin, G. (1968). The tragedy of the commons. *Science, 162*(5364), 1243–1248. Retrieved from http://www.sciencemag.org/cgi/reprint/162/3859/1243.pdf

Health, United States. (2013). Table 107. Retrieved from http://www.ncbi.nlm.nih.gov/books/NBK209225/table/trendtables.t107/?report=objectonly

Horwitz, J. R. (2005). Making profits and providing care: Comparing nonprofit, for-profit, and government hospitals. *Health Affairs, 24*(3), 790–801.

Irving Levin Associates. (2012). *Decade in review: Hospital M&A deal volume increases.* Retrieved from http://www.levinassociates.com/pr2012/pr1202hospital

Kalra, A. D., Fisher, R. S., & Axelrod, P. (2010). Decreased length of stay and cumulative hospitalized days despite increased patient admissions and readmissions in an area of urban poverty. *Journal of General Internal Medicine, 25*(9), 930–935. doi:10.1007/s11606-010-1370-5

Kendall, B. (2012, March 18). Regulators seek to cool hospital-deal fever. *The Wall Street Journal.* Retrieved from http://online.wsj.com/article/SB10001424052702303863404577286071837740832.html

Kocher B., & Emanuel, E. J. (2012). Overcoming the pricing power of hospitals. *Journal of the American Medical Association, 308*(12), 1213–1214. doi:10.1001/2012.jama.11910

Kocher, R., & Sahni, N. R. (2011). Hospitals' race to employ physicians—the logic behind a money-losing proposition. *New England Journal of Medicine, 364*(19), 1790–1793.

Law, S. (1976). *Blue Cross: What went wrong?* New Haven, CT: Yale University Press.

Lee, J. S., Berenson, R. A., Mayes, R., & Gauthier, A. K. (2003). Medicare payment policy: Does cost shifting matter? *Health Affairs.* Retrieved from http://content.healthaffairs.org/content /early/2003/10/08/hlthaff.w3.480.full.pdf

Litvak, E., & Bisognano, M. (2011). More patients, less payment: Increasing hospital efficiency in the aftermath of health reform. *Health Affairs*, *30*(1), 76–80.

Luft, H. S. (1981). *Health maintenance organizations: Dimensions of performance*. New York, NY: John Wiley and Sons.

Mechanic, D. (2011). The "brilliant, persistent" pursuit of health care as a complex social system. *Health Affairs*, *30*(2), 362.

Mitchell, J. M. (2007). *Utilization changes associated with physician ownership of ambulatory surgery centers (ASCs)*. Retrieved from http://ssrn.com /abstract=992622

National Association of Public Hospitals and Health Systems. (2012). *America's safety net hospitals and health systems, 2010: Results of the NAPH annual hospital characteristics survey*. Retrieved from http://essentialhospitals.org/wp-content /uploads/2013/12/NPH214.pdf

Naylor, M. D., Aiken, L. H., Kurtzman, E. T., Olds, D. M., & Hirschman, K. B. (2011). The importance of transitional care in achieving health reform. *Health Affairs*, *30*(4) 746–754.

New York State Department of Health. (2009). *Hospital profile*. Retrieved from http://hospitals. nyhealth.gov/

O'Malley, A. S., Bond, A. M., & Berenson, R. A. (2011). *Issue brief no. 136: Rising hospital employment of physicians: Better quality, higher costs?* Retrieved from http://www.hschange.com /CONTENT/1230/

Qian, X., Russell L. B., Valiyeva, E., & Miller, J. E. (2011). "Quicker and sicker" under Medicare's prospective payment system for hospitals: new evidence on an old issue from a national longitudinal survey. *Bulletin of Economic Research*, *63*(1), 1-27.

Robinson, J. C. (2002). Bond-market skepticism and stock-market exuberance in the hospital industry. *Health Affairs*, *21*(1), 104–117.

Rosenberg, C. E. (1982). From almshouse to hospital: The shaping of Philadelphia General Hospital. *Milbank Memorial Fund Quarterly*, *60*(1), 108–154.

Rosner, D. (1982). *A once charitable enterprise: Hospital and health care in Brooklyn and New York, 1885–1915*. Princeton, NJ: Princeton University Press.

Starr, P. (1982). *The social transformation of American medicine*. New York, NY: Basic Books.

Stevens, R. (1989). *In sickness and in wealth: American hospitals in the twentieth century*. New York, NY: Basic Books.

Tompkins, C. P., Altman, S. H., & and Eilat, E. (2006). The precarious pricing system for hospital services. *Health Affairs*, *25*(1), 45–56.

Werner, R. M., & Dudley, R. A. (2012). Medicare's new hospital value-based purchasing program is likely to have only a small impact on hospital payments. *Health Affairs*, *31*(9), 1932–1939.

CHAPTER 11

Medical Homes and Accountable Care Organizations: Innovation for the Delivery System of the Future

Brenda Helen Sheingold and Joyce A. Hahn

Overview

Historically, healthcare delivery in the United States has not been administered in a systematic manner that promotes alignment of incentives to make care comprehensive, coordinated, and continuous (Enthoven, 2009). *Fragmentation* has been used to characterize this inefficient approach to health care, and it has led to an unfavorable effect on quality, cost, and patient care outcomes (Enthoven, 2009). For the past 15 years, considerable research has been conducted to identify system improvements and provider payment reforms to overcome fragmentation (American Hospital Association [AHA], 2010; Devers & Berenson, 2009).

Objectives

- Describe at least two models that define Accountable Care Organizations (ACOs) and the implications of each model on your own practice.
- Identify at least two challenges and two facilitating factors that impede or support advanced nursing practice in an ACO setting.

- Discuss strategies to overcome the barriers.
- Identify programs that support quality-based payment and reimbursement, encourage provider/payer collaboration, and foster provider performance that meets quality outcome benchmarks.
- Identify strategies and approaches to develop effective and efficient patient-centered care delivery teams for patient-centered medical homes (PCMHs) that serve specific vulnerable or high-risk populations.
- Describe public and private sector efforts to test ACO and PCMH models.

This chapter presents two rapidly evolving models of patient care delivery in the United States that are transforming consumer, patient, academic, and payer expectations in the new millennium. These two practice models are ACOs and PCMHs. Although variations of these models have existed for some time, passage of the Affordable Care Act (ACA) has accelerated their growth through extensive research and testing programs (Gilfillan, 2013).

The origins of both models are similar because they endeavor to respond to a wide range of healthcare system delivery failures. ACOs build on the health maintenance organization (HMO) concept that seeks to improve quality and reduce cost. The strategic difference is that HMOs shift financial risk to providers, and ACOs must also reach quality benchmarks for reimbursement (Frakt & Mayes, 2012). Community health centers were also an important foundation for ACOs because they provided a framework for payment as a reward for improving performance and quality measurement (AHA, 2010). Community health centers are located in medically underserved areas to provide those populations with minimal access to services (Health Resources and Services Administration [HRSA], 2014). Community health centers can

be either public or private nonprofit organizations that can apply for federal grant funds to become a designated Federally Qualified Health Center (HRSA, 2014). The last significant historical factor in our current ACO environment was the 1993 healthcare reform plan, proposed by President Bill Clinton, that required employers to provide health insurance to employees through managed competition, which highlighted HMOs as a mechanism to control costs (Zelman & Berenson, 2007).

The PCMH model is also foundational to the delivery of health care through the ACA. Historically, this model focuses on improved quality that aligns with reimbursement. The difference can be found in terms of its focus on health information technology and evidence-based practice (Arvantes, 2009). Additionally, it employs healthcare teams that are focused or centered on patient needs by offering such services as flexible, lengthened hours for care, proactively employing telephone calls, and patient email (Berenson, Devers, & Burton, 2011).

The overarching goals of these models, such as a reduction in fragmented care, performance-based payments, patient-centered care, and cost savings, serve as the core of modern healthcare delivery systems (Meyer, 2012).

Rationale for New Models

The U.S. healthcare system is historically the most expensive in the world, spending more per capita on health care than any other country (Kaiser Family Foundation, 2011). Recent estimates say that national health expenditures per capita in the United States were $8,953 in 2012, accounting for 17.9% of the gross domestic product (GDP) (Keehan et al., 2012). Traditionally these estimates have been much higher in the United States than in all other nations (Squires, 2012). Despite higher spending, the United States ranks poorly in international comparisons of health system performance (Davis, Schoen, & Stremikis, 2010). In addition, a 2013 study by the National Research Council and the Institute of Medicine demonstrated that out of the top 17 Organisation for Economic Co-operation and Development (OECD) countries, the United States ranked last, due in large part to repetitious patterns of poor health throughout the entire life span (Rubenstein, 2013).

Determinants of poor health are based on a variety of factors that include the incidence of chronic disease, maternal/infant mortality, likelihood of death by violence, smoking, food security, and access to dental and medical care (United Health Foundation, 2013). The need to coordinate healthcare delivery in the United States has been seen as a response to the overall poor health rankings and high costs. Although coordinated care has been on the public agenda for a long time, it has not been a priority of policy makers in Washington, D.C. (Hoffman, 2003). It became a national priority when the ACA was passed by Congress and signed into law by President Obama in 2010. The ACA supports a comprehensive review of healthcare delivery best practices in the United States and brings ACO and PCMH models to the forefront of funded research (U.S. Department of Health and Human Services, 2014).

The Evolution of ACOs and PCMHs

An ACO, as defined by the ACA, refers to a group of providers and suppliers that coordinate services to improve patient care. Medicare is currently one type of ACO financial model that provides incentives to reduce costs and improve the quality of care. One key way that ACOs achieve these objectives is to coordinate care by sharing medical information and data primarily through electronic health records to reduce redundancy and help control costs (Medicare.gov, 2014a). Five types of ACOs are defined and summarized with examples in Table 11-1. It illustrates that ACOs are represented by many organizational paradigms and structures. They all attempt to align financial and practice incentives to ensure quality patient care.

A patient-centered medical home is a model of care that facilitates the coordination of primary care in a cooperative setting of providers that serve the interests of patients (Healthcare Information and Management Systems Society, 2010). The model was originally established in 1967 to provide organized care for pediatric patients and has since evolved to encompass an extensive range of practice that includes families, clinical specialties, and chronic disease management (American Academy of Pediatrics, 2014). The original PCMH concept improved access to health care and progressed with technological advances. Comprehensive care could be provided only by HMOs that

Table 11-1   Snapshot of ACOs in the United States

Type	Characteristics	Examples
Integrated delivery system	• Own hospitals • Sponsor health plans • Salary-based specialty practices • Provide extensive population health care	Kaiser Permanente, Geisinger Health System, Henry Ford Health System, Intermountain Health System
Multispecialty group practice	• Strong affiliation with a hospital (might own one) • Contract with multiple health plans • Physician-led coordinated care	Mayo Clinics (Minnesota, Florida, and Arizona), Cleveland Clinic, Virginia Mason Clinic, Billings Clinic
Physician–hospital organization	• Subset of a hospital staff • Negotiate with health plans • Cost-effective care coordination	Advocate Health System, Middlesex Hospital
Independent practice association	• Individual physician practices contract with health plans • Care coordination varies • Exchange of personal health information varies	Hill Physicians Group, HealthCare Partners
Virtual physician organization	• Independent, small physician practices • Usually located in rural areas • Led by a single physician, foundation, or Medicaid agency	Community Care of North Carolina, Grand Junction Colorado, North Dakota Rural Cooperative Network, Humboldt County California

Source: Data from Shortell, S., Gillies, R., & Wu, F. (2010). United States Innovations in Healthcare Delivery. Public Health Reviews (32)1, 190–212.

owned hospitals; they therefore controlled the transfer of patients or tightly coordinated community health centers and hospitals. Computerization made care coordination possible among providers in diverse locations and helped facilitate the growth of the managed care industry. Combined with the development of a market-driven healthcare system, organizations have been pushed to affiliate as a way to control market share and costs and to address quality issues.

ACOs leverage a wide variety of organizations or integrated care delivery systems and may elect to include a PCMH, which is characterized by five critical elements or core functions, defined by the Agency for Healthcare

Research and Quality (AHRQ) as follows (2014):

- Provides comprehensive care: Organizes care by marshaling a diverse subset of specialists that represent many different professions, such as pharmacists, social workers, nutritionists, physical therapists, occupational therapists, and dentists. This team is usually led by a physician or nurse practitioner (NP).

- Provides patient-centered care: Delivers care that focuses on establishing a relationship with each patient and his or her family. It recognizes and considers the cultural, ethnic, and social differences among patients and incorporates them into care.

- Provides coordinated care: Supervises key transitions that occur at decisive junctures or transfers of care, such as being discharged from the hospital to home or when palliative care services are introduced. Good communication is a requirement to achieve effective coordination.

- Provides accessible services: Offers appointments that are convenient and flexible to suit patient and family preferences. Also offers 24-hour care either by telephone or electronic communication to reduce the overall wait time for patients and families.

- Provides safe care and quality monitoring: Practices evidence-based care that is routinely analyzed to meet standard benchmarks for quality and safety. Values patient engagement and patient satisfaction. Publically shares safety data and quality improvement activities.

The ACO and PCMH care delivery models align with the quality improvement and reimbursement incentives required by ACA. In addition, they conform to the six elements of

high-performing healthcare systems as follows (Shortell et al., 2010):

- Continuity of information
- Care coordination for transitions in care
- System accountability
- Peer review and teamwork
- Easy access to appropriate care
- Continuous innovation

The Innovation Center: Promoting ACO and PCMH Care Delivery Models

The Center for Medicare and Medicaid Innovation (the Innovation Center) was created by Congress to test experimental payment and quality care delivery models that also contain costs (Medicare.gov, 2014b). New initiatives were funded through ACA statutes that expanded services to recipients of Medicare, Medicaid, and the Children's Health Insurance Program (CHIP). The statute provides $10 billion in direct funding for fiscal years 2011–2019 to enable organizations to partner with the Innovation Center for demonstration project testing (Medicare.gov, 2013b). Table 11-2 displays examples of the major types of ACO and PCMH initiatives funded by the Innovation Center. These projects are all efforts to address organizational and financial barriers that have prevented the provision of quality patient care.

Prior to the passage of ACA, the Centers for Medicare and Medicaid Services (CMS) funded initiatives of this type, which were referred to as *demonstration projects*. Since the Innovation Center has been established, the branding of ACO and PCMH initiatives has been changed to *models* or *innovations*, and the term

Table 11-2   Examples of Innovation Center Care: Projects Funded by ACO and PCMH

Business or experimental model	Aim
The Pioneer ACO and Advance Payment ACO models	Align organizational incentives to promote population health, quality, and better outcomes while controlling costs
Bundled Payments for Care Improvement Initiative	Realign quality with incentives for hospitals and postacute care providers
Comprehensive Primary Care Initiative	Support the transformation of primary care practices
Strong Start for Mothers and Newborns Initiative	Evaluate the effectiveness of interventions for expectant mothers who are enrolled in CHIP or Medicaid and are at risk for preterm delivery
State Innovation Model	Provide monetary awards to states that design and test multipayer delivery models and improve quality and health system performance
Health Care Innovation Awards	Improve health and medical care while containing costs for people who are enrolled in Medicare, Medicaid, and CHIP

Source: Data from Gilfillan, R.J. (2013). Congressional Testimony Before the U.S. Senate Committee on Finance. Reforming the Delivery System: The Center for Medicare and Medicaid Innovation. March 20, 2013.

demonstration project is being used less frequently (Berenson & Cafarella, 2012).

It is important to note that the ACA further recognizes the potential of the ACO model to change how care is provided and control costs through the Medicare Shared Savings Program (MSSP). This model is administered by the Center for Medicare within CMS, rather than the Innovation Center. ACOs that are approved by the Center for Medicare will be responsible for a defined group of Medicare beneficiaries. If they succeed in meeting primary care goals and reducing costs below what would otherwise be expected, the cost savings are shared with the ACO. The program initially launched on April 1, 2012, with participation from 27 ACOs; another 106 ACOs were added by January 2013, and another 123 were added in January 2014 (Centers for Medicare and Medicaid Services, 2013).

Military Health Service and Veterans Health Administration PCMH Activity

CMS is not the only governmental agency that envisions medical homes as a way to provide comprehensive, continuous, and quality care. There are four components of the Military Health System (MHS)—Army, Navy (the

Marine Corps is part of the Navy), Air Force, and Coast Guard—under the surgeon general (Military Health System [MHS], 2011). The MHS is an arm of the Department of Defense (DOD), which has a strategic vision to strengthen PCMH health service for more than 9.6 million beneficiaries, including individuals actively on duty, the National Guard and Reserves retirees and their families, and international survivors and former spouses (MHS, 2014).

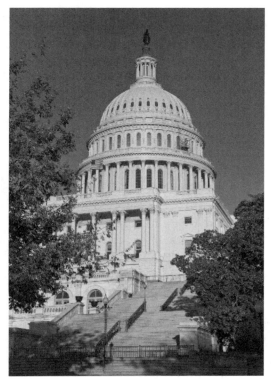

© iStockphoto/Thinkstock

The DOD is transitioning all their primary care centers (there are more than 400 worldwide) to become PCMHs (Agency for Healthcare Research and Quality, 2014).

The Veterans Health Administration (VHA) began transitioning primary care services toward a PCMH model in 2010 for more than 5 million veterans (Rosland et al., 2013). The VHA initiative is called Patient Aligned Care Teams (PACTs) to align with their integrated care delivery models that began in the 1990s (Rosland et al., 2013). The VHS PCMH model follows guidelines established by the National Committee for Quality Assurance.

Development of the National Committee for Quality Assurance Recognition

The National Committee for Quality Assurance (NCQA) was established in 1990 to promote rigorous healthcare quality performance measurement as a key component of the national agenda (National Committee for Quality Assurance [NCQA], 2013). The committee has also assumed an accrediting role and has accredited health plans in all 50 states based on statistical improvement in disease management and population health (NCQA, 2013). Most recently they have started a recognition program for PCMHs.

The recognition program is driven by comprehensive and measurable quality improvement standards. NCQA recognition is a valued accomplishment by consumers and purchasers of healthcare services because of its assurance of high-quality care (NCQA, 2013).

Assessments for NCQA recognition are conducted by independent evaluators. Recognition can be achieved at three levels, based on a sliding scale of 10 scored standards (NCQA, 2013):

- Written standards for patient access and patient communication
- Use of data to show that standards for patient access and communication are met

- Use of paper or electronic charting tools to organize clinical information
- Use of data to identify important diagnoses and conditions in practice
- Adoption and implementation of evidence-based guidelines for three chronic or important conditions
- Active support of patient self-management
- Systematic tracking of tests and follow-up on test results
- Systematic tracking of critical referrals
- Measurement of clinical or service performance
- Performance reporting by physicians based upon the PCMH standards developed by NCQA

Level 1 recognition requires that a PCMH successfully comply with at least five elements. Level 2 or 3 recognition requires compliance with all 10 elements. An overall score determines which level awarded (NCQA, 2013).

Sean Lyon, patient-centered medical home project director of Life Long Care in New London, New Hampshire, was the first person in the nation to achieve NCQA recognition for a nurse-led PCMH. There are now more than 200 NCQH-recognized PCMHs in the nation, and that number is growing rapidly (NCQA, 2013).

Nursing's Role in ACOs

Nurses play an important role in the implementation of the ACA. First, NPs will help address the real possibility of primary care provider shortages caused by an estimated 30 million Americans who, up to now, have been uninsured (Yee, Boukus, Cross, & Samuel, 2013). Utilizing NPs in the primary care workforce would increase the number of primary

care providers. The American Academy of Nurse Practitioners reports that 89% of NPs have been trained in primary care, with more than 75% currently practicing in primary care settings (Yee et al., 2013). An AHRQ report (2012) reported that in 2010, a total of 56,000 NPs practiced primary care in the United States, compared with approximately 209,000 physicians in primary care practice. NP availability would increase the number of available practitioners by more than 25%.

Second, the ACO concept is based on the assertion that coordinated care can improve both patient's health and healthcare quality while decreasing duplication of services, reducing medical errors and complications, and lowering costs (Robert Wood Johnson Foundation, 2011). Nurses working in NP nurse-managed health clinics are demonstrating that nurses working as a team with other healthcare professions within this ACO concept have been improving the healthcare outcomes of patients. A study that looked at the quality of care in 15 of the largest nurse-managed health centers found not only quality measure findings that compared favorably with the national benchmarks, but also high quality demonstrated for chronic disease management (Barkauskas, Pohl, Tanner, Onifade, & Pilon, 2011).

The American Nurses Association (ANA) defined the integral role of nurses in providing patient-centered care when it commented on the CMS-proposed rules for ACOs:

1. Registered Nurses provide care coordination and patient-centered care as a core professional nursing standard of practice
2. Registered Nurses' innovations in care delivery models offer principles and experience to guide successful care coordination and quality improvement,

particularly with high risk and vulnerable populations

3. Registered Nurses are integral to quality of care improvements and their contributions should be recognized and measured

4. Nurse practitioners, clinical nurse specialists, and certified nurse midwives are essential primary care providers

5. Financial and systemic incentives should be required for care coordination to assure that it is properly designed and implemented by qualified healthcare professionals with experience in care coordination. (ANA, 2011, p.2)

Nurses in care coordinator roles will see their roles expand across the continuum of their organizations and out into the community. Quality improvement managers and nurse researchers will demonstrate through evidence-based research findings and data dissemination the link between quality care and cost control measures. Advanced practice nurses—including clinical nurse specialists, nurse midwives, nurse anesthetists, and NPs—with their educational preparation and skill base, are in a position to provide valuable primary care, education, and expertise within ACO settings inclusive of community settings and nurse-managed clinics.

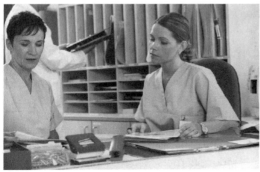

© Jochen Sand/Digital Vision/Thinkstock

Barriers to Independent NP Practice

Despite the scope of services nurses are capable of providing, and need to provide given the ACA, state laws continue to maintain barriers to NP scope of practice by requiring various levels of physician oversight. Some states allow NPs to practice independently, and other states limit NP authority to diagnose, treat, and have prescriptive authority without physician supervision. National policy makers will need to look beyond revising individual state scope of practice laws to grant NPs authority as primary care providers under Medicaid or encourage health plans to pay NPs directly (Yee et al., 2013).

The National Council of State Boards of Nursing developed a consensus model (2008) to provide guidance for states to adopt uniformity in the regulation of advanced practice registered nurse (APRN) roles and scope of practice, with a target completion date of 2015. States with restrictive scope of practice regulations will make it more difficult for NPs to bill both public and private payers and establish independent nursing practices.

In addition to the nursing profession, an Institute of Medicine (IOM) report, *The Future of Nursing: Leading Change, Advancing Health* (2010), recommends that scope-of-practice barriers should be removed and further says that APRNs should be able to practice to the full extent of their education and training. The IOM was established in 1970 and is the health branch of the National Academy of Sciences. Its goal is to generate evidence on which to base healthcare policy (Institute of Medicine, 2014).

Case Study

The Roadmap to an NCQA-Recognized PCMH

Terri Ameri, Danette Alexander, Jean Gargiulo, Juliet Harris-Brown, and Stephanie Stephens

This case study is the result of a project developed by a team of doctor of nursing practice students (class of 2014) at the George Washington University School of Nursing. It is a summary of strategies they developed to support a hypothetical PCMH achieve NCQA recognition. This PCMH would serve a predominantly American Indian population.

The Patient Population

The Navajo tribe represents the largest American Indian tribe in the United States, and they own the land that stretches across the high deserts and forests of north-central Arizona. Traditionally, the Navajos are a matriarchal society, with descent and inheritance determined through one's mother. The Navajo have a strong sense of family allegiance and obligation (Indian Health Services Public Affairs, 2013).

The Navajo Nation economy includes traditional endeavors, such as sheep and cattle herding, fiber production, weaving, jewelry making, and art trading. The reservations operate arts and crafts shops and sell handmade crafts. Other Navajo members work at retail stores and other businesses within the nation's reservation or in nearby towns. Tourism drives the Navajo economy and can often be unpredictable, which results in financial strain and hardship during times of decreased travel (Indian Health Services Public Affairs, 2013).

Navajo spiritual practice is central to daily life. It is believed that restoring balance and harmony to a person's life produces health. Often illness is viewed as a temporary imbalance of harmony or the result of violating a taboo (such as contact with an object that was struck by lightning, exposure to a snake, or contact with the dead). Healing is sought by seeking a certified Hatalii (medicine man) before turning to Western medicine. The Hatalii uses chanting prayers, meditation, and crystals and provides advice to avoid activities for periods of time. In some cases, the Hatalii performs a ceremony to cure the individual from a curse (U.S. National Library of Medicine, 2012).

The provision of medical care to American Indians is challenged by cultural differences in communication, perception of health and illness, and adherence to prescribed treatment. Like other American Indians, the Navajo are challenged by chronic diseases and conditions like diabetes, renal failure, alcoholism, drug abuse, and mental health problems. In addition, Navajos view illness as temporary, which presents barriers to chronic care management such as nonadherence to prescribed treatment and the inability to recognize a chronic illness as a health problem (Indian Health Services Public Affairs, 2013).

The Identification of Leveraging Agents

An adequate assessment and engagement of external agents enhances strategic planning and aids in the development of programs that are specific to and meet the needs of the Navajo population and improve the likelihood of successful PCMH implementation (Moseley, 2009). Arizona is a state with many leveraging agents. A potential PCMH is leveraged and supported by the current legislation related to NP practice, which does not require physician oversight and provides NPs with the authority to prescribe treatment and, admit, discharge, refer, and manage patients independently (Christian & Dower, 2008). These provisions provide support and reduce barriers for independent practice and allow for the establishment of a unique healthcare experience, such as a PCMH. Three key leveraging agents for whom successful engagement is critical for long-term success are the Indian Health Service, public health department, and the University of Arizona. These leveraging agents represent potential partnerships that would be mutually beneficial for each organization and aid in the provision of healthcare services for all.

Meeting National Quality of Care Standards: Institute of Medicine Provisions

Figure 11-1 displays how a PCMH targeted to serve an American Indian population could incorporate the six aims to improve healthcare quality that were identified by the IOM in their landmark report, *Crossing the Quality Chasm* (Institute for Healthcare Improvement, 2011).

A Strengths, Weaknesses, Opportunities, and Threats (SWOT) Analysis

The following is a strengths, weaknesses, opportunities, and threats (SWOT) analysis of the PCMH and recommendations:

Strengths:

- Locate the PCMH within a clinic that already exists and the population is accustomed to visiting

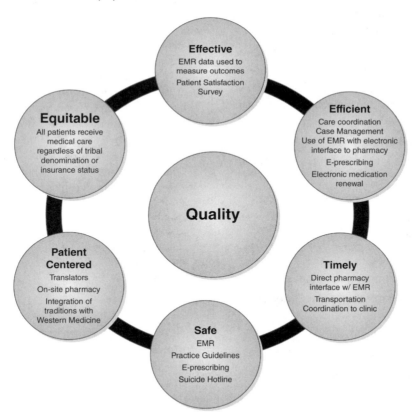

FIGURE 11-1 Aligning patient center medical home model and six aims to improve healthcare quality

- The potential for an Institute for Healthcare Improvement (IHI) partnership currently exists
- Family support
- Support from the University of Arizona School of Nursing
- Arizona Board of Nursing support
- Resources to meet the six IOM aims are located within the Navajo community
- Minimal competition to the PCMH
- Members of the Navajo community can be incorporated into the practice

　Weaknesses:

- Cultural barriers to seeking medical care
- The economy and multiple disparities
- Tribal traditional differences
- Lack of information technology (IT) infrastructure near or on the reservation
- Small clinic to appropriately meet needs of the large population, which is greater than 100,000 individuals

　Opportunities:

- Partnerships with nearby tribes to promote health
- Development of trusting relationships
- Healthcare reform
- Tele-health

　Threats:

- Financial and funding challenges
- Efforts to repeal or dispense with healthcare reform

　Recommendations:

- Commit to secure funding
- Meet with all key stakeholders
- Establish an IT team
- Set goals and objectives for clinics to measure outcomes
- Develop a time line for deliverables

Case Study Questions

- Identify an at-risk, minority, or vulnerable population that lives in your geographic area. What leveraging agents exist in your community to support its access to health care?
- How do the scope of practice laws for NPs in your state affect the health care available to these populations?
- What factors should be considered to ensure their health care meets the IOM six aims?

Case Study References

Christian, S., & Dower, C. (2008). Scope of practice laws in healthcare: Rethinking the role of nurse practitioners. *California Healthcare Foundation, 1*, 1–10.

Indian Health Services Public Affairs. (2013). *Basis for health service*. Retrieved from http://www.ihs.gov/newsroom/factsheets/basisforhealthservices/

Institute for Healthcare Improvement. (2011). *Across the chasm: Six aims for changing the health care system*. Retrieved from http://www.ihi.org/knowledge/Pages/ImprovementStories/AcrosstheChasmSixAimsforChangingtheHealthCareSystem.aspx

Moseley, G. B. (2009). *Managing health care business strategy*. Sudbury, MA: Jones and Bartlett.

U.S. National Library of Medicine. (2012). *Indian health service today*. Retrieved from http://www.nlm.nih.gov/exhibition/if_you_knew/ifyouknew_09.html.

Conclusion

　As the implementation of healthcare reform continues to evolve, ACOs and PCMHs will continue to be evaluated by a variety of government and private entities to ensure the effective delivery of value-based care (Reichard, 2013). PCMHs will undergo similar scrutiny, and the future development of both models will be guided by evidence-based research and

Discussion Questions

1. Identify an at-risk, minority, or vulnerable population that lives in your geographic area. What leveraging agents exist in your community to support their access to health care?
2. How do the scope of practice laws for nurse practitioners in your state affect the health care available to these populations?
3. What factors should be considered to ensure that their health care meets the IOM six aims

process-focused analysis (Geonnotti, Peikes, Wang, & Smith, 2013). This is an advantage for consumers of health care and key stakeholders at all levels, and it will have a lasting effect on nursing practice for the new millennium.

References

Agency for Healthcare Research and Quality. (2012) *Primary Care Workforce Facts and Stats No. 3.* Retrieved from http://www.ahrq.gov/research /findings/factsheets/primary/pcwork3/index .html

Agency for Healthcare Research and Quality. (2014). *Defining the PCMH.* Retrieved from http://www.pcmh.ahrq.gov/portal /server.pt/community/pcmh__home/1483 /pcmh_defining_the_pcmh_v2

American Academy of Pediatrics. (2014). *National Center for Medical Home Implementation.* Retrieved from http://www.medicalhomeinfo.org/

American Hospital Association. (2010). *Accountable Care Organizations synthesis report,* 4. Retrieved from http://www.aha.org/research /cor/content/ACO-Synthesis-Report.pdf

American Nurses Association. (2011). *Comments to CMS on Accountable Care Organizations proposed rule.* Retrieved from http://nursingworld. org/MainMenuCategories/Policy-Advocacy /Positions-and-Resolutions/Issue-Briefs/ACOs /ACO-Rule.pdf

Arvantes, J. (2009). *PCMH likely to form basis of federal health care reform.* Retrieved from http://www.aafp.org/news-now /pcmh/20090217pcmhfedreform.html

Barkauskas, V. H., Pohl, J. M., Tanner, C., Onifade, T., & Pilon, B. (2011). Quality of care in nurse-managed health centers. *Nursing Administration Quarterly, 35*(1), 34–43.

Berenson, B., & Cafarella, N. (2012). *The Center for Medicare and Medicaid Innovation: Timely analysis of immediate health policy issues.* Washington, DC: The Urban Institute.

Berenson, R., Devers, K., & Burton, R. (2011). *Will the patient-centered medical home transform the delivery of health care?* Retrieved from http: //www.rwjf.org/content/dam/farm/reports /reports/2011/rwjf70764

Centers for Medicare and Medicaid Services. (2013). *Medicare shared savings program accountable care organizations start date: April 1, 2012* Retrieved from https://www.cms.gov/Medicare /Medicare-Fee-for-Service-Payment/sharedsav-ingsprogram/Downloads/MSSP-ACOs-List.pdf

Davis, K., Schoen, C., & Stremikis, K. (2010). *Mirror, mirror on the wall: How the performance of the U.S. health care system compares internationally. The Commonwealth Fund Research Update. No. 1400.* Retrieved from http://www.common-wealthfund.org/~/media/Files/Publications /Fund%20Report/2010/Jun/1400_Davis_Mir-ror_Mirror_on_the_wall_2010.pdf

Devers, K., & Berenson, R. (2009). *Can accountable care organizations improve the value of health care by solving the cost and quality quandaries?* Retrieved from http://www.urban.org/Upload-edPDF/411975_acountable_care_orgs.pdf

Enthoven, A. (2009). Integrated delivery systems: The cure for fragmentation. *American Journal of Managed Care,* 15, 284–290.

Frakt, A., & Mayes, R. (2012). Beyond capitation: How new payment experiments seek to find the "sweet spot" in amount of risk providers and payer bear. *Health Affairs, 31*(9), 1951–1958.

Geonnotti, K., Peikes, D., Wang, W., & Smith, J. (2013). *Formative evaluation: Fostering real-time adaptations and refinements to improve the effectiveness of Patient-Centered Medical Home interventions.* Agency for Healthcare Research and Quality. Policy Brief No. 13-0025-EF. Retrieved from http://pcmh.ahrq.gov/page/formative-evaluation-fostering-real-time-adaptions-and-refinements-improve-effectiveness

Gilfillan, R. J. (2013). Congressional testimony before the U.S. Senate Committee on Finance. *Reforming the Delivery System: The Center for Medicare and Medicaid Innovation.* March 20, 2013.

Health Resources and Services Administration. (2014). *What is a health center?* Retrieved from http://bphc.hrsa.gov/about/

Healthcare Information and Management Systems Society. (2010). *Leveraging health IT to achieve ambulatory quality: The patient-centered medical home (PCMH).* Retrieved from http://www.ncqa.org/Portals/0/Public%20Policy/HIMSS_NCQA_PCMH_Factsheet.pdf

Hoffman, B. (2003). Health care reform and social movements in the United States. *American Journal of Public Health, 93*(1), 75–85.

Institute of Medicine (IOM) of the National Academies. (2014, January). *Making a Difference ... Roundtable charter, strategy, tactics, impact.* Released January 2014. Retrieved from: http://www.iom.edu/Activities/Quality/~/media/Files/Activity%20Files/Quality/VSRT/Core%20Documents/Making%20a%20Difference.pdf

Institute of Medicine (IOM) of the National Academies. (2010). The future of nursing: Leading change, advancing health. Released October 5, 2010. Retrieved from http://www.iom.edu/Reports/2010/The-future-of-nursing-leading-change-advancing-health.aspx

Kaiser Family Foundation. (2011). *Snapshots: Health care spending in the United States and selected OECD countries.* Retrieved from http://kff.org/health-costs/issue-brief/snapshots-health-care-spending-in-the-united-states-selected-oecd-countries/

Keehan, S., Cuckler, G., Sisko, A., Madison, A., Smith, S., Lizonitz, J., ... Wolfe, C. (2012). National health expenditure projections: Modest annual growth until coverage expands and economic growth accelerates. *Health Affairs, 31*(7), 1600–1612.

Medicare.gov. (2014a). *Accountable care organizations.* Retrieved from http://www.medicare.gov/manage-your-health/coordinating-your-care/accountable-care-organizations.html

Medicare.gov. (2014b). *Where innovation is happening.* Retrieved from http://innovation.cms.gov/initiatives/map/index.html

Meyer, H. (2012). Many accountable care organizations are now up and running, if not off to the races. *Health Affairs, (31)*11, 2363–2367.

Military Health System. (2011). *Patient centered medical home (PCMH) guide.* Retrieved from http://www.tricare.mil/tma/ocmo/download/MHSPCMHGuide.pdf

Military Health System. (2014). *About MHS.* Retrieved from http://www.health.mil/About_MHS/Health_Care_in_the_MHS.aspx

National Committee for Quality Assurance. (2013). *NCQA patient-centered medical home.* Retrieved from http://www.ncqa.org/portals/0/PCMH%20brochure-web.pdf

National Council of State Boards of Nursing. (2008). *The consensus model for APRN regulation, licensure, accreditation, certification and education.* Retrieved from https://www.ncsbn.org/4213.htm

Reichard, J. (2013). *MedPAC mulls future of ACOs.* Retrieved from http://www.commonwealthfund.org/Newsletters/Washington-Health-Policy-in-Review/2013/Apr/Apr-8-2013/MedPAC-Mulls-Future-of-ACOs.aspx

Robert Wood Johnson Foundation. (2011). *What are Accountable Care Organizations and how could they improve health care quality?* Retrieved from http://www.rwjf.org/en/research-publications

/find-rwjf-research/2011/12
/what-are-accountable-care-organizations-
and-how-could-they-impro.html

Rosland, A., Nelson, K., Sun, H., Dolan, E., Maynard, C., Bryson, C., & Stark, C. (2013). The patient-centered medical home in the Veterans Health Administration. *American Journal of Managed Care*, 19(7), e263–e272.

Rubenstein, G. (2013). *New health rankings: Of 17 nations, U.S. is dead last.* Retrieved from http://www.theatlantic.com/health/archive/2013/01/new-health-rankings-of-17-nations-us-is-dead-last/267045/

Shortell, S., Gillies, R., & Wu, F. (2010). United States innovations in healthcare delivery. *Public Health Reviews*, (32)1, 190–212.

Squires, D. (2012). *Explaining high health care spending in the United States: An international comparison of supply, utilization, prices, and quality.* The Commonwealth Fund Issue Brief. No. 1595.

Vol. 10. Retrieved from http://www.common-wealthfund.org/~/media/files/publications/issue-brief/2012/may/1595_squires_explaining_high_hlt_care_spending_intl_brief.pdf

United Health Foundation. (2013). *America's health rankings.* Retrieved from http://www.americashealthrankings.org/About

U.S. Department of Health and Human Services. (2014). *Key features of the Affordable Care Act.* Retrieved from http://www.hhs.gov/healthcare/facts/timeline/index.html

Yee, T., Boukus, E., Cross, D., & Samuel, D. R. (2013). *Primary care workforce shortages: Nurse practitioner scope-of-practice laws and payment policies* (NIHCR research brief no.13). Retrieved from http://www.nihcr.org/PCP-Workforce-NPs

Zelman, W., & Berenson, R. (2007). *The managed care blues and how to cure them.* Washington, DC: Georgetown University Press.

Healthcare Finance: Understanding the Role of Markets in Government

CHAPTER 12

Healthcare Costs: Follow the Money

Jonathan Engel

Overview

Financing the U.S. healthcare system requires a complex patchwork of public and private third-party payers, as well as cash payments made by consumers for copays, deductibles, out-of-network treatments, and uncovered drugs and services. Providers and manufacturers are aware of inconsistencies in reimbursement and tend to position their goods and services to optimize revenue. This has led to an expensive and cumbersome healthcare system, with overly reliant specialist providers, imaging technologies, surgical procedures, and new drugs. Efforts to change reimbursement will always be imperfect because of fundamental economic inefficiencies in the provision of health care.

Objectives

- Understand the flow of funds within the healthcare system.
- Discuss economic inefficiencies in the production and provision of healthcare services within the framework of a rational market model.
- Learn more about inflationary pressures on the healthcare system.
- Understand the historical development of third-party payments.
- Discuss both failed and successful efforts to rectify abuses and inefficiencies implicit in a system of third-party payment.
- Know more about the critical role of Medicare and Medicaid in paying for health care.
- Understand the fundamental ways in which managed care attempts to rein in costs and rationalize healthcare delivery.
- Learn about the essential nature of risk within an insurance framework and areas in which health insurance is inconsistent with risk distribution.

National Health Spending

Spending in the United States on health care now totals more than $8,000 per capita for an aggregate expenditure of more than $2 trillion, or some 17% of the gross domestic product (GDP). This compares to just over $5,000 per capita in Germany and Canada (the next highest two), and about $3,500 per capita in the United Kingdom (about the lowest in the industrialized world). Canada and Germany devote about 12% of their GDP to healthcare spending, while in the United Kingdom, it hovers around 7.5% (Henry J. Kaiser Foundation, 2010). Although the United Kingdom posts a worse health profile than the United States (lower life expectancy and higher infant mortality, when controlled for recent immigrants), most nations that spend more than 9% of their GDP do as well as or better than the United States. Sweden and Japan, for example, have infant mortality rates around 7 per 1,000 live births, while the United States comes in near 20 per 1,000 live births (United Nations Department of Economic and Social Affairs, 2007). By any meaningful measure of national health profile, the United States is spending substantially more money, both in per capita expenditures and in percentage of GDP, to achieve results no better than, and often worse than, other industrialized countries.

What does the United States have to show for its efforts? In some areas, the United States clearly leads the world and can rightly boast that greater investment has produced superior results. The United States leads the world by a large margin in the success of its biomedical research efforts (both laboratory and clinical), and its training programs in surgical and medical specialties are still unparalleled.

The same cannot be said for primary care and general practice residencies. Although these training programs clearly maintain high standards, other nations have developed greater expertise than the United States in treating patients in more psychologically and socially sensitive ways and in reducing the numbers of invasive surgical procedures. One interesting statistic is that although U.S. citizens stay in the hospital far fewer days each year than Europeans (7 days versus close to 30 days in some countries), the United States spends far more money for each hospital day (World Health Organization, 2014). For Americans, hospitals and, to some degree, physicians' offices and clinics are sites to receive intensive medical and surgical intervention. Other nations view the purpose of their healthcare infrastructure as giving more general care. To this day, the German healthcare system will pay for nearly a week's stay at a spa each year for German citizens. The best that Americans can get out of managed care plans is a modest discount on sports club membership fees. It is not quite the same thing.

The United States health system is expensive for a number of reasons. First, the United States trains more specialists in relation to primary care physicians than other countries, so the system has to absorb both the cost of the extra training and the cost of extra consultations with specialists. Health economists have long been aware of induced demand, in which the mere presence of greater numbers of doctors prompts greater use of their services (Iversen, 2004). Only about 30% of recent medical school graduates go on for training in primary care, including general practice, family practice, pediatrics, internal medicine, and sometimes gynecology (Mutha, Takayama, & O'Neil, 1997). By contrast, most nations push nearly 80% of their medical school graduates into primary care and limit spots in specialty residency programs through national and regional regulations.

Second, the United States has overcapacity in its system. The country has overbuilt hospitals to the point that there is nearly a 30% national vacancy rate of hospital beds (National Center for Health Statistics, 2006). The costs of these beds are borne up front and are later distributed through patient billings over a 10- to 15-year depreciation period. While hospital rooms are functioning, they induce demand insofar as their owners are interested in filling them to quickly recoup their costs.

Third, the United States invests huge amounts of money in novel equipment for diagnosis, treatment, surgery, and convalescence. This cost must be built into ordinary billings. Health economist Henry Aaron believes this is probably the single greatest cost driver in our system (1991). Unless you are a jet fighter pilot, you will probably never be as close to sophisticated machinery as you are when you are admitted to even a modest community hospital. Such developments as artificial skin and organs, genetically engineered drugs, and magnetic resonance imagers give testament to U.S. world-class research and engineering capability, but it costs a great deal without substantially adding to the general health of the population. Americans have gotten used to noninvasive diagnosis and treatment of painful joints, arthritic spines, and inflamed tendons, even though very few patients would be willing to pay for those treatments if faced with an actual bill for services.

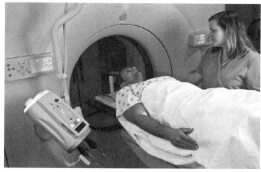

© Mark Kostich/iStockphoto.com

Americans are willing to spend so much on health care in part because the cost is largely hidden. The value of a family insurance policy is between $12,000 and $15,000 per year, yet few employees ask themselves if they are willing to take a $15,000 pay cut for health care. Moreover, virtually all of that cost, when provided by an employer, is tax deductible, meaning that it is subsidized by the federal government to a great degree (the top federal personal income tax rate, as of 2014, is 39%). Moreover, under the terms of the Affordable Care Act (ACA), all employers with more than 50 full-time employees (more than 30 hours per week) must provide comprehensive health insurance to all employees as of January 1, 2014.

Much is changing as the ACA becomes fully implemented. Economists estimate that 29 million currently uninsured Americans will purchase health insurance through either the federal or state health exchanges (many with the help of federal subsidies), or a number of employers that do not currently provide coverage will begin to face steep penalties. Although young people who purchase insurance on the exchanges will experience higher premiums than they did in the past, older and sicker people will see the opposite as the full regulatory weight of the ACA begins to compress the highest premiums to no more than three times the lowest rate.

In a sense, medical care is a public good that needs to be guaranteed because infectious diseases can be spread throughout the population. Given this fact, Americans have a vested interest in seeing their neighbors inoculated against whooping cough and diphtheria, and making sure they have access to a public sewer and public garbage pickup. Back when infectious diseases were still a major health hazard (before antibiotics), the public was much more supportive of school nurses, community clinics, and community inoculations. Now that infectious diseases seem to pose much less of a threat (outside of AIDS), Americans are more likely to assume that their neighbors are responsible for their own states of health.

In a more abstract sense, medical care is still a public good because most people deem it morally unacceptable to live in a community where people die (or at least suffer avoidable health consequences) for lack of access to basic medical care. Most people do not consider a society unjust when rich people can buy fancier cars than poor people, but most people do take exception to a society in which rich children receive smallpox and polio vaccinations but poor children do not. The U.S. government has continually rewritten Medicaid regulations to ensure that children, at the very minimum, are universally covered, as well as pregnant women and people who are permanently disabled, elderly, and severely injured (Engel, 2006). The government also guarantees coverage for U.S. military veterans, civil servants, and American Indians. The ACA guarantees that the last group of uninsured people—young able-bodied men—who were not guaranteed access to either public or private coverage will now be able to purchase reasonably priced insurance. The sole remaining group of uncovered residents—undocumented immigrants—will continue to purchase care through back channels or seek care at public municipal hospitals.

Americans might ask whether 17% of GDP is too much to spend on health care. After all, most Americans do not consider it a problem when a young Wall Street trader spends 80% of his income on a new Porsche—that is, most Americans assume that individuals are capable of allocating their resources however they wish. Why shouldn't people be able to spend their money on buying as much health care as they wish? The answer is, in part, that people are spending the government's money (which is to say, our money) on health care, but the larger problem is that health care does not follow some of the most basic laws of economics that are used to produce and distribute goods.

Physicians

Economic rules fall apart in the most basic transactions between patients and physicians. For one, there is an enormous information gap between doctors and patients. Although the internet has allowed many patients to better educate themselves about the nature and treatment of their conditions, nearly all patients go to a doctor for a diagnosis and treatment plan. Because the doctor simply knows more than patients about their health (often much more), patients essentially throw themselves at the mercy of the doctor in hope that the physician will be honest, competent, and fair concerning pricing.

Second, because every diseased body is slightly different, and every patient has a unique medical history, there is always a degree of uncertainty regarding the outcome of a physician–patient interaction. As a result, no doctor can, in good faith, offer a guarantee concerning a successful surgery or recovery from trauma or flu. This fundamental uncertainty, coupled with the inability of physicians to simply replace the defective service (as might be expected if you are unhappy with your house painter, for example), creates a requirement that the patient reimburse the physician for a good faith effort, not for a guaranteed product or outcome. Consider how unusual this arrangement is in economic life. Can you imagine taking your car to an automotive shop and paying for the mechanic's best efforts, regardless of whether your car is fixed? More likely, if the mechanic couldn't fix the problem, you wouldn't pay, or at least you'd withhold part of the fee. Oncologists, for obvious reasons, can't work this way. You pay them for access to their accumulated wisdom, skill, and judgment, then you both pray for the best.

Third, because demand for medical services fluctuates wildly depending on whether you are sick, the patient–doctor relationship invites price gouging. Suppose you arrive at the local emergency room (ER) hemorrhaging from injuries suffered in a car crash, and before the ER physician starts the blood transfusion, you are informed that this relatively simply procedure will cost $50,000. You're not really in a position to argue. Incidentally, locksmiths face a similar situation when they are called out late at night to get someone into his house when he forgets his key. Ordinarily locksmiths charge $20 to $30, but at 2:00 in the morning on a freezing cold night when you are locked out of your apartment, those same services might be worth $150 to you. The locksmith knows this and elevates the price accordingly. Payment is required up front, in cash, because after your door is unlocked, the locksmith has no more leverage.

For these reasons—information asymmetry, uncertainty of outcome, and opportunity for price gouging—physicians professionalized at an early stage (Stevens, 1998). What does it mean to be a professional? Before the word became grossly diluted in modern corporate speak, it meant that a group of people in a certain trade or business agreed to hold themselves to certain standards of behavior beyond savvy business skills. Professions create ethical standards for themselves, police themselves, and license themselves. Both professionals and clients benefit from professionalization. The profession grants itself some degree of protection from outside competition (only those who have met certain entrance standards are allowed to practice), and customers (patients) can rest assured that the licensed professional will not take advantage of their ignorance or need. If members of the profession refuse to abide by these standards of conduct, they are punished by the profession, possibly stripped of their license, and generally ostracized.

One of the great challenges of constructing fair physician compensation assignments is rewarding the cogitative components of medical practice. The value of an internist, to a large degree, lies in what that individual knows and in how he or she uses information and past experience to arrive at diagnoses, prognoses, and regimens. Unfortunately, it is almost impossible to reward someone for simply sitting and thinking (Hsiao, Braun, & Becker, 1990). Patients will not tolerate it, and insurers fear they are being cheated. Rather, doctors (like all professionals) are rewarded for what they produce or do. This same conundrum exists in other professions as well. Architects are paid for the plans they draft, not the time they spend thinking about the project, despite the fact that much of the drafting has become rote and mechanical and is farmed off to drafting assistants who do it on computers. Lawyers, who offer little beyond their knowledge of the law, get around this problem by charging by the hour rather than by the result. (This, of course, creates other incentive problems, such as encouraging lawyers to be as ineffective as possible with their time.) Academics are rewarded for the volume of material they publish rather than the quality of thought that goes into the material, leading to a plethora of mediocre journal articles and academic monographs that are rarely read or cited. Universities get around these problems by keeping academic salaries low, despite the high-level skills and training required of budding professors.

One of the great breakthroughs of managed care has been capitation payment—that is, paying doctors up front to keep patients healthy, regardless of how much work this entails. By reversing the incentives, doctors are encouraged to practice efficient preventive medicine and refrain from hospitalizing and referring patients. Initially managed care was supposed to totally capitate patients—that is, the primary care doctor would have to pay the specialist and hospital bills when they arose—but this was quickly found to be untenable for all but enormous physician groups. Unfortunately, capitation has failed in many ways. Doctors do not seem to be emphasizing prevention (it turns out that going to the gym and eating your broccoli just doesn't make that big a difference in your medical bills, and quitting smoking actually increases lifetime medical bills since you live longer), and recent studies have shown that the gatekeeping function seems to do more to annoy and antagonize patients than it does to actually keep them away from specialists. Moreover, primary care doctors have become experts at processing patients through their exam rooms at startling speed, further antagonizing patients (although not particularly jeopardizing their health). Capitation has kept patients out of hospitals (which accounts for the nearly flat healthcare inflation in the early 1990s), but it has failed to keep patients away from expensive prescription medications and medical devices. As is usually the case, the only mechanisms that reliably keep people from seeing doctors more and demanding more medicine and devices involve forcing them to pay for it. New drug formularies and copays, in which patients have to pay up to $50 for expensive brand-name drugs, are the most recent response to this type of inflation.

Physicians have also responded to managed care by agglomerating into ever-larger groups. Partnerships of two or three doctors were once standard, but now physician groups of 50, 70, or 100 doctors are not uncommon in heavily populated areas. The intent is twofold: distribute overhead and support staff costs over a larger number of doctors, and create a monopoly, or near monopoly, of a certain type of practice in an area, thus creating better bargaining leverage with managed care plans. If a neurology group has cornered the market on neurology for all of northern New Jersey, then any managed care plan wishing to offer neurology services (which is sort of nonnegotiable) must come to them and pay their price. Fortunately for managed care plans, physician groups of this size frequently split up, and doctors have repeatedly shown themselves to be terrible business people and negotiators. One mark of this is their unwillingness to pay adequately for top-flight management that is needed in a large group; it is not unusual for a medical group with annual revenues of $20 to $30 million to pay its executive director less than $100,000. As is often the case, you get what you pay for.

Hospitals

The modern hospital is a relatively recent creation (Stevens, 1999). Although buildings dedicated to care of the sick have existed since the Middle Ages, these institutions were little more than glorified almshouses where unaffiliated and widowed people convalesced. Medical care was scant, equipment was nonexistent, and nursing care was more spiritual than clinical. It wasn't until the 1930s (and really not until the 1950s) that hospitals became the technologically sophisticated emporiums of surgery, intensive care, and postop that they are today. Despite the fact that hospitals are highly competitive, budget-driven institutions, the majority remain loyal to their nonprofit community origins; few have applied for for-profit status over the past decade, and most continue to provide enormous amounts of care to poor populations—the costs are reimbursed through Medicaid or written off as uncompensated care.

Private hospitals receive operating revenues from private insurance (35%), Medicare (45%), Medicaid (10%), self-paying patients (5%), and philanthropy (5%) (American Hospital Association, 2014). The balance of these numbers fluctuates a good deal. Small rural hospitals tend to have much higher rates of Medicare reimbursement, and inner-city academic medical centers may find that Medicaid revenues approach 70% of their total income. By contrast, a pediatric and maternity hospital in a wealthy suburb may have close to 100% privately insured patients.

Private insurance these days means predominantly managed care contracts. Managed care organizations with large local market shares will either bargain up front for heavily discounted rates that they will indemnify the hospital for (sometimes 60% off book value), or they simply purchase blocks of hospital services up front knowing that on average their subscribers' hospital usage will come out close to the predicted rate. In an effort to negotiate more evenly with payers, hospitals have resorted to the same strategy as physicians—aggregating and merging themselves into networks and systems to try to monopolize power in a particular area. Unfortunately, since the United States has nearly 30% more hospital beds than it currently needs, it is very difficult for a hospital system to absorb enough of the excess capacity to achieve negotiating parity. The mergers have created certain economies of scale in terms of inventory pricing and administrative streamlining, but in the grand race between managed care and hospitals, the payers are probably coming out ahead.

Hospitals spend their operating funds on personnel, supplies, and capital depreciation (and debt service). The personnel, somewhat counter to common knowledge, is everybody but the doctors, although certain physicians—such as anesthesiologists, ER doctors, and pathologists—may have exclusive contracts with a hospital. Doctors, who make up the medical staff of a hospital, don't actually work for the hospital. They are private practitioners who are granted admitting privileges to the hospital. The one exception to this is the house staff in hospitals that have residency programs. These young medical residents provide emergency and critical care for poor patients, and they provide back-up care for the medical staff. The central component of a hospital's personnel is really the nursing staff. Although nursing forces have been augmented in recent years by all sorts of ancillary therapists, nutritionists, social workers, lactation consultants, rehab specialists, and the like, it is the line nurses who in many ways define the major value that a hospital adds to the healthcare system. It is nurses who carry the weight of a hospital's reputation, and it is their responsiveness to physician orders that makes a hospital able to attract competitive, well-reputed physicians to its medical staff. Other personnel worthy of note are the administrative staff, accountants, marketers, orderlies, janitors, cooks, launderers, and maintenance workers.

The supplies (and utilities) include both medical and nonmedical inventory, and both are crucial to a hospital's contribution to the healthcare product. Nonmedical supplies include a huge amount of linens, food, televisions, furniture, office equipment, and the like. Medical equipment ranges from tongue depressors to sophisticated imaging and operating room equipment, and it is the second greatest resource (after nurses) that makes hospitals uniquely situated to add value to the medical transaction. Some healthcare analysts even suggest that a hospital's primary value is in serving as a community depository of biomedical equipment, and certainly the remarkable acceleration in new equipment investment has fueled much of the cost explosion in health care over the past 2 decades. American hospitals are, by world standards, overequipped, with multiple hospitals in a given area competing to outdo one another in a medical arms race of cutting-edge PET scans, MRI machines, catheter labs, and renovated operating rooms (Morris, 2005). The advantage of this race is the total absence of queuing in hospital services. The downside lies in paying nearly double per capita for healthcare services as the rest of the world, with no measurable advantage in longevity, infant mortality, or quality of life.

The fact that a portion of a hospital's operating budget goes to servicing debt is a strikingly new phenomenon that could not really exist before the inauguration of Medicare in 1965. Previous to that year, when hospitals wished to raise money for capital expansion (a new wing, a new building, a major new piece of equipment), they went to their boards and to the larger philanthropic community. With Medicare, hospitals can issue bonds to purchase new buildings and build the cost of debt into their current operating costs and bill the balance back to the government. And since private insurance companies nearly always follow the lead set by the government, private insurance billings soon reflected the increased costs of a debt-financed plant.

Further complicating this scenario is Medicaid, which is the name for state care programs for poor populations. The programs are regulated (and subsidized) by the federal government (more on this later in the chapter). Medicaid programs were brought into existence at the same time as Medicare, with the idea of making public hospitals obsolete. Unfortunately, Medicaid reimbursement rates quickly fell far behind private insurance and Medicare reimbursement, so public hospitals found a new niche in the 1970s and 1980s of caring for Medicaid patients who would be turned away from private hospitals. As managed care contracts began to drive down occupancy rates in the early 1990s, however, Medicaid reimbursement became concomitantly more attractive, and private hospitals began to woo Medicaid patients away from public hospitals (Biles & Abrams, 1998). Medicaid recipients have obviously benefited from this situation because they can now routinely seek care at private hospitals, but public hospitals have been devastated financially because they have lost large chunks of revenue and have been forced to use state and municipal funds to bail them out so they can continue to function.

It should be obvious from this discussion of debt financing that hospitals play fast and loose with the distinction between capital and operating costs, and thus it should come as no surprise that they tend to have rather loose rules in allocating indirect costs. One of the great problems with hospital financial planning is that nearly all costs in a hospital are indirect (outside of tongue depressors and Tylenol). It takes a huge amount of money to open a hospital's doors, but once they're open, the marginal cost of an additional patient is nearly trivial. Nursing, therapy, and equipment need to be allocated to various patients, and often the system for doing so is no more scientific than measuring the square footage of floor space in a particular unit and allocating nursing staffs costs accordingly. Back when generous indemnity plans paid bills unquestioningly, such ambiguous accounting practices allowed hospitals to freely shift money from wealthy, better insured patients to poor and uninsured ones, and thus they remained true to their founding charitable missions. But as managed care has dried up the give in the system, the loose accounting protocols have made it difficult for hospitals to get a handle on their own costs.

This kind of ambiguity can be seen in the failure of many merged hospital systems to achieve financial health. In the late 1980s, hospitals enthusiastically began to merge, assuming that, as in the manufacturing sectors, great economies of scale could be realized from larger institutions. But this simply was not true. Big hospitals have nearly identical costs, per bed, as small hospitals, because within a narrow range, nurse–patient ratios and equipment–patient ratios are fixed. While you can achieve some economies of scale in the kitchen and in nonmedical inventory, for the most part, they are not the major cost drivers in a hospital system. In this sense, health care is similar to education, despite it being a more complex product. If you are running an elementary school, you need one teacher for every 20 children, regardless of whether the school has 50 students or 500 students, and even at the administrative level, there are few economies of scale as the need for assistant principals grows with institution size. The same is true with hospitals. (To continue the analogy, a large school might save a few pennies on ordering pencils and chalk in bulk, just as a large hospital might save a bit on onions and tongue depressors, but it's probably not worth the cost of the merger.)

One solution to holding down hospital costs has been for the government to step in and tell hospitals what they can and cannot build or buy. These types of certificate of need (CON) regulations proliferated in the 1970s and 1980s, and they did succeed in moderately limiting bed expansion (Stevens, 1999). However, hospitals usually managed to game the system and build what they wished to anyway, with the added costs of going through the bureaucracies and offices that oversaw the CON processes. (Most countries heavily regulate hospital building, but it is usually done at a national or provincial level with a global budget over which the many hospitals can fight.) CON regulations are on the decline because the deflationary pressures of managed care have largely superseded their function. Many hospitals have closed in the past decade, and most hospital building these days is for ambulatory care satellite clinics and ambulatory same-day surgical centers, which should reduce costs in the system. Certainly Americans are spending fewer days in the hospital, but each day in a hospital seems more expensive than ever.

A more theoretical approach to hospital cost containment is to treat the hospital not as a community institution, but rather as a job shop for doctors in which doctors are charged for use of the facility. Just as a rock band has to pay for recording studio time (with all the accompanying sound engineers) if they wish to produce an album, so might doctors pay for operating room time, or postop time, or intensive care time, if they deem such services necessary to treating their patients. The doctors would, of course, build these costs into their bills, but such a system would acknowledge the reality that a hospital's true customers are its medical staff, not its patients. Players in the health system—government regulators, physicians, and hospital administrators—are generally not talking about this, though, so it probably will not come to pass. However, such a system would force the primary purchasers of hospital care—the medical staff—to be more cost conscious as they shop around for hospital services, knowing that any savings they accrue could either be passed back to their patients or retained as profit.

Risk and Insurance

Healthcare financing in the United States is conducted almost entirely through third-party agents; that is, most people pay a third party—usually a health insurer or a managed care organization, such as a health maintenance organization (HMO) or preferred provider organization (PPO), or another type of carrier—monthly premiums either out of their own pocket or as part of their compensation package from an employer. The premiums, in turn, pay for healthcare providers, be they doctors, hospitals, diagnostic labs, or pharmacies. Payment arrangement may be through indemnity (retroactive payment for expenses incurred), capitation (up-front payment for estimated average costs), or some combination thereof. As

mentioned previously, third-party payers often purchase services in bulk from hospitals, pharmacy chains, and large physician groups, allowing them to negotiate better terms on behalf of their subscribers. The system promotes overuse (from an economic standpoint) and irresponsible utilization on the part of patients, or overprovision on the part of providers. It is imperfect, frustrating, expensive, and pervasive. It is also probably fundamentally flawed.

Health insurance is actually two products rolled into one: prepaid medical care, and insurance against a catastrophic medical event. The latter is a reasonable product; we cannot predict who will require a $100,000 liver transplant or a million dollars in critical care following a horrible accident. The premium for such coverage (to insure only events that produce medical costs in excess of $5,000, for example) is relatively inexpensive, and of course the cost of one of these events would be catastrophic for most Americans. By contrast, prepaid medical care, which consumes the bulk of our health insurance premiums, makes no sense as an insurable product. Regular medical costs are highly predictable, constant, and affordable for most families. Furthermore, costs are not equally distributed. Older people and people with chronic sicknesses and disabilities spend, consistently, much more each year on regular medical costs than do young healthy people. If we could each buy a separate catastrophic policy (often called major medical, which kicks in only after an annual deductible of several thousand dollars), few young people would voluntarily purchase a comprehensive policy. A 27-year-old would just earmark $1,000 or so each year for a checkup, dental cleaning, some prescription drugs, and maybe a Pap smear. In fact, self-employed young people tend to do just this. The reason most other Americans do not do this is that they have no choice. Most employment carries with it comprehensive health insurance as part of the benefits package, and Americans receive no bonus for refusing the health coverage.

The problem with using a third-party to pay medical costs is that it leads to much higher system utilization, and thus deadweight economic waste. In appealing to a third party to cover medical bills, Americans (and most everybody else in the industrialized world) make themselves utterly insensitive to the price/utility quotient that governs all economic transactions. This means they routinely purchase healthcare services and goods that cost more than the utility they provide, creating a net loss for society. Think about the way you eat when you travel with an expense account. You tend to eat at nicer restaurants than you might otherwise go to, and you order more expensive entrees than usual (or you overlook the prices entirely). In short, you wind up spending more money on dinner than you would if it were your own money. This is not because you don't have enough money to eat this way on your own; it is because when you spend your own money, you consider the other ways you can spend your own money and decide that the same $100 spent on something else (groceries, heating oil, or clothes) will bring you more pleasure than spending it on a nice meal. In short, you maximize the total utility that your money can bring to you.

How much loss does this system create? Nobody knows for sure because there is no good control group, but there are a few isolated pieces of evidence indicating that the loss is substantial. For example, primary care physician visits drop precipitously (as much as 40%) in an HMO when the copayment goes from $0 to $10, suggesting that 40% of the time patients do not value their visit to a general practitioner or internist even

as much as $10 (Cherkin, Grothaus, &Wagner, 1989). When the cost of producing such a visit (in physician time, support staff, equipment amortization, rent, and administration) could easily cost $100, society loses $90 or more in nearly half the primary care visits in the country. Similarly, patients seeking certain sorts of services that are not covered (or are covered incompletely) by most health plans—such as cosmetic surgery, dental work, psychotherapy, Lasik surgery, and fertility treatments—are highly price sensitive, and patients will shop around at length to find a cheaper provider. Although many Americans claim they want the best care money can buy for themselves and their loved ones, this seems to be true only when the money is not their own. When the money is their own, Americans approach the purchase of health services with the same penny-pinching zeal they display at big-box stores.

There are other losses associated with third-party payment as well. Simply administering the system uses nearly one-fifth of our entire healthcare budget annually, due to the Byzantine forms, rules, and regulations that each provider must comply with to win reimbursement for services rendered. Most private physicians today have nearly one full-time staff member per doctor to do nothing but billing work, at a cost of $45,000 per year in salary and benefits. Doctors report spending large portions of their time arguing with managed care companies, utilization oversight professionals, and hospital bursars on behalf of their patients. Furthermore, as managed care pushes people toward certain providers and away from others, we incur losses in utility from suboptimal market flexibility. The system as it stands today is distorted, cumbersome, frustrating to use, and frustrating to work in. It is not a system any of us would design from scratch.

Third-party payment has its uses. Catastrophic medical insurance is a very sensible product, and with the federal government covering everybody older than 65 years through Medicare, the product is a relatively cheap one. Under the ACA, many of the Bronze Plans will have deductibles of more than $6,000 per year (with relatively modest premiums), which may make sense for populations of health consumers who are young and relatively healthy. In addition, the federal government will continue to favor (through tax deductibility) flexible health savings accounts (HSAs), which some employers offer (Dicken, 2008). This type of plan allows you to place money in a special account, tax free, to spend on health purchases, and it is usually provided in conjunction with a catastrophic plan. For a variety of reasons, these plans have not been popular, most likely because of general ignorance.

Managed Care

Managed care is the general term for any sort of oversight in the process in which patients receive either funding for their medical care or the funded care itself. Managed care, as a concept, is as old as industrial health plans from the 1920s. Over the past 80 years, it has periodically received increased interest, as when the Kaiser plans were founded in the 1930s and when the Puget Sound health plans, HIP of New York, and GHA (Washington) were founded in the 1940s and 1950s. Starting around 1980, the federal government began to take a greater interest in the concept, mostly in hopes of holding down healthcare costs, which were rising at frightening speeds. Companies were required to offer at least one managed care option, and Medicare began to offer a managed care choice for reduced copayments in the early 1980s.

The modern age of managed care really began in the mid-1990s; however, in the aftermath of the failed Clinton health bill, employers nationwide began to heavily push their employees into managed care plans in an effort to reduce healthcare costs. At the beginning of the 1990s, fewer than 15% of all Americans who were insured by third-party coverage were being managed, and 85% were receiving indemnity care; by the end of that decade, those percentages had switched. Today, almost all covered Americans receive their health insurance in some sort of managed care package. It has become prohibitively expensive to purchase traditional indemnity insurance, and few people (and even fewer companies) do so. Effectively, managed care is health insurance today.

It might be helpful to dispel a few myths about managed care. First, managed care is not now, nor has it ever been, about ensuring quality; it is about holding down costs. That said, there is little evidence that managed care has actually caused a decline in quality, and for some groups (notably Medicaid recipients), it may have actually improved quality. Second, most Americans do not mind managed care plans. Third, although managed care certainly cuts down on choice, in the fee-for-service age, many Americans didn't have much choice anyway. And fourth, managed care does hold down costs (or at least it did for the first few years). From 1993 to 1996, healthcare inflation dropped from 13% per year to about 4%, suggesting that managed care penetration was undermining the inflationary pressures in the system (Levit, Lazenby, & Braden, 1998). Although healthcare cost inflation returned in the early 2000s, it was probably due more to tight labor markets than to any systemic flaw in managed care.

Managed care works through one or more of several mechanisms:

- Capitation: Capitation pays providers (either physicians or hospitals) a set amount each month for each covered patient. Most patients in any given month will require no care, but a few will require a great deal of care. Capitation provides an incentive to providers to administer as little care as possible, in the most efficient manner possible, because there is no compensation for providing superfluous care. Contrast this with indemnity insurance, in which providers have an incentive to provide as much care as possible, regardless of its redundancy. Many providers work on partial capitation in which basic services are capitated, but specialty referrals are indemnified or on a system of reinsurance in which the costs of patients who require extraordinary amounts of care are indemnified by a subinsurer. Initially capitation was seen as a panacea, but health payment specialists quickly realized that individual physicians and small partnerships could not bear the risk of a few catastrophic patients. Today only very large physician groups, and certain types of specialists (such as obstetricians), work on full capitation; the others are reinsured or work on partial capitation.

- Utilization review: Utilization review (UR) employs a second professional (often an advanced practice nurse) to oversee some of the decision making of the primary provider. The utilization reviewer is employed by the managed care organization (MCO) and must give permission for certain types of referrals, elective procedures, hospitalizations, and nearly all surgeries. UR is effective in holding down costs, but it tends to antagonize physicians (who resent the time spent seeking review). In most MCOs that employ UR, physicians are given license to refer for most common problems and seek review only for major procedures, tests, and hospitalizations.

- Gatekeeping: The use of a primary care provider—who can be an internist, pediatrician, GP, family practitioner, or sometimes a gynecologist—to screen all patient concerns and complaints before access to specialty care can be sought is referred to as gatekeeping. It has become ubiquitous, but it is a relatively new idea in the United States; before about 1990, most insured individuals in the United States could see any specialist and have the visit indemnified, regardless of medical need. Gatekeeping has been remarkably successful in holding down costs because specialty care is one of the greatest single cost drivers in the healthcare system. Unfortunately, gatekeeping is probably the single component of managed care that Americans find most odious, and the majority of Americans now choose a managed care plan—such as a PPO or point-of-service (POS) plan—that allows them some latitude in avoiding a gatekeeper. Gatekeepers work on capitation with extra indemnity for hospital rounds and certain procedures (pediatricians tend to be more heavily indemnified because they have to see their patients so frequently). Not surprisingly, gatekeeping and capitation have created substantial incentives for primary care providers to be highly efficient with their time, and as a result they tend to hire more office help (including clinical help) so they can increase the volume of patients they see each day and keep their income up. It is not unusual today for each full-time primary care provider to employ five or more clinical and clerical staff.

- Bulk purchasing of hospital services: Hospitalization is the largest cost driver in the

U.S. healthcare system, and MCOs have responded by both negotiating substantially reduced hospitalization rates for their members—often half of the published rates for certain Diagnosis-Related Groups (DRGs)—and purchasing covered days up front for their entire local patient population. The latter approach, which is essentially a modified capitation arrangement, creates the same incentives for volume and efficiency in hospitals as it does for physician practices. Hospitals have responded by merging and creating networks so they can control a larger portion of the local hospital market and thus bargain more forcefully on indemnity and capitation rates.

- Creating preferred networks: MCOs selectively sign up doctors who are willing to treat their members at reduced fees, then they offer members a financial incentive to see these doctors (usually by waiving the copayment). Doctors are willing to join the networks out of fear that exclusion will hinder their ability to develop a healthy practice. One substantial concern from patients is whether the doctors in the networks are of lower quality. This is probably not the case because competing MCOs want to demonstrate that they include certain numbers of board-certified specialists or subspecialists. Essentially, a network that registered only subpar doctors would probably fail to satisfy large numbers of patients, who would then complain to their employers and demand a switch to an alternate MCO. In fact, physician quality in networks is rarely a cause of concern for patients; far more frequent are complaints about physician location. The single biggest complaint—the absence of a physician with whom a patient has a preexisting relationship—is not so much a quality issue as an

aesthetic one. Few patients, after all, have the wherewithal to objectively assess the quality of their own physicians.

- Ambulatory care: MCOs try as hard as they can to keep patients out of hospitals because that is the most expensive venue in which to receive care. Consequently, MCOs have pushed patients to receive certain sorts of diagnostic and surgical procedures in outpatient settings—either in physicians' offices or in ambulatory surgical centers. This phenomenon is not so much a managed care strategy as a response of providers to managed care constraints. A hospital, working on capitation or a negotiated contract, has an incentive to provide its services as inexpensively as possible, and thus it may build a freestanding surgical center to move patients through more quickly and efficiently. The hospital receives the same payment for a given procedure regardless of the cost it incurs, so the most effective competitive strategy is to reduce costs.

These six strategies, usually used in some combination, collectively make up managed care. Capitation was initially the great hope of managed care planners, but it was flawed in placing too much financial risk on small providers and groups. UR was effective, but it antagonized the clinical professions. Gatekeeping works too, but it tends to antagonize patients. In fact, all these strategies work to hold down costs, but each has drawbacks. Most MCOs use some combination of the six techniques.

MCOs take on one of several types: HMO, independent practice association (IPA), PPO, and POS plans. HMOs can be of three types: staff, group, or network. The staff HMO is notable in that it is the most highly managed of all, and it was the original template for all managed care. In this arrangement, doctors are all full-time employees of the plan, and patients simply pay a monthly membership fee that covers all services. The disadvantages are the high cost of putting the plan together in the first place and the inability of patients to go outside the plan. Staff model HMOs are rare, but they tend to be the cheapest way to deliver quality healthcare services.

Group and network HMOs employ physicians who work for multiple plans, sometimes as solo practitioners, sometimes as part of a larger physician group. The physicians are paid on partial capitation, with indemnity for specialty referrals. Patients are assigned a primary care provider who serves as a gatekeeper that may incur penalties if too many referrals are made; patients may not go out of network. Large groups sometimes work for the HMO on full capitation if they have adequate specialists in-house to handle most of their referral needs. An IPA is a close cousin to a network HMO in which the doctors bear risk through a shared arrangement; they draw indemnity for all services from a joint fund, but they equally bear the risk that the fund may run out before the end of the year while they are still obligated to provide coverage to the patients.

HMOs are the cheapest form of managed care arrangement, but they are also the most constraining for patients. In response to patient dissatisfaction (and tight labor markets), many employers offer a PPO for an additional monthly fee. A PPO also has a network of physicians who agree to contract on an indemnified basis for reduced reimbursement rates. However, patients may go out of network if they are willing to pay a 30–40% copayment. The strongest allure of PPOs for patients, beyond the ability to go out of network, is the end of the gatekeeper; patients may see any specialist on the roster without a referral. Reducing this

added barrier seems to bring patients enormous satisfaction, and recent studies indicate that it does not seem to promote substantial overutilization.

POS plans are part HMO and part PPO. If patients elect to stay in network, they must use their primary care physician, obtain a referral, and use a network specialist. If patients do this, there is no copayment or a minimal copayment. If patients elect to go out of network, they can dispense with the gatekeeper but must pay a 30–40% copayment. POS plans are attractive to MCOs because they can realize cost savings through the HMO function while granting patients the choice associated with a PPO.

A variety of other arrangements exist, such as physician hospital organizations (PHOs) and various types of networks, but they all use some combination of networks, gatekeeping, negotiated hospital rates, and utilization oversight. Many patients worry that their doctors have a financial incentive to withhold care or referrals, but in fact most primary care providers find they realize savings by referring as long as they do not exceed basic standards set by the MCO.

Managed care is evolving from tight staff model HMOs to loose PPOs, but it is not going away. If there is any revolt against the phenomenon, it is in the turn to cash medicine (either out of pocket or aided by a medical savings account), not in a return to fee-for-service indemnity insurance. We are groping our way toward a highly diversified payment system in which patients receive insurance along a continuum of choice and cost, from HMO, to POS, to PPO, to fee for service (FFS), to medical spending account (MSA), to cash. Poor, young, or healthy patients will choose from the left side of the list, and rich, old, or sick patients will choose from the right. The distinction will be not so much quality, but convenience and freedom, with less constraining plans costing more in either monthly premiums or out-of-pocket copayments and expenses.

Medicaid

Medicaid is not one program but rather 50 separate ones. The 50 programs were established by each state in the aftermath of federal Medicaid legislation (also passed in 1965 as an amendment to the Social Security Act) that provided matching federal funds to all states that established a Medicaid program in compliance with certain federal guidelines (Engel, 2006). In general, the programs had to provide comprehensive hospital and physician services, prescription drugs, eyeglasses, and emergency room care to all women and children who lived under a certain poverty threshold. The programs were required to care for the same population that qualified for Aid to Families with Dependent Children (AFDC), more commonly known as welfare. Since the welfare-reform legislation of 1997, AFDC has no longer existed. The basic poverty thresholds remain, however, albeit somewhat expanded to care for children, pregnant women, and others who previously fell through the cracks. (Note that no state is required to have a Medicaid program, but every state does.)

In addition to caring for poor people, Medicaid also pays for medical care for permanently disabled workers, patients with end-stage renal disease (dialysis treatment), and blind persons, and it pays for long-term care (nursing home) for elderly patients who fall below the poverty line. Medical care for impoverished elderly people is provided through Medicare, but nursing home care is provided through Medicaid. Although Medicaid is perceived by the public to be for poor people, nearly 40% of all Medicaid disbursements go to caring for these other categories of patients, and these categories have been the fastest-growing part of Medicaid since disabilities were more broadly defined under the Americans with Disabilities Act.

The 50 state programs reimburse at different levels, with the programs in the poorest states (Mississippi, Alabama, Arkansas) spending less than half as much per patient as those in the wealthiest and most generous states (New York and California) (American Academy of Pediatrics, 2008). These discrepancies are partially accounted for by different costs of medical and hospital care among states, but not entirely. In general, New York's Medicaid program is viewed as the most generous program in the country, providing the highest quality medical care, prompting some conservative New York voters to suggest that this might be a fruitful area for budget cutting.

Nationally, Medicaid reimbursement rates quickly fell below the customary and prevailing rates paid by Medicare and private insurers, making these patients unattractive to most private hospitals and doctors. As a result, for most of the program's history, Medicaid patients have been shunted to public and municipal hospitals and have had access to only a limited selection of doctors—disproportionately, graduates of foreign medical schools. In addition, the original Medicaid formularies did not pay for regular checkups, meaning that many beneficiaries had no regular physician and relied instead on the local hospital emergency room for routine care. This pattern of care led most analysts to describe the U.S. health system as being two tiered, with private high-quality doctors and hospitals for privately insured patients, and public hospitals and lower quality physicians for Medicaid patients. Such a description is not entirely accurate, however.

Many municipal hospitals, while overcrowded and unattractive, provide first-rate surgical and critical care in certain instances, and many have excellent emergency rooms.

Medicaid is often the single largest line item in a state budget, and governors across the country have pondered ways to reduce its ever-increasing magnitude. In the past 5 years, many states have begun to move Medicaid patients into managed care programs in an effort to save money. The programs have been among the most successful in the history of managed care. Under these programs, Medicaid patients have been assigned regular primary care providers for the first time and are now receiving the type of consistent and preventive care that private patients have long enjoyed. Primary care providers who chiefly see Medicaid patients report that their incomes are rising. This is not so with specialists, however. To make money from Medicaid patients, MCOs have whittled specialty care reimbursement down to meager levels; specialists report that they are paid only 10% as much for Medicaid patients as for privately insured patients, and the arduous task of preapproval for any specialty procedure further deters them from seeking Medicaid patients. Some specialists have stopped seeing Medicaid patients altogether, and others threaten to do so.

On a closing note, one of the oddities of Medicaid is that its inception created the strange American syndrome of the uninsured working class. In our country, the people who receive the worst medical care are not the poor and elderly (they have Medicaid and Medicare), but rather working people just above the poverty line who do not receive insurance from their employers and are unable to purchase it out of pocket. While the ACA initially raised the eligible income level for Medicaid to 133% of the federal poverty level, after multiple challenges by state attorneys general, the Supreme Court ruled that the provision was unconstitutional. As a result, many states are refusing to raise their Medicaid eligibility levels, exacerbating the problem. These people make cash payments for medical care and rely on public hospitals, alternative healers, and over-the-counter treatments. They tend to avoid doctors whenever possible, and as a result exacerbate conditions that could be more easily treated if diagnosed earlier. Currently some 43 million Americans fall into this group, and although some will purchase private subsidized policies through the new health exchanges, as many as 26 million will pay the mandatory $95 penalty and remain uninsured. Their lack of care represents one of the greatest domestic challenges to our nation.

Medicare

The elderly are another story altogether. Anyone aged 65 and older in this country is eligible for Medicare Part A (free hospital insurance) and Medicare Part B (nearly free physician insurance), and nearly 100% of elderly people enroll. More than 90% also enroll in some sort of additional health plan to cover the high deductibles and copays in the Medicare program (which can total up to $2,500 per year). This additional coverage is sometimes obtained through Medicaid (for the elderly poor), but most of the time people buy a private insurance product offered by commercial insurers known as Medigap. The cost of Medigap is frequently covered by employers of individuals who work or by pension plans for retirees (U.S. Department of Health and Human Services, 2008).

Medicare is wildly popular, and it is considered politically untouchable due to the strength of AARP, a lobby that serves the interests of elderly people. The Medicare program, which is the largest single purchaser of healthcare services in the country, sets the standard for reimbursement that the private sector follows. Medicare created DRGs and the Resource Based Relative Value Scale (BRVS), and Medicare sets prevailing rates for hospital services and physician care. The program purchases almost a third of all healthcare services and goods in the country, and it is the single greatest driver of inflation in the healthcare economy. It insures almost all its beneficiaries through indemnity plans (making it an anachronism in today's managed care environment) and has fought vigorously, albeit unsuccessfully, to hold costs down.

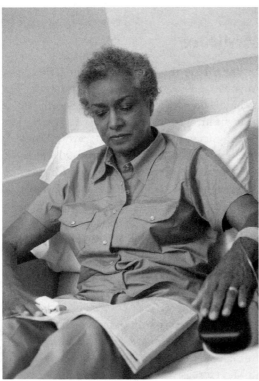

© Monkey Business Images/Dreamstime.com

Elderly people cannot be integrated into commercial programs because they tend to be unemployed, and most private insurance programs are funded through employment; in actuarial terms, they are off the charts. Elderly people simply incur more medical expenses than young people; nearly 50% of all medical costs are incurred in the last year of life, and the majority of chronic afflictions affect people older than 65 years. Thus, the elderly could probably never be integrated into a commercial, profit-driven insurance system, yet our sense of national fealty compels us to make provisions for their care. Of course, the elderly respond to third-party coverage in the same manner as everybody else—by overusing it—and for the elderly, there is a particularly pernicious aspect of the equation in that they tend to value their time at next to nothing (since they don't work) and thus don't mind waiting in a doctor's office. The comprehensive Medigap policies have only exacerbated the situation because they have removed the copayments, deductibles, and hesitation fees that can be highly effective in preventing patients from frivolously obtaining medical care. As a result, we routinely purchase expensive and sophisticated treatment for the very old in this county (bypass surgery on 90-year-olds is not unheard of, and hip replacement for 80-year-olds is relatively common), which contributes to our very high per capita health costs. Congress considered forcing all elderly people into managed care programs about 15 years ago, but Senator Bob Dole led a floor fight to prevent the legislation, and thus today Medicare remains the last bastion of fee-for-service care.

Conclusion

It should be clear that financing America's healthcare system is a complex and often counterintuitive enterprise. The industry defies basic laws of economics: most consumers do not actually pay for their care; most payers do not actually have to market their products to patients; and most providers must prenegotiate reimbursement rates with different payers, creating different pricing scales depending on who is paying the bills. Although elements of these complications can be found in other industries (even hotels negotiate corporate rates with certain large customers), no other industry has all these complicating elements. Furthermore, the landscape changes constantly as state governments rebudget their Medicaid programs; as the federal government reconsiders comprehensive healthcare reform; and as new managed care products evolve and wane to the consternation of consumers. Employers must decide yearly how much of the cost for employee benefits they will pass on to employees, and retirees must choose from a dizzying array of Medigap and prescription drug plans. A number of good pamphlets are available to help consumers navigate these waters, but no one pamphlet or information source can possibly explain them all.

Medical care probably cannot be rationalized until most Americans start paying for it out of pocket—a move that the ACA deliberately avoided. Only market pressures created by out-of-pocket purchases will induce doctors to stop seeking extra training (realizing that few patients will be willing or able to compensate them for their training investment); learn to prescribe lower cost medications, diagnostic tests, and procedures; and learn to market themselves to working-class folk. And who knows—just as Sam Walton discovered, you can make a fortune selling low-cost items to moderate-income individuals if you price them right and move them through at high volume, so some business-savvy doctors may discover that the real money is in delivering flu shots, Pap smears, and throat cultures to the masses at $10 each. But this won't happen as long as someone else pays the bills.

Discussion Questions

1. In what ways does managed care actually manage costs? Does it do so without diminishing the quality of care? If so, how does it accomplish this?
2. Why do we carve out a separate payment program for our elder citizens? In what ways do normal health insurance functions fail as people get older?
3. How does third-party payment distort the market for health care? If it is so distortionary, why does every wealthy country insist on using a third-party intermediary to purchase health care?

References

Aaron, H. (1991.) *Serious and unstable condition.* Washington, DC: Brookings.

American Academy of Pediatrics. (2008). *Medicaid reimbursement survey, 2007/08.* Elk Grove Village, IL : Author.

American Hospital Association. (2014). *Trends affecting hospitals and health systems.* Retrieved from http://www.aha.org/research /reports/tw/chartbook/ch4.shtml

Biles, B., & Abrams, M. (1998). The double bind: Challenges to safety net and teaching hospitals. *Journal of Urban Health, 75*(1), 17–21.

Cherkin, D., Grothaus, L., & Wagner, E. (1989). The effect of office visit copayments on utilization in a health maintenance organization. *Medical Care, 27*(7).

Dicken, J. (2008). *Health savings accounts: Participation increased and was more common among individuals with higher incomes.* U.S. GAO, 4/1/08.

Engel, J. (2006). *Poor people's medicine.* Durham, NC: Duke University Press.

Henry J. Kaiser Foundation. (2010). *Global health facts.* Retrieved from http://kff.org/globaldata/

Hsiao, W. C., Braun P., & Becker, E. R. (1990). *Managing reimbursement in the 1990s.* New York, NY: McGraw-Hill.

Iversen, T. (2004). The effects of a patient shortage on general practitioners' future income and list of patients. *Journal of Health Economics, 23*(4), 673–694.

Levit, K. R., Lazenby, H. C., & Braden, B. R. (1998). National health spending trends in 1996. *Health Affairs, 17*(1), 35–51.

Morris, C. (2005). The economics of health care. *Commonweal, 132*(7), 12–17.

Mutha, S., Takayama, J., & O'Neil, E. H. (1997). Insights into medical students' career choices based on third and fourth-year students' focus-group discussions. *Academic Medicine, 72*, 635–640.

National Center for Health Statistics. (2006). *Hospitals, beds, and occupancy rates, by types of ownership and size of hospitals, 1975–2004.* Washington, DC: Government Printing Office.

Stevens, R. (1998). *American medicine and the public interest.* Berkeley: University of California Press.

Stevens, R. (1999). *In sickness and in wealth.* Baltimore, MD: Johns Hopkins University Press.

United Nations Department of Economic and Social Affairs. (2007). *World population prospects: The 2006 revision* (Working paper no. ESA/PWP.202). New York, NY: Author.

U.S. Department of Health and Human Services, Center for Medicare and Medicaid Services. (2008). *Medigap (supplemental insurance) policies.* Retrieved from http://www.medicare.gov /supplement-other-insurance/medigap/whats-medigap.html

World Health Organization. (2014). *World health statistics.* Retrieved from http://www.who.int /gho/publications/world_health_statistics/en /index.html

CHAPTER 13

Private Health Insurance Market

Joyce A. Hahn and Brenda Helen Sheingold

Overview

Like other developed countries, in the United States, there are both private and public health insurers. What makes the U.S. healthcare system unique is the dominance of private insurers. Private health insurance creates access to healthcare services and thus improves health by protecting individuals from financial loss due to the high cost of medical expenditures. Health insurance covers a broad range of benefit plans that reflect the ways in which health insurance is organized to pay for a wide array of healthcare services. The health insurance plan not only specifies how and where healthcare services will be provided, but also functions as the claims processor by managing payments to providers.

The employer-based private healthcare insurance model gained dominance during World War II. An implicit social contract was developed among the government, employers, and employees to offer health insurance as an employment benefit. With wages frozen, companies had limited financial resources to offer employees. Health insurance benefits provided a competitive advantage when companies recruited and attempted to retain employees. Companies were further encouraged to offer health insurance as an employee benefit because those expenditures were exempt from income tax. This practice laid the groundwork for employer-based health insurance plans (Zhou, 2009). This model has resulted in the United States being one of the only industrialized nations that do not offer universal coverage through some combination of private and public enrollment. The consequence of an employer-based system of health insurance in which employers are not mandated to provide coverage was that employers could choose whether or not to provide coverage and to whom. As healthcare costs rose, there was a steady decline in the percentage of Americans covered by employer-based insurance policies. It is this decline that helps explain the pressure to address the rising number of uninsured individuals through the Affordable Care Act (ACA).

This chapter will provide an overview of the private health insurance industry in the United States, beginning with the historical evolution of private insurance and managed care, the identification of key federal laws and their impact on the insurance industry, and the rise of consumer-driven health care and the empowerment of the healthcare consumer. The impact of the ACA will be examined at this dynamic time in healthcare history.

Objectives

- Explain the historical evolution of private health insurance and managed care into a healthcare industry.
- Identify the key federal laws and their impact on the insurance industry.
- Identify the key federal laws that protect individuals who are enrolled in private insurance.
- Understand consumer-driven health care and the empowerment of the healthcare consumer.
- Examine the impact of the ACA on the private insurance industry.
- Explore the emerging opportunities for nursing practice within the private insurance market.

History of U.S. Health Insurance Reform

The first insurance plans became available in the United States during the Civil War. These early accident insurance plans covered personal injury related to travel by rail or steamboat. They paved the way for more inclusive plans that covered illness and injury and were the precursor to disability plans. The first group policy that gave comprehensive benefits was offered by Massachusetts Health Insurance of Boston in 1847. The first group plans that worked with healthcare providers were the predecessors of the fee-based contracts of today's modern health insurance plans (Zhou, 2009).

Prior to the 1920s, Americans distrusted the quality of medical care received in hospitals, and patients were treated at home by their families and were attended by family physicians. Medical advances, such as the development of X-ray

technology, blood pressure monitoring devices, and the identification of disease-causing organisms, increased confidence in the healthcare system. By the 1920s, the demand for physicians exceeded the number of qualified doctors (HealthInsurance.net, 2014). More important, the cost of health care began to rise given the increased use of technologically based services that were provided in medical facilities.

The economic reality of the Great Depression brought home the impact of rising healthcare costs. Hospitals faced falling revenues because individuals could not afford the cost of care. Health insurance was created as a way to finance the costs. In 1929, Dr. Justin Ford Kimball of Baylor University in Texas introduced a medical insurance plan called the Baylor Plan to allow teachers to prepay $0.50 per month for 21 days of semiprivate hospitalization at Baylor Hospital. Rather than have each hospital compete for employer contracts, the

American Hospital Association (AHA) hired Rufus Rorem to promote hospital prepayment and seek the necessary enabling legislation to create a special class of nonprofit corporations that could sell hospital insurance. In 1934, New York became the first state to offer such hospital insurance coverage. These plans were promoted by the AHA. In 1938, the Blue Cross Commission of the AHA began a formal approval process for plans, and only those endorsed plans could use the Blue Cross symbol and name (Michigan Association of Health Plans, n.d.). This was the origin of Blue Cross, which was a hospital-driven insurance plan. Blue Shield followed as physicians were pressured to offer an insurance product, and it was organized under the auspices of the American Medical Association (Blue Cross Blue Shield, 2014; Zhou, 2009). When private insurance companies understood that health insurance was a potentially viable product, they began to compete with Blue Cross for business and controlled more than 50% of the market by the 1960s. The success of the private plans resulted from their lower costs. Blue Cross offered a service contract—a fixed quantity of service for a fixed price. Private insurers offered indemnity plans—a cash amount toward a particular medical service. Ultimately Blue Cross was forced to offer indemnity plans to remain competitive.

Starting in the 1930s, another way of organizing and financing healthcare delivery was introduced: health maintenance organizations (HMOs). Henry Kaiser, an American entrepreneur who owned shipyards and factories on the West Coast, began to offer his employees the opportunity to prepay for health care for a few cents a day (Kaiser Permanente, 2014). This unique employer-based health insurance system not only evolved into the largest HMO in the world but also established the foundation for many government and private healthcare payment innovations that followed (Kaiser Permanente, 2014). In addition to Kaiser, which was organized by a major business, HMOs were organized in other parts of the country by other stakeholders. Group Health Cooperative in Puget Sound was organized by members of the Grange, the Aero-Mechanics Union, and local supply and food cooperatives. Health Insurance Plan (HIP) is an example of a government-managed care plan that was organized when Fiorello LaGuardia was mayor of New York City (HealthPlanOne, 2014).

Within the HMO paradigm, patient care is coordinated by a primary doctor who cares for the patient and determines if a referral to a specialist within a provider network is required (HealthInsurance.net, 2014). HMO enrollees are entitled to comprehensive and continuous service for a fixed payment. Until the 1970s, HMOs comprised a limited part of the market and met stiff competition from local medical societies. In 1970, the federal government recognized the potential of HMOs as a way to control costs and improve the quality of care. In the 1980s, the same potential was recognized by the private insurance industry. What had been organized under the umbrella of nonprofit organizations like Kaiser was now being organized by the private insurance industry. The term *managed care* replaced the term *health maintenance organization*. What is important about the growth of managed care in the late 1980s is that it was a progressive strategy to provide access, a business strategy to control costs, a government strategy to control costs and achieve access, and a political strategy to avoid national health insurance.

Health Insurance Plans

Today nearly 150 million Americans rely on their employers for health benefits. Employers provide health insurance plans as a benefit package for employees. Those plans, also known as private health insurance, are varied and include traditional indemnity insurance or a variety of models that fall under the heading of managed care plans, such as HMO, preferred provider organization (PPO), point of service (POS), consumer-driven health plan (CDHP), high-deductible health plan (HDHP), health savings account (HSA), health reimbursement account (HRA), or flexible spending account (FSA).

Indemnity Insurance

Indemnity plans make a fixed cash payment toward a particular medical expense based on what services are covered and what reimbursement method is used by the insurance company. An insured person decides when and from whom to seek healthcare services. If the services are covered under the plan, the provider submits a claim after services have been provided. In this model, the individual carries the risk of covering the cost of his or her care (Fernandez, 2011). Examples of some historical key innovative approaches to healthcare insurance are provided in Table 13-1.

HMO

Healthcare service delivery and financing are integrated under managed care. In the original HMOs, individuals joined group practices where their insurance premiums provided the budget to cover the cost of operating the group. Physicians were typically salaried, so their costs were known. With the growth of managed care, organizations

prospectively controlled costs by restricting enrollees to access in-network providers who agreed to accept a discounted fee-for-service payment. Enrollees needed primary care physician approval to access specialty care, a process known as gatekeeping. Precertification was required for routine in-hospital care. Disease management or care management services coordinated care for enrollees with certain medical conditions. A distinguishing feature of the managed care approach is the emphasis on preventive health and quality assurance processes (Fernandez, 2011).

PPO

A PPO offers individuals a hybrid policy that combines the benefits of indemnity and managed care. The PPO enters into contractual arrangements with providers and creates provider networks. If a patient uses a preferred provider, the cost of the provider's services are heavily discounted. If a patient uses an out-of-network provider, the PPO will cover a portion of out-of-network charges depending on the plan. PPOs have an out-of-pocket deductible for the enrollee (U.S. Government, 2002).

POS

A POS plan is another hybrid form that loosens the gatekeeping restrictions imposed by HMOs. *Point of service* reflects the ability of enrollees to decide which provider they will see without prior authorization from a primary care provider. The rules are generally similar to an HMO in that patients can see an out-of-network provider for a fee (U.S. Government, 2002).

CDHP

CDHPs are one of the most recent innovations in the insurance market. They seek to control

Table 13-1   Historical Time Line of Payment Reform Efforts

Year	Reform	Goal	Sponsor
1934	Blue Cross	Designed to reimburse hospitals for expenditures; the blue cross symbol was derived from the Greek cross	American Hospital Association (AHA)
1935	Social Security	Strengthened public health services; a provision to include health insurance was omitted because of physician opposition	President Franklin D. Roosevelt
1939	Blue Shield	Offered reimbursement to physicians	American Medical Association (AMA)
1965	Title XVIII of the Social Security Act—Medicare	Covered health expenditures for aging or disabled Americans	President Lyndon Baines Johnson
1965	Title XIX of the Social Security Act—Medicaid	Covered health expenditures for impoverished Americans	President Lyndon Baines Johnson
1985	Consolidated Omnibus Budget Reconciliation Act (COBRA)	Provided continuous coverage for healthcare expenditures when coverage from a group health plan concludes	President Ronald Reagan
1993	Health Security Act	Provided universal healthcare coverage; never voted on by Congress	President William Clinton
1996	Health Insurance Portability and Accountability Act (HIPAA)	Prevented insurance companies from denying coverage due to pre-existing conditions	Senator Edward Kennedy, Senator Nancy Kassenbaum
1997	Children's Health Insurance Program (CHIP)	Provided coverage for healthcare expenditures for children from low-income families whose income is too high to qualify for Medicaid	Senator Edward Kennedy, Senator Orrin Hatch
2010	Affordable Care Act (ACA)	Provided coverage options for healthcare expenditures for all Americans as of January 2014	President Barack Obama

Sources: Data from American Public Health Association (2014); Blue Cross Blue Shield (2014); Patel & Rushefsky (1999); SASid (2007); Sultz & Young (2009).

costs by empowering healthcare consumers to make personal decisions about their coverage. As healthcare expenditures and insurance plan premiums have increased, both employers and employees have sought alternatives to high-cost insurance coverage. The theory behind CDHPs is twofold. First, there is an overuse of services because individuals do not know the cost of services and do not carry substantial financial risk in terms of being responsible for paying for services. Second, healthcare consumers become better educated about personal healthcare services and costs. Because consumers are at risk, they will make more cost-effective decisions about the care they receive. One concern, however, is that patient care is typically driven by physicians, and patients do not have adequate information to discern between cost and quality.

A CDHP is a combination of a high-deductible plan with a pretax payment account, as described in Table 13-2.

HDHP

An HDHP has a lower premium and a higher deductible that the insured must pay before receiving coverage. These plans provide catastrophic coverage and guard against major medical costs. The lower premiums translate into cost savings for both the employer and the employee. An important feature that distinguishes an HDHP from a traditional plan is the ability for the enrolled person to open an HSA.

HSA

HSAs were created by Congress in 2003 so individuals who were covered by HDHPs could receive tax-preferred treatment of money saved for medical expenses. An HSA is the account holder's individual account and can be used to pay for qualified medical and pharmacy expenses. The account can be funded by the employer or employee with pretax dollars up to a statutory limit, which varies yearly. An HSA plan includes a deductible, but enrollees can use their HSA to pay for out-of-pocket expenses before they meet the deductible. All deposits to an HSA become the property of the policyholder, regardless of the source of the deposit. Funds deposited but not withdrawn each year will carry over into the next year. If the

Table 13-2   Comparison of Pretax Savings Plans

Type of account	Pretax employee contribution allowed	Employer contribution allowed	Rollover allowed	Account must be linked with HDHP
Health savings account (HSA)	Yes	Yes	Yes	Yes
Health reimbursement arrangement (HRA)	No contribution allowed from the employee	Yes	Yes	No
Flexible spending account (FSA)	Yes	Yes	No	No

Source: Data from U.S. Department of Labor (2010). Bureau of Labor Statistics. Compensation and Working Conditions. Consumer- Driven Health Care: What is It and What does it mean for employees and employers? Retrieved from http://www.bls.gov/opub/cwc/cm20101019ar01p1.htm

policyholder ends the HSA-eligible insurance coverage, he or she loses eligibility to deposit further funds, but funds already in the HSA remain available for use (U.S. Department of the Treasury, 2013).

HRA

An HRA account can be funded only by an employer. No pretax dollars from the employee can be added to the account. Money in the HRA can be used only for medical expenses. Any unused funds will roll over from one year to the next. It is not necessary for an employee to be enrolled in an HDHP to participate (U.S. Bureau of Labor Statistics, 2010).

FSA

An FSA allows employees to have their employers set aside pretax dollars from their wages to pay for out-of-pocket medical expenses. These expenses can include insurance copayments and deductibles, qualified prescription drugs, and medical devices. There is no carry-over of unused FSA funds; you either use it or lose it. After January 2013, only $2,500 may be set aside in an FSA (Healthcare.gov, 2014a).

Employer-Sponsored Health Insurance

In 2012, a little more than 50% of employers offered their employees health insurance. In 2013, the data remained static, additionally reporting that more than 95% of firms with 50 or more employees offered health insurance, and only 35% of firms with fewer than 50 employees did so (Kaiser Family Foundation, 2013b). Employers decide the benefits to be offered and the structure of payment. Thus, there is no uniformity among plans. Plans have different copays and deductibles, and they offer different benefits, such as prescription coverage.

Employer-sponsored family coverage cost as much as $16,351 in 2013, which was up 4% from 2012. Employer-sponsored health insurance is financed both through employers who shoulder the larger burden of the premium and employees who pay the remainder of the premium. As the cost of health insurance has risen, employers have shifted a larger percentage of the costs to employees, who now pay an average of $4,565 toward their premium (Kaiser Family Foundation, 2013a). To further control the cost of health insurance, employers are increasing cost sharing for services. Employees in many small companies, for example, must pay annual deductibles of $2,000 or more. Small companies with many low-wage employees (defined as those earning $23,000 or less per year) require employees to pay $1,363 more for health insurance, on average, than employees who work for companies with fewer low-wage earners (Ducat, 2013). This makes it difficult for the working poor to afford healthcare insurance.

Health insurance plans are administered by private and nonprofit companies; some well-known plans are Aetna, Cigna, United Health Care, and Blue Cross and Blue Shield. Employers send premiums directly to the insurance company, a system known as group market health insurance. The premium is a set fee for the employer, based on estimates of the costs that will be incurred by a particular group of employees. The cost of the premium is typically divided between the employer and the employees, with employees paying an ever-increasing percentage. The insurance company provides underwriting and claims processing services, negotiates agreements with providers, processes payments to providers, and negotiates agreements with providers. Many larger employers, in an effort to contain costs, choose to be self-insured. They negotiate agreements with providers, and the employer sets aside funds to pay for health benefits directly. In this case, the employer contracts with a third party to administer the insurance plan (Fernandez, 2011).

Private Plans

Individuals who cannot access health insurance through their employer can purchase individual insurance plans; these are private plans that are not part of a group. This market covers people who are self-employed or work part time, or people who are otherwise unable to obtain insurance through an employer. Private plans are administered by insurance companies, and individuals assume responsibility for the full cost of the premium. These plans are typically very costly because rates are based on the health status of the individual named on the plan. The ACA is designed to address some of the problems in both the employer and the individual health insurance markets as a way to ensure that more individuals can purchase health insurance at an affordable cost (Fernandez, 2011).

Laws and Regulations Impacting the Provision of Health Insurance

Health insurance regulations address the benefits that must be offered, the individuals to whom the insurance is made available, and the insurers' responsibilities to plan enrollees. The U.S. federalism system makes the regulation of the health insurance market quite complicated. In most cases, health insurance regulation is the primary responsibility of the

states, as established in the 1945 McCarran-Ferguson Act. Individual states have established standards and regulations. Fully insured plans (that is, employer-sponsored plans) are subject to state requirements. Self-insured plans are not subject to state insurance regulation. State insurance regulations typically require a richer set of benefits, such as prenatal care and well-child care, than plans that are offered by companies that self-insure. Because these companies are not regulated, they can change the benefits package whenever it suits them.

All health insurance plans are subject to federal laws. There are three federal laws that have a significant impact on how health insurance is provided:

- Employee Retirement Income Security Act of 1974 (ERISA, P.L. 93-406)
- Health Insurance Portability and Accountability Act of 1996 (HIPAA, P.L. 104-191)
- Affordable Care Act (ACA, P.L. 111-148)

ERISA

ERISA is a federal law that sets minimum standards for employer-sponsored benefits. Companies that self-insure are subject to regulation under ERISA because the services are defined as an employer-sponsored benefit. This law requires health plans to provide participants with information regarding plan features, participant rights to establish a grievance through an appeals process, and adequate disclosure of the plan's financial activities. ERISA preempts state laws that relate to employee benefit plans. Self-insured health plans are exempt from state laws under ERISA because health care is defined as an employer benefit, not insurance (U.S. Department of Labor, 2013a).

HIPAA

This federal act is an amendment to ERISA that provides protections for working Americans and their families who have preexisting medical conditions. The provisions in HIPAA established federal requirements for private and public employer-sponsored health plan insurers. This legislation permits individuals to continue health insurance after a loss of employment or job change. Additional HIPAA provisions address patient privacy of identifiable medical information and electronic transmission of health information (U.S. Department of Labor, 2013b).

ACA

This federal healthcare reform act includes private insurance provisions that mandate new requirements on individuals, employers, and health plans; restructures the private health insurance market; sets minimum standards for healthcare coverage; and provides financial assistance to individuals and small businesses in certain circumstances (WhiteHouse.gov, 2014).

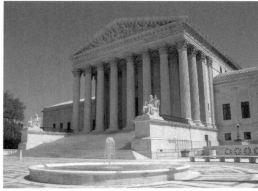

© Jason Maehl/ShutterStock, Inc.

Health Reform Changes That Impact Private Insurers

The ACA and the healthcare provisions of the Health Care and Education Reconciliation Act (HCERA) were signed into law by President Obama on March 23, 2010. On June 28, 2012, the Supreme Count rendered a final decision to uphold the healthcare law (Supreme Court of the United States, 2012). Significant private health insurance market reforms within the ACA are intended to improve consumer protections, including oversight of premiums, access, coverage, and clearer communication between insurers and enrollees.

The ACA requires all Americans to have health insurance, which is known as the individual mandate, beginning January 1, 2014, or they will face penalties. Insurance can be obtained in several ways. Individuals can purchase insurance through state or federal exchanges. Individuals who cannot afford the cost of insurance can apply for a federal subsidy. Insurance is also available through employers. The ACA does not require employers to provide insurance coverage to their employees, but it does impose penalties on employers that have at least 50 full-time equivalent employees and do not provide coverage (Chaikind, Fernandez, Newsom, & Peterson, 2010). In addition, eligibility for federal programs, such a Medicaid and State Children's Insurance Program (SCHIP), has been expanded.

ACA and Its Impact on Employers

Large employers will be subject to penalties of $2,000 per year multiplied by the number of employees minus 30 (Kaiser Family Foundation, 2013a) if they do not offer minimum and affordable health coverage. Their employees will be eligible to purchase insurance through the exchanges. Employers are required to cover only full-time employees. Employers that currently offer a health plan to their part-time employees (less than 30 hours per week) may decide to drop part-time eligibility for insurance plans. Similarly, employers that currently sponsor retiree health plans may choose to terminate those plans and send this group into the state health insurance marketplace. It is not known how many large employers will opt to pay the penalty and direct their employees to the insurance exchanges. Small employers, many of whom did not offer health insurance, are not subject to penalties. To encourage small businesses to purchase health insurance for their employees, employers with 50–100 employees can purchase coverage through the Small Business Health Options Program. Employers with fewer than 25 employees are eligible for a tax credit to offset the cost of insurance.

All the changes under the ACA apply to new insurance plans. Some of the changes do not impact older plans that are called *grandfathered* plans. If the private insurance plan was in existence before the ACA became law on March 23, 2010, it is a grandfathered plan. This is important because persons who are covered under such plans do not have the same level of protection as people in plans that were organized after that date. A grandfathered plan changes status only when a major change, such as reducing benefits or increasing out-of-pocket costs, occurs. Insurance plans must inform enrollees if they are grandfathered and provide them with contact information to ask questions. The consumer coverage reforms are summarized in Table 13-3.

Table 13-3   Consumer Protections under ACA

All health plans must:
- End lifetime limits on coverage
- End arbitrary cancellation of health coverage
- Cover adult children up to age 26
- Provide a Summary of Benefits and Coverage (SBC), a short, easy-to-understand summary of what a plan covers and the costs
- Hold insurance companies accountable to spend premiums on health care, not administrative costs and bonuses

Grandfathered plans do not have to:
- Cover preventive care for free
- Guarantee participants' right to appeal
- Protect participants' choice of doctors and access to emergency care
- Be held accountable through rate review for excessive premium increases

In addition, grandfathered *individual* health insurance plans that people buy themselves—those not provided by an employer—*do not* have to end yearly limits on coverage or cover people if they have a preexisting health condition.

Source: Modified from U.S. Department of Health and Human Services (2013b). What if I have a grandfathered health insurance plan? Retrieved from https://www.healthcare.gov/what-if-i-have-a-grandfathered-health-plan/

Group Plans and Individual Plans That Are Not Grandfathered

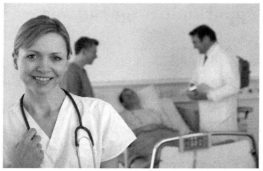

© iStockphoto/Thinkstock

Group plans and insurers are prohibited from excluding coverage for preexisting health conditions. They may not put lifetime limits on essential health benefits (EHB), which include emergency services, hospitalization, maternal and newborn care, mental health and substance abuse disorder services, prescription drugs, laboratory services, preventive and wellness services, chronic disease management, and pediatric services, to include oral and vision care. Plans can only charge a higher premium based on the plan level benefits of the individual or family insurance plan, age, tobacco use, and geographic rating area (set by each state). Group and individual market plans must provide insurance to everyone who applies, and they must guarantee the ability to renew health insurance regardless of changes in health or the amount of health services that will be required (Chaikind et al., 2010).

State Health Insurance Marketplaces

Private health insurers can also sell their insurance products on the state health insurance exchanges, which are marketplaces where individuals who are not covered by employer-sponsored plans and small businesses with fewer than 100 employees can choose affordable, comprehensive health coverage that meets or exceeds a set of minimum benefit standards. The state exchange insurance plans must be offered at four tiers designed from the lowest premium (Bronze Plan) to the highest premium (Platinum Plan). Government-sponsored premiums and subsidies will be available to make coverage affordable (Hahn, Sheingold, & Ott, 2013).

Private Insurance Industry Response to ACA

ACA and Its Impact on the Cost of Health Insurance

The ultimate impact of the ACA on the cost of health insurance is unknown. Many provisions of the healthcare law will make insurance coverage more affordable to individuals, including premium and cost-sharing subsidies, depending on income and rate restrictions on health plans for individuals and small businesses. Newer innovative benefit designs that are being developed by health plans are also designed to control costs. These include wellness programs to encourage healthy living, incentives to choose lower cost generic drugs, and the availability of high-value networks to increase quality care (O'Connor, 2013).

At the same time, it is suggested that the ACA will increase health insurance premiums and the cost of premiums to select individuals. The expansion of coverage will include both healthy people and those who are less healthy but could not afford healthcare services. It will also include persons whose employers have terminated coverage because it did not meet the minimum requirements set by the ACA and persons who had policies that do not meet the minimum benefit standards set by law. As a result, some persons will experience higher premium costs. The Obama administration has already received pushback on this issue.

Private Insurer Initiatives to Transform Health Care

The private insurer industry is responding to the ACA by becoming proactive and adjusting their business models to move from underwriting risk to managing populations. They are changing from insurance carriers to consumer health solution companies. Insurer websites are describing best practices and their goals of improving access to high-quality, affordable care. Personalized care and care coordination through Accountable Care Organizations (ACOs) and medical homes are highlighted. Insurers are also empowering consumers with online and mobile device apps to gain access to extensive provider networks, which demonstrates technological advances. Apps are available for physicians and are meant to assist doctors with meaningful use, workflow management, and clinical support (Monitini, 2012). Wellness and prevention programs, including stress-reduction programs, free cholesterol screenings, hypertension education and monitoring, and tobacco cessation

programs, are being reimbursed. Patient satisfaction is the ultimate goal.

Opportunities for Nursing

The evolving healthcare policy environment is a remarkable opportunity for nurses to demonstrate the quality and value of nursing. Nurse leaders, nurse practitioners, and nurse researchers are in a unique position to demonstrate clinical outcomes, identify wasteful practices, and eliminate inappropriate care (Hahn et al., 2013). Nurse executives have the opportunity to lead their organizations into becoming ACOs by utilizing quality improvement outcomes founded on evidence-based care (Cady, 2012). Researchers will find that the current healthcare environment provides an opportunity to validate nursing's value to healthcare and demonstrate links between quality patient outcomes and care coordination strategies. Nursing case managers will find employment opportunities in private insurance companies as nurse coordinators, navigators, and transition to care specialists that assist patients and families through the continuum of care. Nurses will also be involved in the design and implementation of health information technology in their workplaces as consumers and healthcare providers embrace

Table 13-4   Nurse Employment Opportunities

Opportunities for nurses in the private insurance industry	Scope of role
Nurse coordinators	Responsible for interprofessional coordination of skilled nursing care. Also serves as a patient advocate and facilitates communication among all stakeholders. Champions healthcare quality by supervising compliance with the Minimum Data Set (MDS) and Resident Assessment Instrument (RAI) requirements.

Nurse navigators	Facilitates patient empowerment as a coach, tutor, and direct care provider. Skilled in overcoming system barriers to comprehensive care with a variety of interprofessional team members.
Transitional care specialists	Oversees care when a patient is relocated, transferred, or transitioned due to a change in the type of care required. This model primarily applies to the management of complex chronic medical conditions. The goal is to promote the flow of information and ease the patient's and family's adjustment to a new situation.
Nurse information specialists	These specialists are usually registered nurses with graduate degrees. They construct, execute, and administer data systems that support healthcare quality through electronic medical records and outcomes analyses. They often deliver educational programs to clinicians and monitor trends.

Sources: Data from American Association of Nurse Assessment Coordination (2011); Care Transitions Program (2013); Desimini et al. (2011); Nelson (2013).

technology (Paradis, Wood, & Cramer, 2009). These evolving roles are explained in more detail in Table 13-4.

Nursing has a tradition of providing a voice and leadership in the healthcare reform arena from the perspective of both patients and consumers (Hahn et al., 2013).

Quality Patient Care and Care Coordination Strategies

The current healthcare reform environment provides an opportunity for nurses to participate as leaders in care coordination and promote positive quality patient health outcomes. The ACA contains provisions that support the measurement of effective patient care transitions, support health delivery redesign with payment innovations to foster evidence-based transitional care, support integrated models that hold providers accountable across patient episodes of care, and establish public reporting and payment disincentives for

avoidable hospital readmissions (Naylor & Sochalski, 2010). Master's prepared nurses— that is, advanced practice registered nurses (APRNs)—have been proposing and researching innovative transitional models of patient care that focus on primary care, chronic care management, care coordination, and wellness. The Transitional Care Model (TCM) developed by Mary Naylor and researchers at the University of Pennsylvania has been successful in demonstrating positive outcomes related to the triad of patient access to care, quality of care, and cost.

Naylor, who is Robert Wood Johnson Foundation's Interdisciplinary Nursing Quality Research Initiative director and a professor at the University of Pennsylvania School of Nursing, designed the evidence-based TCM to enhance the quality of life for patients and their families. The model involves care by APRNs serving as the primary care coordinator to reduce hospital readmissions and promote positive health outcomes (Robert

Wood Johnson Foundation, 2013). The APRN will perform an in-hospital assessment of the patient and collaborate with the patient's care team to develop an evidence-based discharge care plan that is designed to meet the expectations of the patient, caregiver, and healthcare providers. Beginning with a visit within the first 24 hours after hospital discharge, the transitional care nurse (TCN) makes regular home visits and is available through telephone support for an average of 2 months after discharge. The TCN facilitates continuity of medical care among the hospital and primary care providers in the community. Patient and family engagement is a cornerstone of this model; it connects the patient, family caregivers, and healthcare providers as members of the care team (Robert Wood Johnson Foundation, 2013; University of Pennsylvania, 2013).

Naylor reported increased patient satisfaction, physical functioning, and quality of life with the TCM model (Naylor et al, 2009). Improved healthcare quality outcomes at a lower cost have been demonstrated in National Institutes of Health (NIH) trials, including a drop in readmission rates within 6 weeks by 57% (Naylor et al., 1994) and a 50% reduction in readmission rates within 6 months (Naylor et al., 1999). Naylor and her team of researchers partnered with Aetna Corporation and Kaiser Permanente Health Plan to translate research into practice. Throughout research and practice testing, the model has been proven to provide improved quality of care at lower cost by reducing the number of hospital readmissions. TCM was the basis for a new Medicare benefit for hospital discharge planning (University of Pennsylvania, 2013).

For decades, another dynamic nursing leader has been setting the example of expert care coordination while meeting the needs of childbearing women in the urban healthcare arena. Ruth Watson Lubic is credited with establishing two certified birth centers: the Maternity Center Association in New York City and the Family Health and Childbirthing Center in Washington, D.C. Prenatal and labor and delivery care is provided at these centers for low-risk pregnancies. The cost savings are significant for childbearing women, the Cesarean rate was reduced in 2005 compared with the rest of the city (15% versus 28%), and the rates of premature and low-birth rate infants were significantly reduced. This resulted in a cost savings of $1.2 million. Such a nurse-driven innovation, if expanded to a nationwide model, could potentially save almost $13 billion for Medicaid-funded deliveries (Nickitas, 2011). Lubic's legacy lives on in Washington, D.C., with the Family Health and Childbirthing Center reporting their yearly 2012 statistics demonstrating a Cesarean section rate of 18%, which is significantly below the 2012 national Cesarean section rate average of 34%. The Center has been successful in decreasing premature infant births and reported a 5% premature infant rate in 2012 (Community of Hope, 2013).

Conclusion

Private insurers continue to hold the largest insurance market share, with 150 million Americans participating in private health plans. For most Americans, healthcare insurance remains a benefit from their employers. Key federal legislation has shaped the healthcare industry, and the most recent healthcare reform legislation, the ACA, is changing the way private insurers conduct business. Consumer empowerment and legislative reforms are instrumental in changing the private insurer business models from underwriting risk to managing populations. The ACA is providing new opportunities for nurses to demonstrate quality outcomes through evidence-based practice and research and to provide patient services as navigators and clinical coordinators, and for APRNs to provide and bill for patient care.

Discussion Questions

1. Describe the difference between employer-sponsored health insurance plans and private (nongroup) plans.
2. Explain some of the features all health plans must offer as of January 2014. What are some of the exceptions for grandfathered plans?
3. Conduct an internet search of the insurance marketplace for your state. What are some of the features that you and your family will benefit from the most?
4. Describe the new nursing opportunities and roles that are evolving as the ACA is being implemented.

References

American Association of Nurse Assessment Coordination. (2011). *Defining the role of nurse assessment coordinators: Beyond paperwork and reimbursement.* Retrieved from http://www .aanac.org/docs/white-papers/the-role-of-the-nurse-assessment-coordinator-(april-2011).pdf?sfvrsn=2

American Public Health Association. (2014). *ACA basics and background.* Retrieved from http: //www.apha.org/advocacy/Health+Reform /ACAbasics/

Blue Cross Blue Shield. (2014). *About Blue Cross Blue Shield Association.* Retrieved from http: //www.bcbs.com/about-the-association/

Cady, R. F. (2012). Health care reform after the Supreme Court ruling: Implications for nurse executives. *JONA's Healthcare, Law, Ethics, and Regulation, 14*(3), 81–84.

Care Transitions Program. (2013). *Health care services for improving quality and safety during care hand-offs.* Retrieved from http://www.caretransitions.org/definitions.asp

Chaikind, H., Fernandez, B., Newsom, M., & Peterson, C. L. (2010). *Private health insurance provisions in the Patient Protection and Affordable Care Act (PPACA).* Retrieved from http://www .fas.org/sgp/crs/misc/R43048.pdf

Community of Hope (2013). *Family Health and Birth Center.* Retrieved from http://www.communityofhopedc.org/fhbc

Desimini, E., Kennedy, J., Helsley, M., Shiner, K., Denton, C., Rice, T., . . . Lewis, M. (2011, September/October). Making the case for nurse navigators: Benefits, outcomes and return on investment. *Oncology Issues, 26–33.*

Ducat, S. (2013). *Employer-sponsored family health premiums rise a modest 4 percent in 2013, national benchmark employer survey finds.* Retrieved from http://www.healthaffairs.org /press/2013_08_20.php

Fernandez, B. (2011). *Health insurance: A primer.* Retrieved from http://www.law.uh.edu/faculty

/jmantel/health-regulatory-process/Fernandez-CRSReportforCongress-Health%20Insurance-APrimer.pdf

Hahn, J. A., Sheingold, B. H., & Ott, K. M. (2013). Demystifying state health insurance marketplaces. *Nursing Economic$, 31*(3), 119–127.

Healthcare.gov. (2014a). *Glossary. Flexible spending accounts.* Retrieved from https://www.healthcare.gov/glossary/flexible-spending-account-FSA/

Healthcare.gov. (2014b). *What if I have a grandfathered health insurance plan?* Retrieved from https://www.healthcare.gov/what-if-i-have-a-grandfathered-health-plan/

HealthInsurance.net. (2014). *History of health insurance.* Retrieved from http://www.healthinsurance.net/history-of-health-insurance.html

HealthPlanOne. (2014). *HIP.* Retrieved from http://www.healthplanone.com/healthinsurancecarriers/hip/

Kaiser Family Foundation. (2013a). *Employer responsibility under the Affordable Care Act.* Retrieved from http://kff.org/infographic/employer-responsibility-under-the-affordable-care-act/

Kaiser Family Foundation. (2013b). *Percent of private sector establishments that offer health insurance to employees.* Retrieved from http://kff.org/other/state-indicator/percent-of-firms-offering-coverage/

Kaiser Permanente. (2014). *Our history.* Retrieved from http://xnet.kp.org/newscenter/aboutkp/historyofkp.html

Michigan Association of Health Plans. (n.d.). *Blue Cross and Blue Shield: A historical compilation.* Retrieved from http://consumersunion.org/wp-content/uploads/2013/03/yourhealthdollar.org_blue-cross-history-compilation.pdf

Monitini, L. (2012). *A tale of two keynotes: Futurist Joe Flower and Aetna's Mark Bertoli.* Retrieved from http://thehealthcareblog.com/blog/2012/10/09/a-tale-of-two-keynotes-futurist-joe-flower- and-aetna%E2%80%99s-mark-bertoli/

Naylor, M. D., Brooten, D., Campbell, R., Jacobsen, B. Mezey, M., Pauly, M., & Schwartz. J. S. (1999). Comprehensive discharge planning and home follow-up of hospitalized elders: A randomized controlled trial. *Journal of the American Medical Association, 28*(7), 613–620.

Naylor, M. D., Brooten, D., Jones, R., Lavizzo-Mourey, R., Mezey, M, & Pauly, M. (1994). Comprehensive discharge planning for the hospitalized elderly: A randomized clinical trial. *Annals of Internal Medicine, 120*(12), 999–1006.

Naylor, M. D., Feldman, P. H., Keating, S., Koren, M. J., Kurtzman, E. T., Maccoy, M. C., & Krakauer, R. (2009). Translating research into practice: Transitional care for older adults. *Journal of Evaluation in Clinical Practice 15*(16), 1164–1170.

Naylor, M. D., & Sochalsi, J. A. (2010). Scaling up: Bringing the transitional care model into the mainstream. *The Commonwealth Fund.* Retrieved from http://www.commonwealthfund.org/Publications/Issue-Briefs/2010/Nov/Scaling-Up-Transitional-Care.aspx

Nelson, B. (2013). *Health information technology: Where do nurses fit in?* Retrieved from http://nursing.advanceweb.com/Student-and-New-Grad-Center/Career-Counseling/Health-Information-Technology-Where-Do-Nurses-Fit-In.aspx

Nickitas, D. M. (2011). Nurses. In D. M. Nickitas, D. J. Middaugh, & N. Aries (Eds.), *Policy and politics* (p. 93). Sudbury, MA: Jones & Bartlett Learning.

O'Connor, J. T. (2013). *Comprehensive assessment of ACA factors that will affect individual market premiums in 2014.* Retrieved from http://www.ahip.org/MillimanReportACA04252013/

Paradis, M., Wood, J., & Cramer, M. (2009). A policy analysis of health care reform: Implications for nurses. *Nursing Economic$, 27*(5), 281–287.

Patel, K., & Rushefshy, M. (1999). *Health care politics and policy in America* (2nd ed.). New York, NY: M. E. Sharpe.

Robert Wood Johnson Foundation (2013). *The transitional care model. The future of nursing.* Retrieved from http://www.nursing.upenn.edu/media/transitionalcare/Pages/default.aspx

SASid. (2007). *COBRA law information*. Retrieved from http://www.cobrainsurance.com/COBRA_Law.htm

Sultz, H. A., & Young, K. M. (2009). *Health care USA: Understanding its organization and delivery* (6th ed.). Frederick, MD: Aspen.

Supreme Court of the United States. (2012). National Federation of Independent Business et al. v. Sebelius, Secretary of Health and Human Services, et al. Retrieved from http://www.supremecourt.gov/opinions/11pdf/11-393c3a2.pdf

University of Pennsylvania. (2013). *Transitional care model*. Penn State Nursing. Retrieved from http://www.nursing.upenn.edu/media/transitionalcare/Pages/default.aspx

U.S. Bureau of Labor Statistics. (2010). *Compensation and working conditions. Consumer-driven health care: What is it and what does it mean for employees and employers?* Retrieved from http://www.bls.gov/opub/cwc/cm20101019ar01p1.htm

U.S. Department of Labor. (2013a). *Health plans and benefits: Employment Retirement Income Security Act*. Retrieved from http://www.dol.gov/dol/topic/health-plans/erisa.htm#doltopics

U.S. Department of Labor. (2013b). *Health plans and benefits: Health Insurance Portability and Accountability Act*. Retrieved from http://www.dol.gov/dol/topic/health-plans/portability.htm

U.S. Department of the Treasury. (2013). *Resource center: Health Savings Accounts (HSAs)*. Retrieved from http://www.treasury.gov/resource-center/faqs/Taxes/Pages/Health-Savings-Accounts.aspx

U.S. Government. (2002). *Interdepartmental Committee on Employment-based Health Insurance Surveys. Definitions of health insurance terms*. Retrieved from http://www.bls.gov/ncs/ebs/sp/healthterms.pdf

WhiteHouse.gov. (2014). *Health care that works for Americans*. Retrieved from http://www.whitehouse.gov/healthreform/healthcare-overview

Zhou, K. (2009). The history of medical insurance in the United States. *Yale Journal of Medicine and Law, 6*(1), 38–39. Retrieved from http://www.yalemedlaw.com/issues/vol6-issue1.pdf

CHAPTER 14

Medicare: From Protector to Innovator

Lucas Pauls

Overview

In 1965, President Johnson signed Medicare and Medicaid into law to protect two vulnerable populations: the old and the poor, respectively. At first, despite its massive size, Medicare passively protected those vulnerable populations, and other at-risk populations were added over time. As costs rose at startling rates and threatened Medicare's solvency, it was slowly forced to emerge as the key driver of the U.S. healthcare system. Medicare still faces many financial challenges, and it will for many years. It has recently, and most assertively under the Affordable Care Act (ACA), asserted itself as the dominant player in healthcare reform. Medicare's history highlights common tensions in U.S. policy and will continue to both reflect and lead policy discussions in the future.

Objectives

- Understand the history of Medicare enactment and the evolution of the program.
- Explain the structure of Medicare, including who is eligible and the covered benefits.
- Discuss Medicare's role in protecting seniors.
- Analyze Medicare's role in influencing the larger U.S. healthcare system.
- Assess Medicare's future financial challenges.
- Discuss the changes to Medicare with the implementation of the ACA.

A casual observer to the lead up, passing, and aftermath of the ACA can tell you that the government's role in U.S. health care is a politically charged topic. It has been so for almost a century. The policy and politics surrounding the government's role in health care involves such themes as federalism versus states' rights, special interests versus societal interests, government versus the market, and individualism versus collectivism.

Fifty million Americans are covered under Medicare, the federal insurance program for people aged 65 years and older and many younger people with long-term disabilities. Federal spending for Medicare accounts for 1 of every 5 dollars spent on health care and represents 16% of the federal budget (Kaiser Family Foundation, 2012b). In 2012, the Medicare budget was $536 billion (more than $11,000 per recipient), and with expected growth in prices, services, and especially the number of people covered as the baby boomers age, it is expected to balloon further (Congressional Budget Office [CBO], 2013).

Even with the very significant federal outlay, Medicare does not provide blanket coverage. Long-term care is usually not covered, and most other care requires copays, deductibles, and other out-of-pocket requirements. The covered elderly shoulder a substantial healthcare burden. On average, people older than age 65 use 15% of their household income to pay for services not covered or partially covered by Medicare—three times the share of spending in non-Medicare households.

Most people aged 65 years and older are entitled to Medicare Part A if they or their spouse are eligible for Social Security payments and have made payroll tax contributions for 10 or more years. Also covered are people younger than age 65 with permanent disabilities. Nonelderly people who receive Social Security Disability Insurance (SSDI) generally become eligible for Medicare after a 2-year waiting period, and people who are diagnosed with end-stage renal disease (ESRD) and amyotrophic lateral sclerosis (ALS) become eligible for Medicare with no to minimal waiting periods.

During its near half century, the original Medicare has been amended and profoundly changed:

- In 1972, the entitlement was expanded beyond the elderly to include people with permanent disabilities.

- During the 1980s, an inflation-inducing cost-based hospital payment system was replaced by a case-based system, called Diagnosis-Related Groups (DRGs), that depended on each patient's diagnosis and severity of illness.

- Prescription drug coverage was added in 2003 along with partial private Medicare Advantage plans.

- Expansions and changes were made in 2010 as an integral part of the ACA.

Medicare is a federally financed and administered behemoth, and thus its history is fraught with policy and politics on the grandest scale. Medicare, along with its fraternal twin, Medicaid, grew out of Social Security in 1965 as integral parts of the welfare safety net. However, the mere magnitude of Medicare now makes it a driver, if a reluctant one, of healthcare trends and policy. As Medicare goes, the rest of health care follows. More recently, with the enactment of the ACA, the United States has the tools it needs to harness the size of Medicare so it can be a payment innovator and a key tool to protect the financial and physical well-being of the elderly.

Structure of Medicare Today

Medicare is a federal universal healthcare entitlement program for people aged 65 years and older regardless of income or health status and for people younger than age 65 who have long-term disabilities. Medicare added people with ESRD in 1972 and people with ALS in 2001. In 2012, 50 million people were covered under Medicare (CBO, 2013). To be eligible for Medicare, you must also meet the work requirements. Simply stated, you have to pay into Medicare by working (or your spouse must work) for 40 quarters (10 years).

Medicare is split into four parts—Parts A through D. Parts A and B were established as part of Title XVIII of the Social Security Act in 1965. Part A covers hospital bills, skilled nursing facilities, and home health and hospice services, and it is compulsory. Part A is funded by an income tax of 2.9% that is split between employers and employees, with higher percentages for high earners. Part A accounted for 36% of Medicare expenses and covered 50 million people in 2012.

Part B is a voluntary, opt-out arrangement that covers physician services. It accounts for 27% of Medicare expenses and is funded through general revenue and enrollee-paid premiums with mild progressive tiers based on income. In 2012, 46 million people were enrolled in Part B (CBO, 2013).

Part C is also known as Medicare Advantage. These are private plans that Medicare enrollees can opt in to. They cover both hospital and physician services (Parts A and B) and frequently include a prescription benefit. They are financed by general funds and enrollee premiums. Premiums are typically equal to Part B premiums, but they may be higher depending on the coverage level of the plan. Part C as it exists today was enacted in the Balanced Budget Act of 1997 in an attempt to control costs through market competition among plans. However, Medicare Advantage plans have not performed as intended and typically cost 9–13% more than standard Medicare. In 2012, 13 million people were enrolled in Part C, which accounted for 24% of Medicare spending (Kaiser Family Foundation, 2010).

Part D is a prescription drug plan that was established in the Medicare Modernization Act of 2003 and rolled out in 2006. Private plans contract directly with Medicare to provide this benefit and are financed through general revenue, state payments, and enrollee premiums (separate from Part B premiums). In 2012, 37 million people were enrolled in one of these private prescription plans and accounted for 10% of Medicare expenditures. Each private plan can either offer the standard benefit or a benefit that is actuarially equivalent. Nearly 90% of plans offer an equivalent package, but all plans include high cost sharing (deductibles, copays, or coinsurance), and most plans include the infamous doughnut hole where enrollees pay 100% of their drug costs after the total drug costs reach $2,830 and before the total drug costs reach $6,440, when plan coverage kicks back in. The ACA is scheduled to gradually fill in the doughnut hole by 2020 (Kaiser Family Foundation, 2010).

Medicare has significant gaps in care—most significantly, long-term healthcare coverage—and includes large out-of-pocket expenses. Enrollees have historically filled these gaps and paid these expenses in a variety of ways, such as employer-based insurance, private plans called Medigap, the use of more generous Medicare Advantage plans, and Medicaid. In 2007, only 11% of enrollees used standard Medicare without some sort of gap protection (Kaiser Family Foundation, 2010).

Box 14-1   Medicare Overview

Coverage type; date instituted; dollars spent; financing scheme:

- Part A: Hospital-based coverage; 1965; 36%; 2.9% payroll tax
- Part B: Physician-based coverage; 1965; 27%; general funds and premiums paid by enrollees
- Part C: Medicare Advantage private plans inclusive of hospital and physician coverage (some include drug coverage); 1997; 24%; general funds and premiums paid by enrollees (varies by plan)
- Part D: Prescription plan; 2003; 10%; general funds and participant cost sharing

Source: Data from Kaiser Family Foundation (2010).

National Health Insurance

The United States has struggled to adopt national health insurance for many reasons, including the inherent constitutional-based divided nature of our government; the influence of special interests; and an American ideology of independence, self-reliance, limited government, and market principles. Incongruently, Medicare is an overwhelmingly popular federal health insurance program, even among those that are opposed to universal health care ("New York Times/CBS News," 2011). How do we as a society resist the concepts of universal health care for so long but hold so dearly to Medicare, a near-universal program for the elderly?

The creation of Medicare in 1965 can be understood in the context of two competing ideas. On one hand, there have been repeated efforts to create a national health insurance program since 1912 and Theodore Roosevelt's platform on the Bull Moose Party. Each effort was soundly defeated, and national health insurance was pulled off the public agenda given the opposition by the medical profession and the expansion of employer-based insurance starting in the late 1940s, which made universal coverage through the market seem possible. The counterbalance was the rising cost of health care and the exclusion of the elderly and the poor from benefits. On one hand, hospitals that historically had opposed any move toward national health insurance were suddenly finding themselves bearing the financial brunt of patients who could not pay for increasingly expensive services. On the other hand, the elderly, who lost access to health benefits upon retirement through no fault of their own, were finding themselves bankrupted by the cost of medical care in their old age. As a result, by the late 1950s, health insurance for the elderly was put back on the public agenda because it addressed multiple interests. Advocates of national health insurance saw it as the first step toward a more inclusive program. Hospitals saw it as a means to pay for services that had been attributed to bad debt. Democrats saw such as programs as responsive to the demands of civil rights activists, and Republicans understood the need to take action, even in a limited way.

Box 14-2   Timeline of Medicare: Major Dates

- 1934 and 1938: Healthcare coverage was proposed and dropped during President Franklin Delano Roosevelt's administration.
- 1945: President Truman advocated for a national health insurance plan.
- 1960: The Kerr-Mills bill was passed and provided money to states to pay for medical services for the elderly poor.
- 1965: Medicare Parts A and B were created under Title XVIII of the Social Security Act.
- 1972: President Nixon signed the Social Security Amendments of 1972, which provided benefits to those with long-term disabilities who were younger than age 65 and to individuals with ESRD.
- 1980s: A series of changes were added to control Medicare spending, including DRGs, in which hospital payments were established based on medical conditions. Hospice became a covered benefit.
- 1988–1989: The Medicare Catastrophic Care Act was passed and repealed. It capped out-of-pocket spending and added an outpatient drug benefit, but it collapsed under backlash regarding increased premiums and an increased progressive tax finance scheme. A provision that Medicaid would pay Medicare premiums for participants with incomes lower than 100% of the federal poverty level survived.
- 1997: Medicare Part C was established through the Balanced Budget Act of 1997.
- 2001: People with ALS became eligible for Medicare benefits, regardless of age.
- 2003: Medicare Part D was established through the Medicare Modernization Act of 2003.
- 2010: The ACA was enacted.

Source: Data from Kaiser Family Foundation, (2012c).

Passage of Medicare

The passage of any large bill through the constitutionally divided and substantially immovable political process takes the convergence of many factors. In 1965, several key events aligned:

1. After President John F. Kennedy's assassination in 1963 and President Lyndon B. Johnson's landslide victory in 1964 over the staunchly conservative Barry Goldwater, the liberal policy agenda was given a strong headwind. Along with a Democratic House and Senate, the will and, more important, votes to enact President Johnson's agenda were present. Medicare was among President Johnson's top priorities. He moved quickly and took advantage of the cyclical open window that is characteristic of the beginning of most presidential terms. President Johnson proposed his bill (HR-1 in the House and S-1 in the Senate) on January 4, 1965 (Brown, 1996).

2. The elderly had been identified as a vulnerable group for more than a decade. In 1959, 35.2% of Americans older than age 65 years were living below the poverty line, compared with 17% of Americans younger than age 65. Moreover, in 1964, slightly more than 50% of elderly Americans did not have health insurance coverage (Health Care Financing Administration, 2000). The existing patchwork of coverage left the elderly exposed, and the increased cost of insurance left many of them without the means to access medical services. Both the elderly themselves and their children faced a growing liability.

3. During the 1960s, there was a national awakening to the needs of minorities and the poor. The civil rights movement exposed poverty in America, and the Great Society programs arose to address these issues. The Civil Rights Act of 1964 was passed 12 months before Medicare, and Title VI of the Civil Rights Act outlawed discrimination at any institution that receives federal funding. Privately, Medicare was seen as a vehicle to advance civil rights (Brown, 1996), and publicly it was a bill to protect a vulnerable, deserving, and often impoverished population. Although Medicare is an entitlement program, the elderly were seen as a deserving population. The work requirement reinforced this notion. The moral incentive to extend civil protections in 1964, and then financial protections through Medicare, to a vulnerable deserving population brought strength to a historically weak constituency.

4. The U.S. economy was strong in 1965, and budgetary concerns produced little anxiety. The government was running a surplus. Antitax sentiment was relatively weak. Healthcare costs, though increasing rapidly, were not so insurmountable that they were seen as a national crisis, but they increased fast enough that the financial burden to the elderly was increasingly real (Brown, 1996). Rising personal costs were seen as an incentive to action, unlike today, when concern over the budget often trumps everything else.

5. The leadership in the Executive Branch, House, and Senate did not overreach. Their policies clearly considered the medical professions' political muscle and the difficult history of healthcare expansion. They also believed that incremental steps were a realistic path to national health insurance, so they did not see the need for, and they did not propose, universal coverage (Brown, 1996).

President Johnson's proposal in 1965 was the central pillar of his Great Society and had three main goals. First, he would increase the Social Security cash benefit. Second, he would create hospital-only insurance for the elderly. His plan did not include financing for outpatient physician services to avoid the opposition of medical professionals, most notably the American Medical Association (AMA), which had a long history of opposing government intervention in medical care. Third, he would improve medical assistance to the poor. The bill was first considered in the Ways and Means Committee in January 1965. In addition to President Johnson's compulsory hospital insurance proposal, two alternative proposals were being considered. The first proposal, surprisingly offered by the AMA and referred to as Eldercare, offered hospital and physician services on a voluntary means-tested basis as an alternative to compulsory programs, and the program would be controlled at the state level. The second alternative proposal before Representative Wilbur Mills (D-AR), chairman of the Ways and Means Committee, was offered by the Republican leadership and was a voluntary, subsidized physician package. In what turned out to be a shrewd and surprising move, Representative Mills combined President Johnson's compulsory hospital insurance (Part A) with the Republican voluntary and subsidized physician coverage (Part B). He also took the AMA's Eldercare concept of using a state-level, means-tested formula to expand coverage to the poor (Medicaid) to complete the three-pronged bill (Starr, 1982). The House approved the bill on March 29, 1965, in a 313 to 115 vote. The Senate passed the bill on July 9, 1965, in a 68 to 21 vote. President Johnson signed Title XVIII of the Social Security Act on July 30, 1965, which established Medicare and Medicaid. When Medicare passed, President Johnson (1965) said the following:

> No longer will older Americans be denied the healing miracle of modern medicine. No longer will illness crush and destroy the savings they have so carefully put away over a lifetime so they might enjoy dignity in their later years. No longer will young families see their own incomes, and their own hopes, eaten away simply because they are carrying out their deep moral obligations. (p. 811)

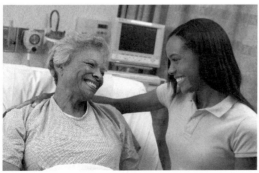

© BananaStock/Thinkstock

When it came to the broader questions of the government's role in health care and federalism, Medicare and Medicaid were a great compromise that settled very little. Title XVIII of the Social Security Act gave a little to both sides of the federalism debate. Medicare clearly answered that the federal government has a strong role to play. Medicaid argued for state authority. For national health insurance advocates, the passage of Medicare and Medicaid was seen as a first step toward that goal. Those who favor a limited government role in health care saw its passage as strengthening the welfare safety net and repudiating further encroachment by the federal government.

Implementation

Medicare coverage began on July 1, 1966—11 months after it passed. Part A was a well-understood policy before enactment. The American Hospital Association (AHA) was a willing partner both prior to enactment and during implementation. Part B was a complete surprise to the administration, and implementation needed to start from scratch. In 11 months, the Department of Health, Education, and Welfare (HEW) had to inform, engage, and enroll 8 million people. For Part A, this involved the same administrative process already in place under the Social Security benefits. For Part B, this involved back-and-forth conversations between HEW and 8 million potential participants regarding the benefits and the premiums. Further, payment policy and procedures, including the enforcement of the Civil Rights Act, were established among HEW, payment intermediaries, and providers. On an administrative level, the implementation was as remarkable as the enactment itself (National Academy of Social Insurance, 2001).

A Changed Landscape

Medicare and Medicaid extended financial and political protections to vulnerable populations. In 1963, 53% of Americans aged 65 years and older had insurance against hospital costs (Moon, 1996). By 1970, this rate had increased to 97%. In 1965, 35% of Americans older than age 65 lived in poverty. By 1974, the poverty rate for this group had dropped to 15% (Health Care Financing Administration, 2000). Medicare and Medicaid also played a crucial role in ending racial segregation in healthcare settings for people of all ages. With federal funding now flowing to almost every corner of the healthcare system, the entirety of the health system fell under the purview of the Civil Rights Act. Of course, Medicare cannot be credited with every gain, but certainly it played a crucial role in ensuring the financial stability of older Americans and in assisting the transformation of the healthcare industry into a more race-blind community (Quadagno, 2000).

Spiraling Costs

As healthcare access grew, costs also rose dramatically. The growth rate for the 7 years prior to Medicare passage averaged 3.2%, followed by a 5-year average of 7.9% (Starr, 1982). In 1967, Medicare spent $3 billion; it spent $50 billion by 1980, $211 billion by 1997, and more than $500 billion in 2012 (CBO, 2013; Health Care Financing Administration, 2000). Medicare's mere size and its role in covering the most expensive population makes unwinding its role in health inflation from the myriad of inflationary factors almost impossible. It is certainly true that healthcare costs have been escalating for reasons outside of Medicare's purview, including advancements

in technology, an aging population, the rise of long-term chronic conditions, the deteriorating health of society, provider specialization, and many other factors. But the steep rise in healthcare costs must be understood as a political choice to build a wall separating Medicare from the relationship between providers and their patients that reinforced the retrospective fee-for-service model, stymied public and private payer innovation, and led to an escalation of prices. Ultimately, medical providers prospered due to a larger pool of paying patients and favorable payments.

Medicare was designed strictly to be a payer of care. It was explicitly understood during implementation that Medicare was not in the business of reforming care or the payment of care (National Academy of Social Insurance, 2001). Provisions in the legislation allowed hospitals to choose an intermediary private carrier to administer the payment—in most cases, Blue Cross plans with deep hospital roots—as a buffer between federal payments and providers. The same buffer concept held true of Part B and physicians, with Blue Shield being the common intermediary. Explanations for using intermediaries could include the expertise and efficiency of private payers or that it was a compromise to obtain the support of special interests, but intermediaries certainly protected the healthcare industry from the intrusion of the federal government into health services and created a role for health insurance providers in new government programs.

Furthermore, Medicare explicitly and significantly decided to pay on the basis of costs rather than using its purchasing power to negotiate rates. The hospital costs included capital projects and depreciation—a decidedly favorable arrangement for hospitals (Starr, 1982). Further, institutions and providers established their own costs, thereby holding Medicare hostage to their reimbursement demands. As long as the customary fees were reasonable compared with peers, Medicare paid the bill. As providers pushed their usual and customary fees higher and higher, the reasonability of high fees became ever more reasonable (Starr, 1982). Hospitals did not manage to a budget as most businesses require, but they seek reimbursement for their costs no matter how inflated they are. Ultimately, implementation followed two simple ideas: Americans needed more medical services than they could afford or the market demanded, and physicians and hospitals were best equipped to organize and structure all aspects of health delivery (Starr, 1982).

Cost Controls

In 1967, costs were not a primary concern, and it can be argued that cost-control mechanisms were traded for increased access and political support from the healthcare industry. By the 1970s, the politics that improved medical access and focused on vulnerable populations reversed course because of concern over price, excessive services, and large inefficiencies. During Medicare's creation, the strategy was accommodation to the medical community, but 5 years later, in the face of mounting bills, attention turned toward regulation and cost controls. The original hope of reformers to incrementally build on Medicare and Medicaid was stymied by the increasing focus on budgets and spiraling costs.

In response to rising costs, Medicare began to look for cost-control mechanisms, but the reforms were underwhelming. In 1972, Medicare established Professional Standards Review Organizations (PSROs), which retrospectively reviewed medical necessity and the appropriateness of the provided healthcare services. However, their ability to control costs was minimal (Bhatia, Blackstck, Nelson, & Ng, 2000). Under President Nixon's urging, the Social Security Amendments of 1972 formalized a managed care option. However, by 1979, only 34 regional managed care options under Medicare were available. The managed care option in Medicare was more symbolic than practical (Zaraboza, 2000). Throughout the 1970s, additional cost control measures, including revived pushes for national health insurance, were proposed and debated, but few gained traction. What was clear was that fee for service, especially on a cost basis, was not a workable long-term plan and that other payment models would need to be tested. Exactly how to do this was unknown.

By 1983, healthcare costs in general, and Medicare expenditures specifically, were continuing in an inflationary spiral. The retrospective payment system adopted in 1966 was seen as a main culprit in the rising costs. Advancing technology paired with a payment system that pays costs and offers no resistance to increasing technology expenses regardless of effectiveness is an often maligned duo. Eighteen years after Medicare enactment, Congress passed the Social Security Amendments of 1983, which instructed Medicare and Medicaid to pay hospitals through a prospective payment system (PPS) as a first counter to escalating prices and in stark contrast to Medicare's beginnings.

A prospective payment system is a per-case reimbursement structure under which inpatient admission cases are divided into relatively homogeneous categories called Diagnosis-Related Groups (DRGs). In the DRG payment system, Medicare pays hospitals a flat rate per case for inpatient hospital care so that efficient hospitals are rewarded for their efficiency and inefficient hospitals have an incentive to become more efficient (Gottlober, 2001). No longer was Medicare reimbursing the hospitals' costs. DRG rates were meant to set averages for bundled hospital, nonphysician care for a specific diagnosis, including nursing, room and board, and ancillary services. DRGs do not cover services under Part B or follow-up care after hospital discharge. The intermediary system remained intact, and their new job was to use the Medicare grouper algorithm to decode the diagnoses and assign the proper DRG to claims. The price paid per DRG is based on the average charges for a given collection of services, which are used to calculate the weight of a DRG. The weight of a DRG plus other adjustment factors—including a geographically specific wage index, medical education factor, and disproportionate share factor (care to hospitals that service low-income, uninsured, and Medicaid populations)—increase or decrease the payment from a hospital's base case rate. Simply stated, if a case is expected to require more intensive services, the weight is larger and a higher DRG payment will follow.

The Social Security Amendments of 1983 accomplished several important changes. Primarily, Medicare payments moved from strictly a cost basis to an expected cost basis, which, even if minimally, put some pressure on hospitals to rein in their costs. Specifically, DRGs provide hospitals incentives to provide less intensive care and to shorten the length of stay. On the flip side, hospitals have an incentive to increase admissions and discharges quickly to raise the possibility that costs will be shifted to less acute settings (i.e., skilled nursing facilities or home health) or that readmission rates will increase. Further, there was concern that DRGs would stifle advances in medical technology. PSROs were reconstituted to monitor this behavior. Ultimately, DRGs

reduced the length of stay between 20% and 25% (Cutler, 1999), and no significant adverse health quality issues arose. Readmission rates remained constant, and discharge patterns did not change dramatically as feared (Davis, 1988). By 1987, New York State mandated that all payers would reimburse on a DRG basis. DRG payments for Medicare and all payer DRGs for the general population became increasingly the norm for public and private payers. Most significantly, the PPS system placed some risk on hospitals for the first time, changing the power structure between hospitals and payers.

The PPS system did not change payments to physicians. Medicare paid physicians based on their usual and customary fees, which are directly related to the doctors' charges. It was not until 1989, 34 years after its enactment, that Medicare shifted from its initial payment structure through the Omnibus Reconciliation Act of 1989 to the resource-based relative value scale (RBRVS). Relative value units (RVUs) are calculated using three components: physician work (54%), practice expense (41%), and malpractice costs (5%). A geographical cost inflation factor is added based on the location of the service. The AMA assigns RVUs to each Current Procedure Terminology (CPT) code in a relatively secret process—a process from which the AMA receives an estimated $70 million annually through licensing fees (Roy, 2011). Payers using RBRVS negotiate a price for a single RVU. Each CPT is reimbursed based on the amount of RVUs assigned. The RBRVS system does not insert risk or incentivize for efficiency like DRGs did on the hospital side, but it did unlink payments from physician charges for the first time. The major criticism of RBRVS is that it does not incentivize evidence-based medicine and continues the practice of paying for volume over quality of services.

The other significant change resulting from the Social Security Amendments of 1983 was Medicare's increased reliance on data and the mandate for Medicare to use outside expertise to maintain the PPS. Today Medicare uses one private company, 3M, and an expert panel called MedPAC (formerly ProPAC, which started in 1986). The role of 3M is to make recommendations for restructuring and adding new DRGs based on changes in health care. MedPAC takes a broader view and offers expert recommendations on DRG methodologies or how to improve quality of care for a specific subpopulation (Gottlober, 2001). The insertion of outside expertise, especially MedPAC, brought a level of professional input into what could be a purely political forum, and it set a precedent for the ACA.

Medicare Catastrophic Care Act of 1988

Even though the cost issue was not resolved, politics toward the middle of the 1980s allowed an opening for the expansion of Medicare. The Medicare Catastrophic Care Act (MCCA) of 1988 was the first expansion of Medicare since 1972. In 1987, President Reagan sent the MCCA of 1988 to Congress with a similar sentiment as President Johnson's on the enactment of Medicare in 1965:

> I am asking Congress to help give Americans that last full measure of security to provide a health insurance plan that fights the fear of catastrophic illness ... For too long, many of our senior citizens have been faced with making an intolerable choice, a choice between bankruptcy and death. (Reagan, 1987)

The MCCA of 1988 was meant to be a significant expansion of Medicare, but maybe its title promised too much. The MCCA filled financial gaps when an enrollee had an extended hospital stay and capped physician out-of-pocket copays. It also added a prescription drug benefit and protected a spouse's home from insurmountable medical bills usually due to long-term care. The MCCA's title implied a promise to protect against the biggest financial risk seniors face—long-term care—and it did not fulfill this wish. The MCCA filled gaps that few people hit and provided benefits that many elderly already had obtained through supplemental coverage—sometimes provided by a previous employer at little cost to the enrollee.

By 1989, a strong grassroots swell against the MCCA climaxed with the very public and vocal protests against Representative Dan Rostenkowski of Illinois after a community meeting in which elderly people chased and beat his car with picket signs. Elderly people were upset, partially due to misinformation resulting from the complexity of the healthcare delivery system and from deliberately misleading campaigns, but mainly due to the fact that the Medicare expansion was to be financed, as President Reagan insisted, by the elderly only, and specifically by wealthier elderly people who did not need or want this new coverage (Rice, Desmond, & Gabel, 1990). The mounting costs of health care had made the task of finding politically tolerable financing schemes nearly impossible. By November 1989, the MCCA was repealed under the political weight of the Medicare beneficiaries' dissatisfaction and left a political timidity to alter Medicare in any way.

Medicare+Choice

The politics of the 1990s led to passage of the Balanced Budget Act (BBA) of 1997. As it related to health care, the threat confronting Medicare was insolvency. Insolvency happens when the trust funds that pay the Medicare bills cannot cover expenses. Since Medicare's inception, the insolvency date has been reported on an annual basis, and occasional legislative action has delayed this date on several occasions (Figure 14-1).

With a threat of insolvency in 4–5 years, the BBA cut Medicare expenditures by an estimated $116 billion over 5 years ($393.8 billion over 10 years), with most of this savings coming from a slowing of the growth rates used to calculate provider payments and changing the payment methodology for skilled nursing facilities, home health agencies, and other service categories. Further, premiums were projected to increase from $60 per month in 2007 to $105 per month for Part B to provide

increased revenue (O'Sullivan et al., 1997). The third major change was the creation of Part C—Medicare+Choice. Part C was designed to provide market competition among various types of private plans and give private insurers access to millions of new customers.

Since 1972, Medicare supported managed care plans, but the BBA of 1997 opened up Medicare to all types of private plans—preferred provider organizations (PPOs), fee for service, and high-deductible plans. Initial participation in these plans was meager, and they were often unavailable in rural areas. The Medicare Modernization Act of 2003 renamed Part C plans Medicare Advantage and infused life into the plans by making the funding equations even more generous. From 2003 to 2010, the enrollment in Medicare Advantage more than doubled, from 5.3 million to 11.1 million (Kaiser Family Foundation, 2012a). The generosity lavished onto Medicare Advantage plans, based on a geographically specific benchmarking system, also made them more costly, resulting

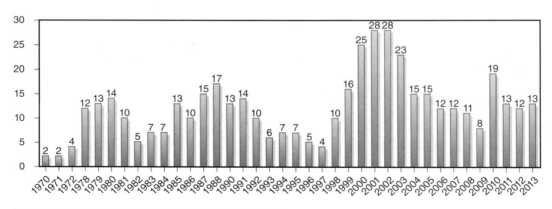

Source: Intermediate projections of various Medicare Trustees report, 1970-2013.
Note: No specific estimates were provided by the Trustees for years 1973-1977 and 1989.

FIGURE 14-1 Projected number of years until HI insolvency

Reproduced from Davis, P. (2013). *Medicare: Insolvency projections.* Congressional Research Service. https://www.fas.org/sgp/crs/misc/RS20946.pdf

in Medicare paying 108% of traditional fee for service Medicare to Medicare Advantage plans (Kaiser Family Foundation, 2012a). The extra expense may be understated because there is considerable debate about whether Medicare Advantage plans skim the Medicare pool for healthier enrollees, making the aggregate population less expensive (McWilliams, 2012), or whether they manage care in ways that improve health (Landon, 2012). What is empirically true is that up to the implementation of the ACA, Medicare Advantage plans, on average, cost Medicare more per enrollee than traditional fee-for-service Medicare.

Prescription Drugs and Medicare

One of the obvious omissions in Medicare benefits until 2003 was the lack of prescription drug coverage. Although a prescription plan was attached to several policy proposals since Medicare's inception, no such bill ever passed, with the exception of the short-lived MCCA of 1988. Underlying each missed opportunity was the escalating costs of Medicare. Too often administrations were so focused on limiting costs (such as President Reagan in 1983) that the idea of adding additional costs seemed overreaching. Under the MCCA of 1988, the weight of the financing scheme doomed the prescription benefit. The pharmaceutical companies often opposed coverage, fearing overregulation and price controls that could accompany government intervention. The increased regulations and cost controls associated with President Clinton's healthcare reform package in 1993 were strong enough to outweigh the promise of an increased customer pool (Oliver, Lee, & Lipton, 2004).

By 2001, a new opening emerged. The combination of budgetary surpluses and flat Medicare trends between 1998 and 2001 following the Balanced Budget Act of 1997 temporarily relieved pressure on Medicare. Further, prescription drug costs were escalating at an unprecedented pace, placing an increasing burden on elderly people who did not have other prescription coverage and forcing employers and Medicare+Choice plans to drop prescription coverage for retirees. Both Medicare's ability to cover these benefits, if only fleeting and shortsighted, and the need for prescription coverage were present. Although a trillion-dollar tax break and a recession in 2001 ate up the budget surplus, the momentum for a prescription benefit was well established. Political roadblocks, accentuated by the administration's focus on the war on terror, prevented further movement for 2 more years as the Bush administration and a very partisan Congress fought over the size (how generous), scope (means tested or universal), and delivery mechanism (run through the states or the federal government). The Bush administration wanted a small, means-tested, block grant program run through the states by private plans, diminishing the federal government's role in Medicare while handing over large functions to private insurers. The Senate, narrowly controlled by Democrats, preferred no benefit over a benefit that they deemed would introduce destructive concepts to the Medicare program.

By 2003, Republicans gained control of Congress, and it was clear that the Bush administration would pursue a prescription drug plan that was linked to a broader overhaul of Medicare, including mechanisms to incentivize beneficiaries to leave fee-for-service Medicare. However, the administration ultimately decided to let Congress write up the legislation under a framework of the administration's choosing—$400 billion over 10 years, a means-tested prescription fixed-credit discount drug program to all beneficiaries, and a requirement for enrollees to use Medicare+Choice plans to receive prescription benefits beyond catastrophic coverage. This last provision was envisioned as a means to move people away from traditional Medicare and into Medicare+Choice. Following quick passage in the Senate and an arm-twisting, one-vote margin in the House of Representatives, a new structure of the prescription benefit appeared in June 2003. The legislation kept the $400 billion price tag but eliminated the incentives to leave traditional Medicare because legislators from rural states were concerned about the availability of private options in their regions. Bill Tauzin (R-LA) said, "You couldn't move my mother out of [fee-for-service] Medicare with a bulldozer. She trusts in it, believes in it. It's served her well" (Oliver et al., 2004, p. 311). When it came down to it, legislators feared the political backlash from any policy that undermined traditional Medicare.

However, there was a larger structural problem. The general framework that emerged was for private prescription-only plans to be offered to standard Medicare beneficiaries, but there were significant concerns about this approach. Foremost, the $400 billion budget was only a fraction of what the Congressional Budget Office (CBO) projected seniors would spend on prescription drugs, making any offered plan very bare bones with high cost sharing. The $400 billion budget was a practical ceiling that allowed the legislation to run through the budget reconciliation process and avoid the prospect of a filibuster in the Senate. A larger budget would require an improbable 60-vote tally in the Senate. There was a real concern

that with voluntary enrollment and high cost sharing, only beneficiaries with known high prescription costs would enroll, thereby contaminating the pool—a phenomenon called adverse selection (Oliver et al., 2004). It was unknown whether private plans would enter the market under these conditions. Further, the private plan model diced the Medicare population into small subgroups that purposefully limited Medicare from leveraging its size to gain significant cost controls.

The final bill that came out of the conference was structured around a requirement for Medicare enrollees to either maintain their current prescription coverage or enroll in Part D to limit adverse selection. Coverage would require a premium, deductible, and coinsurance, which would provide some limited coverage up front, followed by a sizeable gap in coverage before significant catastrophic coverage would begin. The bill prevented the Centers for Medicare and Medicaid Services (CMS), previously the Health Care Financing Administration, from negotiating prices, which allowed pharmaceutical companies to expand profitable deals with their current purchasers (Kaiser Family Foundation, 2010). The concept of infusing Medicare with market competition through increased enrollment in Medicare+Choice was transformed into something closer to a corporate handout while at the same time preventing CMS from negotiating rates, outlawing reimportation of drugs at lower costs, and any other form of cost controls (Oliver et al., 2004). The final approach gave premium support to poorer beneficiaries who did not previously have prescription benefits, and it favored the pharmaceutical companies, who just gained millions of paying customers without the threat of increased regulation or cost controls.

The politics leading up to the vote flipped the norms of the past 70 years, forcing Democrats to vote against a large entitlement expansion and forcing Republicans to support such an expansion without the meaningful market competition most of them craved. After exhausting all of their political capital during the legislative buildup, the Bush administration had no choice but to support the final legislation even if it was missing its most prized features. Defeat of the Medicare Modernization Act would have been a huge political setback. Democrats who were still wary of a private gutting of Medicare but coveted the prescription benefit were split in their thinking. The legislation squeaked through during an extended late-night, vote-wringing, often questioned roll call. The legislation that emerged, the Medicare Modernization Act of 2003, ultimately seemed to please very few. As things turned out, it was the perfect example of destructive compromise whereby each party seemed more intent on the other's defeat than constructing legislation that built on key elements from each party's agenda.

ACA and Accountable Care Organizations

When Medicare was passed in 1965, some of its proponents saw it as the first step toward national health insurance. It took Congress until 2010 to respond by passing the ACA. The ACA is a complicated and multifaceted bill with a wild and controversial history that touches all aspects of health care. It has been touched by all three branches of government and was adopted energetically by only some states and was derailed and obstructed by many others. It is a welcome answer to many blatant weaknesses in the U.S. healthcare system, and simultaneously it is vilified by many people and politicians. It deserves a deeper telling than presented here from historical, political, and policy standpoints. It is also an evolving story. The final effects of the ACA will not be known for many years, and even then they will likely be debated. Its history involves partisan and regional politics, constitutional questions, and, as of this writing, there are still vigilant attempts to deny funding and repeal its mandates.

In relation to Medicare, and in simplistic overgeneralizations, the ACA does the following (Kaiser Family Foundation, 2011):

- Leaves Medicare benefits intact so beneficiaries will not see a decrease in benefits.
- Gradually fills the Medicare Part D coverage gap by 2020. Today Part D includes a 100% coinsurance during the gap. By 2020, covered drugs will include a 20% coinsurance.
- Alters the payment model to Medicare Advantage programs to lower costs in high-cost areas and increase costs in low-costs areas. It also adds bonus payments to plans with high-quality performance.
- Reduces annual payment increases to inpatient hospitals and other facilities.
- Establishes a Payment Advisory Board that is designed to advise Congress of a set of reforms, under legislative guidelines, if CMS does not meet moderate spending targets.

The ACA also improves public transparency of quality performance metrics by making quality measures for hospitals and physicians public. Hospital Compare and the still-developing Physician Compare tools on Medicare's website allow patients to research and select providers that provide the highest quality care (Centers for Medicare and Medicaid Services, 2013).

To further advance quality improvement, the ACA established an Innovation Center that will test and evaluate payment reforms within Medicare and will run several pilot programs to test innovative approaches to payment structures and delivery systems. One such pilot program widens the bundle under a fixed payment to include all services from facilities and physicians 3 days prior to an admission and 30 days after a discharge. A second program tests the cost effectiveness of providing high-risk beneficiaries primary care services in their homes (Kaiser Family Foundation, 2011).

The ACA uses Medicare as a driver of payment reform and improved quality. It establishes value-based payment models whereby Medicare pays more for good outcomes and does not pay for some poor outcomes, especially outcomes that never should occur—descriptively called *never events*. Although the ACA does not mandate private payers to change their business models, it does instruct CMS to move away from fee for service and move toward global, performance-based payment models via Accountable Care Organizations (ACOs).

The ACA is accelerating a large restructuring of the healthcare delivery system through ACOs, which are large groups of providers—often hospitals and physician groups that must include primary care—that come together to form a large network to better coordinate care delivery across multiple care settings. At face value, ACOs sound much like managed care, and in theory they will function in similar ways, with strong financial incentives to keep patients healthy and coordinate care to achieve lower costs. The major difference is that patients are not assigned nor restrained by the ACO like they would be in a managed care plan. Patients have the freedom to choose their care providers. The onus is on the ACO to not only coordinate patients' care, but also to get the patient's buy-in so the patient willingly complies with the ACO's treatment plan. This forces the ACO to not only provide a high level of cost-efficient care, but also to provide a high level of customer service. The patient must be willing to come back and stick with the ACO. CMS incentivizes ACOs by allowing them to share in the savings they produce. On a high level, benchmarks for expected costs under a fee-for-service model are set for patients who are attributed to an ACO. If an ACO beats these benchmarks, the ACO and Medicare split the savings. If the ACO misses the benchmark, the ACO shares the risk to varying degrees, depending on the ACO arrangement. The ACO model maintains the fee-for-service model of care but inserts incentives for improved outcomes and cost-efficient practice patterns.

The feared downside of the ACO is the forced consolidation of medical groups and hospitals. As hospitals merge and buy up medical practices, they can demand more in payments and can funnel more care into higher revenue settings. This is especially true in areas with only one dominant provider group. Rural regions seem especially at risk, but examples have been seen in large urban areas as well. Even in situations when the ACO payment model limits Medicare's liability from this risk, other payers without the size and clout of Medicare are certainly at risk of price inflation due to consolidation (Gold, 2013).

Unlike its beginnings, when Medicare was specifically designed to not use its size and muscle to transform care, the ACA, and specifically the ACO payment model, allows CMS to lead and transform care delivery. Throughout Medicare's history, it has been reluctant to encroach on the providers' domain and thus has been too often a mere payer and not an innovator. There have been exceptions, such as DRGs in 1980s, but these have been few compared to instances when Medicare specifically chose not to interfere. For example, Medicare does not negotiate prescription prices. Under the ACA, CMS has become the 800-pound gorilla, using its weight to force providers to move away from a lucrative fee-for-service payment model. Variants of ACOs have begun emerging from large private insurers in a direct response to Medicare. For example, by 2014, Cigna's goal was to have 100 ACOs up and running (Cigna, 2013). The ultimate success of the ACA, especially with promised near-universal coverage, will depend on the ability to moderate healthcare costs both for Medicare and for other payers. The payment reform models being tested in Medicare are the most promising opportunities today to both manage costs and improve care.

Conclusion

Medicare rose out of the national health insurance movement and provides universal care for people aged 65 years and older and people with long-term disabilities. It has morphed from being the largest payer of healthcare services at its enactment in 1965 and a crucial pillar of the U.S. safety net to an industry innovator. Medicare, from day one,

has lifted millions of seniors out of poverty and provided some level of financial protection to seniors and their children. Today, Medicare is acting more as an innovator of payment reform under the ACA. The success of CMS in changing incentives, driving quality improvements, and managing costs will be one of the most significant factors in the success of the ACA and, in a larger context, in the success of managing the federal deficit and maintaining the economy as a whole. Health care absorbs 18% of the gross domestic product, and before 2010, this percentage was expected to increase, further threatening the growth of other economic sectors. To the extent that CMS, as the largest purchaser of healthcare services, can reform the healthcare delivery system through payment incentives, the long-term economy will either expand or stagnate. Further, as Medicare enrollments increase, its long-term solvency, without other major reform, is dependent on improved cost trends. Medicare holds an important role of protector and financial support to millions of senior Americans, and, as the largest healthcare payer at the center of the U.S. healthcare delivery system, it may do much to determine our economic future and our ability to live up to the finest ideals our nation has always inspired.

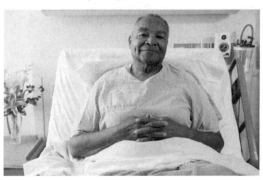

© Monkey Business/Thinkstock

Discussion Questions

1. Describe the four parts of Medicare as they are today—who is eligible, what is covered, and what coverage gaps remain.
2. Trace the history of Medicare and highlight times when Medicare took an assertive role in healthcare transformation and times when it purposefully avoided such a role.
3. What are Medicare's biggest challenges today? How is Medicare tackling these challenges, and which vulnerabilities remain insufficiently addressed?
4. Even though many envisioned the enactment of Medicare as a stepping stone to universal health care, why did it take 45 years for the enactment of the ACA?
5. What does it say about U.S. politics that the ACA—despite Medicare beneficiaries' positive views of Medicare and its success in protecting a costly and vulnerable population—did not extend Medicare as a mechanism to obtain universal coverage?

References

Bhatia, A., Blackstock, S., Nelson, R., Ng, T. (2000). Evolution of quality review programs for Medicare: Quality assurance to quality improvement. *Health Care Financing Review*, *22*(1), 69–74.

Brown, L. (1996). *The politics of Medicare and health reform, then and now.* Retrieved from http://ftp.ssa.gov/history/pdf/PoliticsMedicareReform.pdf

Centers for Medicare and Medicaid Services. (2013). *Hospital compare.* Retrieved from http://www.medicare.gov/hospitalcompare/search.html

Cigna. (2013). *Accountable Care Organizations (ACO).* Retrieved from http://newsroom.cigna.com/KnowledgeCenter/ACO/

Congressional Budget Office. (2013). *CBO's February 2013 Medicare baseline.* Retrieved from http://www.cbo.gov/sites/default/files/cbofiles/attachments/43894_Medicare2.pdf

Cutler, D. (1999). *The anatomy of health insurance.* Retrieved from http://www.nber.org/papers/w7176.pdf

Davis, C. K. (1988). The impact of DRG's on the cost and quality of health care in the United States. *Health Policy, 9*, 117–131.

Gold, J. (2013). *FAQ on ACO's: Accountable Care Organizations, explained.* Retrieved from http://www.kaiserhealthnews.org/stories/2011/january/13/aco-accountable-care-organization-faq.aspx

Gottlober, P. (2001). *Medicare hospital prospective payment system: How DRG rates are calculated and updated.* Retrieved from http://oig.hhs.gov/oei/reports/oei-09-00-00200.pdf

Health Care Financing Administration. (2000). *Medicare 2000: 35 years of improving American's health and security.* Retrieved from http://www.cms.gov/Research-Statistics-Data-and-Systems/Statistics-Trends-and-Reports/TheChartSeries/downloads/35chartbk.pdf

Johnson, L. B. (1965). Public Papers of the Presidents of the United States (Vol. 11, entry 394, pp. 811-815). Washington, DC: Government Printing Office.

Kaiser Family Foundation. (2010). *Medicare: A primer.* Retrieved from http://kaiserfamilyfoundation.files.wordpress.com/2013/01/7615-03.pdf

Kaiser Family Foundation. (2011). *Focus on health reform.* Retrieved from http://kaiserfamilyfoundation.files.wordpress.com/2011/04/8061-021.pdf

Kaiser Family Foundation. (2012a). *Medicare Advantage fact sheet.* Retrieved from http://kff .org/medicare/fact-sheet /medicare-advantage-fact-sheet/

Kaiser Family Foundation. (2012b). *Medicare at a glance.* Retrieved from http://kff.org/medicare /fact-sheet/medicare-at-a-glance-fact-sheet/

Kaiser Family Foundation. (2012c). *The story of Medicare: A timeline.* Retrieved from http://kff .org/medicare/video /the-story-of-medicare-a-timeline/

Landon, B. (2012). *Analysis of Medicare Advantage HMOs compared with traditional Medicare shows lower use of many services during 2003–09.* Retrieved from http://content.healthaffairs .org/content/31/12/2609.abstract

McWilliams, M. (2012). *New risk-adjustment system was associated with reduced favorable selection in Medicare Advantage.* Retrieved from http:// content.healthaffairs.org/content/31/12/2630. abstract

Moon, M. (1996). *What Medicare has meant to older Americans.* Retrieved from http://ssa.gov /history/pdf/WhatMedicareMeant.pdf

National Academy of Social Insurance. (2001). *Reflections on implementing Medicare.* Retrieved from http://www.nasi.org/usr_doc /med_report_reflections.pdf

New York Times/CBS News Poll: 2012 Republicans, Obama and the Economy. (2011, April 21). *The New York Times.* Retrieved from http://www .nytimes.com/interactive/2011/04/22/us /politics/20110422-poll-republicans-economy .html?_r=0

Oliver, T., Lee, P., Lipton, H. (2004). *A political history of Medicare and prescription drug coverage.* Retrieved from http://amcp.org /WorkArea/DownloadAsset.aspx?id=11196

O'Sullivan, J, Franco, C., Fuchs, B., Lyke, B., Price, R., & Swendiman, K. (1997). *Medicare provisions in the Balanced Budget Act of 1997.* Retrieved from http://greenbook.waysandmeans.house .gov/sites/greenbook.waysandmeans.house .gov/files/2011/images/l97-802_gb.pdf

Quadagno, J. (2000). Promoting civil rights through the welfare state: How Medicare integrated southern hospitals. *Social Problems, 47*(1), 68–89. Retrieved from http://www.jstor.org /discover/10.2307/3097152?uid=2&uid=4& sid=21102697047173

Reagan, R. (1987). *Text of statements by Reagan and White House.* Retrieved from http: //www.nytimes.com/1987/02/13/us/text-of- statements-by-reagan-and-white-house .html?pagewanted=2&src=pm

Rice, T., Desmond, K., & Gabel, J. (1990). *The Medicare Catastrophic Coverage Act: A post-mortem.* Retrieved from http://content .healthaffairs.org/content/9/3/75.full.pdf

Roy, A. (2011). *Why the American Medical Association had 72 million reasons to shrink doctor's pay.* Retrieved from http://www.forbes.com /sites/theapothecary/2011/11/28/why-the- american-medical-association-had-72-million- reasons-to-help-shrink-doctors-pay/

Starr, P. (1982). *The social transformation of American medicine: The rise of sovereign profession and the making of a vast industry.* New York, NY: Basic Books.

Zaraboza, C. (2000). Milestones in Medicare managed care. *Health Care Financing Review, 22*(1), 61–67.

CHAPTER 15

Medicaid and the Financing of Care for Vulnerable Populations: A Story of Misconceptions

Barbara Caress and Nancy Aries*

Overview

Unlike any other country in the world, access to health care in the United States is based on social attributes such as employment, disability, age, and parentage. This has resulted in tremendous inequities in health insurance enrollment and the level of benefits received. Medicare was a breakthrough in terms of opening eligibility to all elderly persons. At the time, it was assumed that Medicare would be the first step to universal coverage, but this has not happened. Instead there is Medicaid, Medicare's poor cousin. The federal government sets a loose set of parameters regarding services and eligibility and matches the states' payments for services. Although many people think Medicaid covers all poor and vulnerable people, because the population is categorized by social characteristics and states have the option to determine income cutoffs for eligibility, that is not true. Many persons living in poverty are not eligible for services. However, Medicaid is the major source of support for elderly persons and those with disabilities because it covers services such as long-term care, including nursing homes and home health care that are not covered by Medicare. As passed, the Affordable Care Act (ACA) would have created a more seamless system of financing for the poor, but the Supreme Court decision in 2012 allowed states to choose

*The authors want to thank Cathy Schoen, Senior Vice President for Policy, Research, and Evaluation at the Commonwealth Fund, who generously gave her time to explain her understanding of the causes and impacts resulting from disparities in access and cost of care for vulnerable populations.

whether or not to participate. Only 27 states are participating in the Medicaid expansion, and Vermont is the only state to take full advantage of the law. Vermont will provide universal coverage starting in 2017. The experience of Vermont demonstrates that patients and the persons who work in healthcare settings can have access to and receive the care they deserve.

Objectives

- Consider why access to health care is more limited in the United States than other industrialized nations.
- Explain how Medicaid can be a safety net but not cover all persons who live in poverty.
- Analyze the critical role Medicaid plays in supporting long-term care for the elderly and disabled.
- Describe why Medicaid is actually 50 different state programs.
- Assess how the Supreme Court's decision related to the ACA will slow progress toward eliminating a two-class system of care.

Introduction

Unlike other countries, America has created a healthcare system in which access to care is based on social criteria. There is private insurance for many productive members of society, although a declining percentage of the workforce receives employer-based health insurance benefits (State Health Access Data Assistance Center, 2013). The elderly receive health insurance through the government-sponsored Medicare program. Having worked throughout their lifetimes, they are viewed as deserving of benefits to which they contributed while employed. The government also pays for the most vulnerable, low-income populations who had been eligible for income support. Historically this has included children, their parents, the disabled, and the elderly.

The different modes of access to health care, however, do not ensure that every American has access to health insurance and health services. There are still large groups in the population who are left out because they are uninsured or underinsured (Kaiser Commission on Medicaid and the Uninsured, 2013b). They are unemployed people who do not have small children. They are families who make slightly more than the cutoffs for Medicaid but not enough to pay for private insurance. They are working persons whose employers do not provide health insurance, or whose employers do provide health insurance but the coverage is not adequate to pay for expensive medical procedures. They are the population that the ACA was intended to reach.

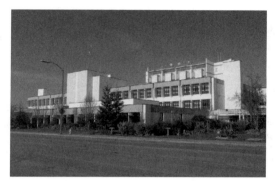

© Hank Shiffman/ShutterStock, Inc.

Gaps in coverage meant that a series of programs were developed to ensure that there was some minimal floor of health care for all persons. The public hospital system is a case in point. Most large cities have at least one large public hospital that cares for the poor (Starr, 1982). In the 1960s, a large number of community health centers were built in low-income rural areas, and then in urban communities, to serve persons who had no other access to care (Sardell, 1988). Public health departments organize clinics for persons with communicable diseases, such as AIDS, and other programs for special populations and services, such as school-based care or family planning (Rosenbaum, 2011).

The patchwork ways in which access to health care has been defined created a tremendous variety of programs and disparities related to access and quality of care, none of which is well understood. People with excellent health insurance and limited out-of-pocket obligations can generally get care from a wide range of providers who participate in their network. However, Medicaid recipients in many states have access to an extremely small list of providers because low reimbursement rates result in their nonparticipation. And uninsured people have only as much

access as they can afford to pay out-of-pocket. Where people live also matters in terms of their health outcomes. Academic medical centers tend to be located in urban areas and make it easier for persons needing complex care to access these services than persons who live several hours away (Schwamm, 2014). These differences are further aggravated by differences among states. Although disparities exist between rich and poor, white and black, educated and noneducated, urban and rural, it is also true that a low-income person in a top-performing state on the Commonwealth Fund scorecard may fare better than advantaged populations in low-performing states (Schoen, Radley et al., 2013).

This chapter will examine how care is financed for vulnerable populations and the consequences of these organizational choices. The chapter begins with a comparison of the United States with other developed nations. Such a comparison is critical to understanding how the choice to determine access based on social criteria leads to worse health outcomes. Next, the chapter will review the Medicaid program because it is the primary source of care for low-income populations. It will consider the populations served by Medicaid, the high costs of Medicaid, and the significance of Medicaid being a federally mandated and state-implemented program. This means there is no one Medicaid program; rather, there are 50 different programs with 50 sets of outcomes. Medicaid, however, is not all inclusive in terms of access to health care for poor and vulnerable populations, so the chapter will consider other care options available to these populations. The discussion would not be complete without an examination of the ACA and its potential to eliminate the health status disparities among the populations being served.

Health Outcomes in the United States in Relation to 10 Developed Nations

Most Americans assume that the United States has the best healthcare system in the world. This is true for many persons, but it is also true that millions of Americans receive subpar care. To understand the variance that exists in the United States, a good place to begin is by examining the United States in comparison with other developed nations. While there are many differences among these healthcare systems, the fact that the United States is the only nation to define access to care based on social classifications impacts both access to and affordability of care. A study of health system performance thus becomes a way to demonstrate the extent to which different modes of access have resulted in disparate outcomes.

Every year, the Commonwealth Fund conducts an annual survey of 11 developed nations concerning access to and affordability of care (Schoen, Osborn, Squires, & Doty, 2013). Table 15-1 highlights some findings from the 2013 survey. First to consider is the percentage of adults who did not see a doctor when they were sick or did not get recommended care because of cost. In the United Kingdom, only 4% of respondents reported not seeing a doctor because of cost, whereas 32% of respondents in the United States reported not seeing a doctor. The U.S. percentage is further broken down between insured and uninsured respondents, a categorization that is not necessary for other countries. For uninsured persons in the United States, 58% reported not seeing a doctor. The next closest response was 20% each in the Netherlands and New Zealand, which is approximately the same response as that of insured persons in the United States.

The second indicator to consider is out-of-pocket spending. In Sweden, only 2% reported having spent more than $1,000 out of pocket. Of the other nine developed nations being compared with the United States, the highest percentage of persons who reported out-of-pocket expenses in excess of $1,000 was persons in Australia, with 25%. In the United States, 41% of respondents spent more than $1,000 out of pocket. Interestingly, this percentage does not vary greatly between the insured (42%) and the uninsured (39%). All Americans are confronted with high out-of-pocket expenses. This can be attributed to the fact that the United States is the least regulated country in terms of limiting out-of-pocket spending.

Fewer respondents from the United States reported seeing a doctor or nurse when they needed care on the same day compared with other developed countries. Seventy-six percent of Germans reported same-day care. This was comparable with insured people in the United States, where 73% received same-day care. However, only 35% of uninsured Americans reported receiving same-day care. Inversely, it is possible to consider the percentage of people who waited 6 or more days. In this case, 40% of uninsured people reported delays in care of 6 or more days, but only 5% of persons in New Zealand reported such delays.

The last point to consider is per capita spending on health insurance. The United States has the most complex system of care, which is evident in the per capita spending on the administration of health insurance. The cost in the 10 comparison nations ranged from a low of $35 per person in Norway to a high of $277 per person in France. In the United States, $606 was spent per person. This is more than twice as much as France, the next highest country.

Table 15-1   Adult Access and Affordability of Care in the United States and 10 Other Countries

	Percentage of adults who:				
Nation	Did not see a doctor when sick or did not get recommended care because of cost	Had $1,000 or more in out-of-pocket medical spending	Saw a doctor or nurse the last time they needed care — Same day or next day	Waited 6 days or more	Per capita spending on health insurance administration, 2011
Australia	14	25	58	14	$70
Canada	8	14	41	33	$148
France	14	7	57	16	$277
Germany	10	11	76	15	$237
Netherlands	20	7	63	14	$199
New Zealand	20	9	72	5	$128
Norway	8	17	52	28	$35
Sweden	4	2	58	22	$55
Switzerland	10	24	Not obtained	Not obtained	$266
United Kingdom	4	3	52	16	Not available
United States	32	41	48	26	$606
Insured all year	21	42	73	21	Not available
Uninsured	58	39	36	40	Not available

Source: Data from Schoen, C., Osborn, R. Squires, D., & Doty, M. (2013a). Access, affordability, and insurance complexity are often worse in the United States compared to ten other countries. Health Affairs. 32;12, 1–11.

The importance of considering the United States in the context of other developed nations is to demonstrate the variance that exists and to suggest that the differences can be attributed in part to the complexity of the healthcare system in the United States and the limited access of persons to care due to the distribution of health insurance based on social characteristics such as employment, income, disability, and family relations.

Populations Served by Medicaid

Medicaid is the primary safety net insurer of low-income persons younger than age 65 years who have no other access to care. The common assumption is that Medicaid is a program for poor children and their parents. Their need for services is distorted by the rhetorical claims that the program is dominated by persons who are abusing the intentions of the program to serve women and children who are truly in need. Sadly, this misperception causes an incorrect depiction of the Medicaid program. The reality is that Medicaid overwhelmingly serves disabled and elderly populations.

Health spending for elderly persons is rarely associated with Medicaid because it is mistakenly assumed that their healthcare services are paid solely by Medicare. Medicare payments, however, stop at the door of acute care recovery. Thus, the long-term care services needed by low-income elderly are paid by Medicaid. The reasons go back to the original alignment of Medicaid in the 1960s with welfare programs. While medicine and Medicare were limited to the treatment of diseases that could be impacted by the intervention of healthcare providers, Medicaid was understood to be part of the social welfare system that covered a range of services that fall at the intersection of medical care and social services, including nursing homes, intermediate care facilities, mental health facilities, and home health and personal care (Rosenbaum, 2009). When cash support provided by Social Security was not adequate to cover these services, they were classified as a health-related service and thus fell under the eligibility guidelines for Medicaid (Brown & Sparer, 2003).

Nonelderly disabled persons are also an invisible Medicaid population (Vladeck, 2003). This is a heterogeneous group that has traditionally been served by other state agencies but whose care is increasingly paid for by Medicaid. Included in this group are physically disabled children and adults, developmentally disabled adults, the mentally ill,

and persons with AIDS and substance abuse problems.

Eligibility rules have changed over time to extend services to larger groups of low-income persons, but the basic structure of the program remains the same. Children are generally people aged 18 years and younger. During the past 2 decades, eligibility for this group has been expanded to families with incomes less than 133% of the federal poverty level. Adults are categorized as persons aged 19–64 years. This group has also been extended beyond mothers who receive welfare benefits to include parents of eligible children younger than age 18 years, pregnant women, and a small number of people who are eligible through the Breast and Cervical Cancer Prevention and Treatment Act of 2000. The original categorization of the aged, blind, and disabled is now broken into two groups: persons aged 65 years and older and disabled persons, and persons younger than age 65 years who have physical, mental, or emotional conditions that prevent them from performing the activities of daily living.

When comparing the percentage of Medicaid enrollees by enrollment group, Medicaid can be understood as a program for poor children and women because they comprise more than three-quarters of all Medicaid recipients. Forty-nine percent of enrollees are children, and 27% are adults. Less than 10% of enrollees are elderly, and only 15% are disabled. Medicaid payments by enrollment group give a much clearer understanding of the program's scope because the percentage of payment is not correlated with the percentage of enrollment. Children comprise 49% of enrollments but only 21%

Table 15-2 Medicaid Enrollment and Distribution of Payment by Enrollment Group, Fiscal Year 2010

	Distribution of Medicaid enrollees by enrollment group	Distribution of Medicaid payments by enrollment group
Aged	9%	22%
Disabled	15%	42%
Adult	27%	15%
Children	49%	21%
Total	100%	100%
	Enrollees = 66,390,542	Expenditures = $81,507,921,594

Source: Data from Kaiser Family Foundation (2014).

of spending. Health care for children is not a costly endeavor. For the most part, children are healthy. Even adults account for a smaller percentage of spending than enrollment. Looking at Table 15-2, it is obvious that the preponderance of Medicaid expenditures are for services to the disabled and elderly. Spending on the disabled is nearly three times greater than the percentage of disabled people who are enrolled in Medicaid. Disabled individuals account for 15% of enrollees and 42% of Medicaid spending. Spending on the elderly is nearly 2.5 times greater than the percentage of elderly on Medicaid. The elderly account for 9% of all enrollees and 22% of spending. Taken together, the disabled and elderly are less than a quarter of enrollees but incur almost three quarters of program spending.

Medicaid Is 50 Different State Programs

Another common misconception about Medicaid is that knowing how it works in one state can be generalized to the other 49 states and the District of Columbia. This could not be further from the truth. Medicaid, like Medicare, was enacted in 1965 during Lyndon Johnson's presidency. Medicare is a federally mandated and operated program of health insurance for the elderly, but Medicaid is a residual program linked to public assistance. It was never meant to cover all poor people. The federal program provided states with general guidance about the populations that would be eligible for services and the range of services that states were either mandated to provide or had the option to provide. The implementation of these guidelines was to be determined by the states. It was assumed that states were in the best position to identify exactly who should receive care, what services would be included in the benefits package, and payment rates for services. During the past half century, Medicaid has evolved into 50 different programs in terms of the populations served, the services provided, and provider payments. Although more than 60 million Americans received Medicaid prior to implementation of the ACA, only by looking at the evolution of state programs can the vast need for health care of low-income persons be understood.

Medicaid eligibility is determined in two ways. Broadly, it covers three distinct populations: elderly, disabled people who receive federally assisted income maintenance through Supplemental Security Income (SSI), and low-income families and children who meet the 1996 eligibility requirements for Aid to Families with Dependent Children (AFDC). Medicaid also covers some related groups that do not receive cash assistance but whose income puts them close to the poverty level. These groups include children, pregnant women, certain Medicare beneficiaries, and recipients of adoption and foster care services. Such broad eligibility criteria initially resulted in relatively standard eligibility guidelines across states. When Medicaid was first passed, states covered most eligible persons at income cutoffs close to the poverty line. Over the past 50 years, the income cutoffs have dropped to very low levels in many states. When Temporary Assistance to Needy Families replaced AFDC in 1996, Congress required states to implement a new Medicaid eligibility category for low-income families and set the minimum income standard at the same level as had been in effect in state welfare programs. In most states, the income level is so low that many parents who work at low-paying jobs that do not provide health insurance cannot qualify for Medicaid. At the same time, Congress expanded eligibility for low-income children so they would have access to services (Families USA, 2000).

The unequal nature of eligibility for Medicaid is demonstrated in Table 15-3, which shows income eligibility for Medicaid and the Children's Health Insurance Program (CHIP) as a percentage of the federal poverty level in 2013. Federal law requires that children aged 6–18 years be covered at the poverty level, or 100%. However, states have the discretion to extend eligibility to more children. Fourteen states fund children at the poverty level, and two states and the District of Columbia set income eligibility for children at 300% of the poverty level. The remaining 36 states fall somewhere in between. The eligibility levels for working parents are more stark. Five states (Arkansas, Alabama, Indiana, Louisiana, and Texas) set eligibility at or below 25% of the federal poverty level. The federal poverty level for a household of three in 2014 is $19,790 (Families USA, 2014). Twenty-five percent of the federal poverty level for a family is $4,948. This means that practically no low-income working parents are eligible for Medicaid in these five states. Sixteen states set the income eligibility below 50% of the federal poverty level. Twenty-eight states set the income eligibility below 75% of the federal poverty level, and 33 states set the income eligibility below 100% of the federal poverty level. Only 18 states set the eligibility cutoffs at or above the federal poverty level, with Minnesota setting the cutoff at 215% of the poverty level. The tremendous variation among states regarding income eligibility is inversely related to the number and percentage of working parents who are uninsured by state (Schoen, Radley et al., 2013).

Table 15-3   Income Eligibility for Medicaid/CHIP as a Percentage of Federal Poverty Level, 2013

	Children (aged 6–18 years)	Working parents (aged 18–64 years)		Children (aged 6–18 years)	Working parents (aged 18–64 years)
Alabama	100	23	Montana	133	54
Alaska	175	78	Nebraska	200	58
Arizona	100	106	Nevada	100	84
Arkansas	200	15	New Hampshire	300	47
California	100	106			
Colorado	133	106	New Jersey	133	200
Connecticut	185	191	New Mexico	285	85
Delaware	100	120	New York	133	150
District of Columbia	300	206	North Carolina	100	47
			North Dakota	100	57
Florida	100	56	Ohio	200	96
Georgia	100	48	Oklahoma	185	51
Hawaii	300	133	Oregon	100	39
Idaho	133	37	Pennsylvania	100	58
Illinois	133	139	Rhode Island	250	181
Indiana	150	24	South Carolina	200	89
Iowa	133	70	South Dakota	140	50
Kansas	100	31	Tennessee	100	122
Kentucky	150	57	Texas	100	25
Louisiana	200	24	Utah	100	42
Maine	150	200	Vermont	225	191
Maryland	300	122	Virginia	133	30
Massachusetts	150	133	Washington	200	71
Michigan	150	64	West Virginia	100	31
Minnesota	275	215	Wisconsin	150	200
Mississippi	100	29	Wyoming	100	50
Missouri	150	35			

Source: Data from Schoen, C., Radley, D., Riley, P., Lippa, J., Berenson, J., Dermody, C., & Shih, A. (2013b). Health care in the two Americas. New York: The Commonwealth Fund., Exhibit 27.

Medicaid Costs and Variation by State

Medicaid is also expensive. In fiscal year 2012, it covered over 65 million persons at a cost of $421 billion (Kaiser Commission on Medicaid and the Uninsured, 2013a). The costs of Medicaid are covered by federal, state, and local governments. The federal share is based on average per capita income for each state relative to the national average. It ranges from 50% in 14 states (including New York, California, and North Dakota) to more than 70% in 10 states and the District of Columbia (including Mississippi, West Virginia, and Kentucky) (Kaiser Commission on Medicaid and the Uninsured, 2014). As of 2012, the state and local share for all of Medicaid was $183 million (45%) of total spending (Martin, Harman, Whittle, Catlin, & National Health Expenditure Team, 2014). Despite federal support, Medicaid is often the largest part of state budgets and it is countercyclical, meaning Medicaid enrollment expands when the economy contracts, which puts state legislatures under tremendous pressure to make cuts to the Medicaid budget in times of fiscal austerity as they seek to lower taxes and control state spending (Sommers & Epstein, 2011).

The higher costs of Medicaid can be attributed to the elderly and disabled. What few people understand is that Medicaid is the safety net for middle-class persons who go bankrupt in old age due to the costs of long-term care. As a result, Medicaid is a major institutional payer for nursing homes and home care. In 2012, Medicaid accounted for 46% of nursing home and 73% of home health or personal care expenditures (Centers for Medicare and Medicaid Services, 2014). Medicare spending accounts for a smaller portion of these expenditures because its payments are limited to acute care and the recovery of persons from incidents associated with these acute episodes. Medicaid, however, is more inclusive because it pays for the long-term care of persons with chronic conditions. The more inclusive definition of services results from Medicaid historically being part of the social welfare system of this country.

Medicaid expenditures also reflect the ways that the 50 states have chosen to define covered services and payment rates. Even though the federal government pays the majority of costs, spending decisions are made at a local level. States have discretion about what optional services to provide in addition to those mandated by the federal government and how to structure payment rates. Table 15-4 provides data for the five states that pay the least per beneficiary for Medicaid services and the five states that pay the most per beneficiary by enrollment group. There are tremendous variations among payments by the lowest paying states and the highest paying states. The difference is least pronounced for children because they do not use a high volume of expensive healthcare services. California pays $1,567 per child, and Alaska pays $4,666 per child. The larger differentials in payments for services can be found among the elderly and disabled. New Mexico has the lowest payment for the elderly ($5,247), and Alaska pays four times more ($21,286). The differences are slightly greater in terms of payments for the disabled; Alabama pays $7,020 per beneficiary, and Connecticut pays $32,954.

Low payment rates can impact both access to and quality of services. Many physicians do not accept Medicaid patients because the payment is so low (Zuckerman, McFeeters, Cunningham, & Nichols, 2004).

Table 15-4   Average Per Capita Medicaid Payments by Enrollment Group, Fiscal Year 2009

				Five Lowest Spending States				
State	**Children**	**State**	**Adults**	**State**	**Elderly**	**State**	**Disabled**
California	$1,567	California	$1,073	New Mexico	$5,247	Alabama	$7,020
Florida	$1,627	Arkansas	$1,237	Tennessee	$7,484	Georgia	$8,999
Georgia	$1,811	Alabama	$2,035	Florida	$7,917	Mississippi	$9,697
Ohio	$1,838	Iowa	$2,109	Nevada	$8,117	Tennessee	$9,826
Indiana	$1,896	Maine	$2,126	Georgia	$8,183	Kentucky	$10,430
				Five Highest Spending States				
State	**Children**	**State**	**Adults**	**State**	**Elderly**	**State**	**Disabled**
Rhode Island	$3,584	Rhode Island	$4,569	Alaska	$21,286	Washington DC	$23,140
Maine	$3,879	Delaware	$4,578	Wash DC	$22,094	Alaska	$25,793
New Mexico	$3,936	New Jersey	$4,817	New York	$22,494	Minnesota	$26,402
Massachusetts	$4,098	New Mexico	$5,215	Montana	$22,823	New York	$29,881
Alaska	$4,666	Alaska	$5,916	Connecticut	$24,761	Connecticut	$32,954

Source: Data from Snyder, L., Rudowitz, R., Garfield, R., & Gordon, T. (Revised November 2012). Why does Medicaid spending vary across states: A chart book of factors driving state spending. Kaiser Commission on Medicaid and the Uninsured.

In Princeton, New Jersey, almost no physicians take Medicaid patients (Kitchenman, 2014). This means that children who are eligible for Medicaid in that area cannot easily make an appointment with a physician if they need one. Likewise, poor payment rates impact working conditions and the quality of care (Grabowski, Angelelli, & Mor, 2004). Interviews with nursing home aides in Mississippi revealed a situation in which the aides, who are low paid, took it upon themselves to bring food to residents and cover for one another while they took soiled sheets to the laundromat so residents would not lie in their own feces (C. Schoen, personal interview, October 20, 2013). Although it is assumed that these institutions meet a minimum standard of care because they are reimbursed by Medicaid, they do not.

Low payment also results in perverse incentives where program eligibility can overlap. Such is the case for elderly people who are eligible for Medicare and Medicaid due to their financial circumstances. These persons are referred to as dual eligible. Regulators are less concerned with the overall cost of a person's care than with controlling the individual budget for which they are responsible. In the case of dual eligible persons, Medicare prefers that Medicaid pay, and Medicaid prefers that Medicare pay, even though the federal government pays most of both expenditures. For nursing homes, this means that an elderly patient who has been hospitalized is admitted to the nursing home under Medicare, and Medicare is a good payer. When that person becomes a long-term patient, he or she becomes a Medicaid patient. When the same person is hospitalized, some states put a hold on the bed, and Medicaid continues to pay the nursing home for the days that the patient spends in the hospital. When that individual returns to the nursing home, he or she once again becomes a Medicare patient. The incentives are such that nursing homes are not penalized for hospitalizations. In fact, they are paid when a resident is hospitalized, and then they receive the higher reimbursement rate when that same resident is discharged back to their care (C. Schoen, personal interview, October 20, 2013).

Medicaid Is 50 Different Programs with 50 Different Outcomes

The result of Medicaid being 50 different programs is that there can be 50 different outcomes, depending on the state. In fact, the lowest income persons in the highest performing states can have better health outcomes than the national medium and even a number of more advantaged populations in low-performing states (Schoen, Radley,

et al., 2013). This finding comes from a scorecard developed by the Commonwealth Fund that uses income to define vulnerability. It identifies 30 indicators of healthcare system performance that include prevention and treatment, avoidable hospitalizations, and healthy lives. For each indicator, the vulnerable population was compared with a high-income population, then each state's performance was compared with the other 49 states and the District of Columbia.

The surprising result is that for 24 out of 30 indicators, the low-income population fared better than the national average, and for 14 indicators, the low-income population fared better than the advantaged population in lagging states (Schoen, Radley et al., 2013). Several examples of such differences can be found in Table 15-5, which compare the experiences of low-income persons across states and demonstrates how variable this can be. The categories are defined generally, but they have real impacts on individuals' lives. One example is potentially avoidable hospitalizations from respiratory disease. Many nursing home residents are frail and have dementia. Unless the staff is actively involved, pneumonia can easily manifest. Another diagnosis, septicemia, is the second most prevalent among Medicaid recipients. In some nursing homes, 25–30% of the residents are regularly hospitalized for septicemia and bed sores (C. Schoen, personal interview, October 20, 2013). If the nursing homes had offered decent primary care, many, but not all, of these cases could have been avoided. However, as previously described, incentives are not in place to improve care.

Table 15-5   Number of States in Which the Low-Income/Vulnerable Rate Is Better Than the National Average

Indicator	National average Number of states	Advantaged population in lagging states Number of states
Access and affordability		
Percentage of children aged 0–18 who are uninsured	12	10
Prevention and treatment		
Percentage of children with both a medical and dental preventive care visit in the past year	5	0
Percentage of patients hospitalized for heart failure or pneumonia who received recommended care	18	0
Potentially avoidable hospital use		
Hospital admissions for pediatric asthma per 100,000 children	9	11
Potentially avoidable hospitalizations from respiratory disease per 100,000 adults	4	6
Medicare 30-day hospital readmissions as a percentage of admissions	10	23
Healthy lives		
Infant mortality deaths per 1,000 live births	8	8
Percentage of adults who are obese (body mass index ≥ 30)	3	21
Percentage of adults aged 18–64 who have lost six or more teeth because of tooth decay, infection, or gum disease	3	3

Source: Data from Schoen, C., Radley, D., Riley, P., Lippa, J., Berenson, J., Dermody, C., & Shih, A. (2013b). Health care in the two Americas. New York: The Commonwealth Fund., Exhibit 53.

Care Options for the Uninsured

In addition to Medicaid, there are several federal programs that provide health care to vulnerable populations regardless of insurance status. Like insurance, social categories are used to determine eligibility for services. In some cases, services are available to an entire class of citizens, such as veterans. In other cases, services are available to those who live within a catchment area where there is a funded provider, such as a rural health center. Federal support is also given to hospitals to help subsidize the cost of care to the uninsured through programs such as Medicaid's Disproportionate Share Hospital allotment. There is no easy way to classify these programs, which were organized to address the gaps in access. They increase the patchwork of services available to vulnerable populations (Duke Center for Health Policies and Inequalities Research, 2014).

The first group of programs to consider consists of those identified as categorical entitlement programs, meaning that they provide relatively comprehensive health care to specially designated populations, usually in government-sponsored facilities. The three populations whose needs are considered outside the mainstream medical care system and whose rights are protected under the Constitution are veterans, American Indians and Native Alaskans, and prisoners. Health services for veterans are provided by the Department of Veterans Affairs. The Indian Health Service is run by the Department of Health and Human Services. Federal and state officials are obligated by law to provide medical care to inmates who have no other source of care.

In addition to categorical programs, the federal government has made funding available to health centers that serve populations with special needs. The first of these programs, community health centers, were funded as part of the War on Poverty. Over the past 50 years, additional programs were created as new groups were identified as needing services. The second group of programs falls under the heading of primary care programs. They were initially funded in whole or in part by federal grants. Later, these programs began to rely on Medicaid and other third-party revenue

to cover costs. In addition, these programs are typically designated sites where young health professionals can participate in loan forgiveness programs. The ACA allocated an additional $11 billion to support primary care centers, including federally qualified health centers, community health centers, rural health centers, migrant health centers, and healthcare centers for the homeless.

Besides targeting population groups, the federal, state, and local governments also cooperate in providing a fairly wide range of categorical treatment programs targeted at particular health problems or illnesses. The best known are a number of programs related to maternal and child health. These include the federally funded Maternal and Child Health block grant programs, and the Women, Infants, and Children (WIC) program, which is provided through local health departments. In addition, family planning is available through Title X of the Public Health Service Act. State public health departments, with a combination of state and federal dollars, provide dental health services; services for persons with communicable diseases ranging from sexually transmitted diseases to tuberculosis; chronic disease management; developmental and behavioral health; and school health programs.

Last are a number of programs that support institutions providing services to low-income, vulnerable populations. Among these are the Disproportionate Share Hospital payments made by both Medicare and Medicaid to hospitals that serve indigent patients. These funds are heavily concentrated in large urban hospitals and academic medical centers. Another program is the National Health Service Corps, which provides loan repayment programs for primary care practitioners who practice for 2 years in a medically underserved community.

Another example is payments made through the Graduate Medical Education program to teaching hospitals to support interns and residents. As already noted, these hospitals tend to serve a large number of indigent patients, so it becomes another pathway for supporting their care.

The Impact of the ACA

Prior to passage of the ACA, the United States had come a long way in addressing the problems of child health through the State Child Health Insurance Program (SCHIP). This program, which gave states the option as to how it would be organized, set the floor for child eligibility for health insurance at 138% of the poverty level. The ACA gave states the opportunity to further eliminate disparities between high- and low-income populations by expanding public coverage, subsidizing the purchase of private insurance, setting minimum standards for benefits, and regulating such things as out-of-pocket expenses.

The expansion of Medicaid is a linchpin of the ACA. With its passage, Congress changed Medicaid from a 50-state checkerboard of eligibility rules to a single national standard for very-low-income legal residents. Any uninsured adult living in a family with an income less than 138% of the poverty line would be entitled to minimal coverage ($15,415 for an individual and $26,344 for a family of three in 2014). About $1.028 billion was budgeted to be spent over 10 years to enroll 12–17 million new Medicaid and SCHIP recipients. The federal government was directed to fund 100% of the cost of expansion through 2016, and 90% after that. Depending on the state option, newly eligible people may receive the same benefit package as the state's traditional Medicaid program

or a special expansion package, but in no case can the benefits be less than the 10 essential benefits offered on healthcare exchanges to other ACA participants.

The program as described was cut short by a U.S. Supreme Court decision in 2012. Twenty-four states joined a petition filed by Florida challenging the constitutionality of the ACA's Medicaid expansion. If a state wished to continue to receive the traditional federal funding match for its Medicaid program according the ACA, it was required to accept the expansion—funding, eligibility, and benefit design. In a variety of split decisions, the Supreme Court found that the requirement was a coercive overstep of federal authority and declared that linking current funding with future funding was unconstitutional. Rather than the Medicaid expansion being mandatory, the court made it optional. Each state was permitted to decide whether to participate (Jost & Rosenbaum, 2012).

As of April 2014, 27 states (including Washington D.C.) had opted into the Medicaid expansion, the legislatures in 5 states were still deciding, and 19 had declined participation (Kaiser Family Foundation, 2014) (Figure 15-1). Approximately 4.8 million people are caught in a coverage gap. They are deemed too poor to pay any part of a premium for subsidized private coverage, and they are categorically ineligible for help from the state in which they live.

Although the court made expansion a state option, it left in place a number of ACA elements that are designed to have an impact on the way care is provided to both insured and uninsured persons (Grossman, Witgert, & Hess, 2012). Among the most important is new models of integrated care, including Accountable Care Organizations (ACOs), Community

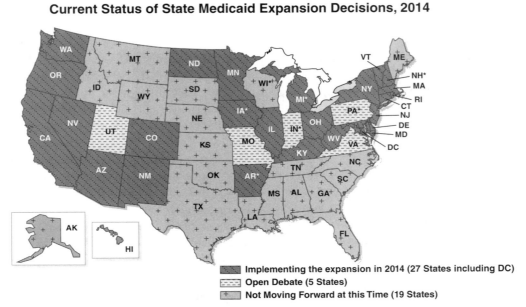

Current Status of State Medicaid Expansion Decisions, 2014

Implementing the expansion in 2014 (27 States including DC)
Open Debate (5 States)
Not Moving Forward at this Time (19 States)

Notes: Data are as of March 26, 2014. *AR and IA have approved waivers for Medicaid expansion. MI has an approved waiver for expansion and plans to implement in Apr. 2014. IN and PA have pending waivers for alternative Medicaid expansions. WI amended its Medicaid state plan and existing waiver to cover adults up to 100% FPL, but did not adopt the expansion. NH has passed legislation approving the Medicaid expansion in Mar, 2014; the legislation calls for the expansion to begin July 2014.
Sources: States implementing in 2014 and not moving forward at this time are based on data from CMS here. States noted as "Open Debate" are based on KCMU analysis of State of the State Addresses, recent public statements made by the Governor, issuance of waiver proposals or passage of a Medicaid expansion bill in at least one chamber of the legislature.

FIGURE 15-1 Current status of state Medicaid expansion decisions, 2014

Data from: The Kaiser Family Foundation, Current Status of Medicaid Expansion Decisions, http://kff.org /health-reform/slide/current-status-of-the-medicaid-expansion-decision/

Care Networks, and nonprofit co-op plans; significantly increased support for community health centers; support for research into and publication of quality standards and report cards; substantial support for workforce training; and greater support for the National Health Service Corps (Riley, Berenson, & Carmody, 2012).

Even if the court had not invalidated the state Medicaid expansion mandate, there would still be millions of people without insurance coverage. The Urban Institute estimated that there would be more than 19 million people in this group, most of whom would be exempt from the ACA mandate because they are undocumented immigrants, very-low-income people who are eligible for Medicaid but are not enrolled, or other low-income people who could not find affordable insurance options (Buettgens & Hall, 2011).

State Alternatives to Medicaid Expansion

Even with passage of the ACA, there will be 50 different options for expanding coverage.

A number of states that rejected Medicaid expansion are experimenting with state-specific alternatives. Among them are Arkansas, Iowa, Michigan, and Pennsylvania, each of which has applied for a funding waiver that would leverage federal Medicaid expansion money for non-Medicaid programs. Arkansas, Iowa, and Pennsylvania have requested funding to permit the state to enroll very poor residents in private health insurance that is offered on their state exchanges. Each state would extend benefits to parents and guardians, and childless adults, in families with incomes below 138% of the federal standard. These four states have asked for permission to impose a variety of Medicaid programs that prohibit cost sharing, but include a small premium ranging from 2% of family income (Michigan) to a flat $35 per month for family coverage (Pennsylvania). In addition, some of the plans include modest doctor visit copays. If the plans are approved by the Centers for Medicare and Medicaid Services, these four customized plans would extend coverage to an estimated 1.4 million people (Garber & Collins, 2014).

The most ambitious ACA-inspired expansion plan is underway in Vermont. Green Mountain Care (H. 202), created by the state legislature in 2011, envisions a Vermont single-payer health insurance benefit funded by a combination of federal ACA subsidies, traditional Medicaid funds, and state taxes. In 2017, if the state receives federal approval, Green Mountain Care would replace traditional insurance plans and Medicaid with a single plan managed by a state-appointed entity that would provide near universal benefits to virtually every resident of the state. The state entity would regulate both benefits and expenses. As

Vermont Governor Shumlin wrote in a Huffington Post blog, "Under the plan, single payer coverage will be a right and not a privilege, and will not be connected to employment . . . This is groundbreaking. But our success in guaranteeing coverage depends on our ability to control health care costs, so our plan is focused squarely on that goal" (Marcy, 2011, para. 4).

How Does the United States Cover Its Most Vulnerable Residents?

Since the very early days, local, state, and federal governments have grappled with ways to provide care for those who cannot afford or cannot access care for themselves. The United States began down the road of universal, one-class care with provisions of the Social Security Act, which not only identified the elderly as a special needs group but also identified a number of other special needs populations, including mothers and children, the disabled, and the blind. Since 1935, the nation has come a long way in creating a floor for all its citizens, but, as is evident from passage of the ACA and its implementation, there is still a long way to go. In his very last speech, at the dedication of a new building for the U.S. Department of Health and Human Services (at the time it was the Department of Health, Education, and Welfare), former vice president and senator Hubert H. Humphrey said, "The moral test of government is how that government treats those who are in the dawn of life, the children; those who are in the twilight of life, the elderly; those who are in the shadows of life; the sick, the needy and the handicapped." Those words are now inscribed in the portal of the building as a reminder to each of us about what a society owes its citizens.

Discussion Questions

1. What does it mean to say Medicaid is 50 different programs?
2. In what ways do financing mechanisms for the care of vulnerable populations contribute to a two-class care system?
3. How will the ACA help eliminate some of the variation that currently exists among states in terms of the access, quality, and cost of care?
4. Which group or groups of people still have inadequate insurance coverage?

References

Brown, L. D., & Sparer, M. S. (2003). Poor program's progress: The unanticipated politics of Medicaid policy. *Health Affairs, 22*(1), 31–44.

Buettgens, M., & Hall, M. A. (2011). *Who will be uninsured after health care reform?* Retrieved from http://www.urban.org /uploadedpdf/1001520-Uninsured-After-Health-Insurance-Reform.pdf

Centers for Medicare and Medicaid Services. (2014). *National health expenditures by type of service and source of funds, CY 1960–2012.* Retrieved from http://www.cms.gov/Research-Statistics-Data-and-Systems/Statistics-Trends-and-Reports/NationalHealthExpendData /NationalHealthAccountsHistorical.html

Duke Center for Health Policies and Inequalities Research. (2014). *U.S. health policy gateway.* Retrieved from http://ushealthpolicygateway. com/vi-key-health-policy-issues-financing-and-delivery/h-public-medical-programs/

Families USA. (2000). *Go directly to work, do not collect health insurance: Low-income parents lose Medicaid.* Washington, DC: Families USA Publication.

Families USA. (2014). *Federal poverty guidelines.* Retrieved from http://familiesusa.org/product /federal-poverty-guidelines

Garber, T., & Collins, S. R. (2014). *The Affordable Care Act's Medicaid expansion: Alternative state approaches.* Retrieved from http: //www.commonwealthfund.org/Blog/2014 /Mar/Medicaid-Expansion-Alternative-State-Approaches.aspx

Grabowski, D. C., Angelelli, J. J., & Mor, V. (2004). Medicaid payment and risk-adjusted nursing home quality measures. *Health Affairs, 23*(5), 243–252. Retrieved from http://content. healthaffairs.org/content/23/5/243.full

Grossman, L., Witgert, K., & Hess, C. (2012). *Toward meeting the needs of vulnerable populations: Issues for policymakers' consideration in integrating a safety net into health care reform implementation.* Retrieved from http://www .nashp.org/sites/default/files/safety.net_.hcr_ .pdf

Jost, T. S., & Rosenbaum, S. (2012). The Supreme Court and the future of Medicaid. *New England Journal of Medicine, 367*, 983–985. Retrieved from http://www.nejm.org/doi/full/10.1056 /NEJMp1208219

Kaiser Commission on Medicaid and the Uninsured. (2013a). *Issue brief: Medicaid enrollment, 2012 data snap shot.* Retrieved from http://kaiserfamily-foundation.files.wordpress.com/2013/08/8050-06-medicaid-enrollment.pdf

Kaiser Commission on Medicaid and the Uninsured. (2013b). *The uninsured: A primer: Key facts about insurance on the eve of health reform.* Retrieved from http: //kaiserfamilyfoundation.files.wordpress .com/2013/10/7451-09-the-uninsured-a-primer-key-facts-about-health-insurance.pdf

Kaiser Commission on Medicaid and the Uninsured. (2014). *Federal and state share of Medicaid spending: Timeframe 2012.* Retrieved from http://kff.org/medicaid/state-indicator/federalstate-share-of-spending/

Kaiser Family Foundation. (2014). *Distribution of Medicaid payments by enrollment group, FY2010.* Retrieved from http://kff.org/medicaid/state-indicator/payments-by-enrollment-group/

Kitchenman, A. (2014). Profile: *Princeton economist makes national mark with insights on health care.* Retrieved from http://www.njspotlight.com/stories/14/04/19/profile-princeton-economist-makes-national-mark-with-insights-on-health-care-issues/

Marcy, J. (2011). *Vermont edges towards single payer health care.* Retrieved from http://www.kaiserhealthnews.org/stories/2011/october/02/vermont-single-payer-health-care.aspx

Martin, A. B., Harman, M., Whittle, L., Catlin, A., & National Health Expenditure Team. (2014). National health spending in 2012: Rate of health spending growth remained low for the fourth consecutive year. *Health Affairs, 33*(1), 67–77.

Riley, P., Berenson, J., & Carmody, C. (2012). *How the Affordable Care Act supports a high-performance safety net.* Retrieved from http://www.commonwealthfund.org/Blog/2012/Jan/Affordable-Care-Act-Safety-Net.aspx

Rosenbaum, S. (2009). Medicaid and national health reform. *New England Journal of Medicine, 361*, 2009–2012. Retrieved from http://www.nejm.org/doi/pdf/10.1056/NEJMp0909449

Rosenbaum, S. (2011). Medicaid and access to health care—a proposal for continued inaction? *New England Journal of Medicine, 365*, 102–104. Retrieved from http://www.nejm.org/search?q=title%3AMedicaid&date=past10Years#qs=%3Fq%3Dtitle%253AMedicaid%26date%3Dpast10Years%26page%3D2

Sardell, A. (1988). *The U.S. experiment in social medicine: The community health center program,* 1965–1986. Pittsburgh, PA: University of Pittsburgh Press.

Schoen, C., Osborn, R., Squires, D., & Doty, M. (2013). Access, affordability, and insurance complexity are often worse in the United States compared to ten other countries. *Health Affairs, 32*(12), 1–11.

Schoen, C., Radley, D., Riley, P., Lippa, J., Berenson, J., Dermody, C., & Shih, A. (2013). *Health care in the two Americas.* New York, NY: The Commonwealth Fund.

Schwamm, L. H. (2014). Telehealth: Seven strategies to successfully implement disruptive technology and transform health care. *Health Affairs, 33*(2), 200–206.

Snyder, L., Rudowitz, R., Garfield, R., & Gordon, T. (2012). *Why does Medicaid spending vary across states: A chart book of factors driving state spending.* Retrieved from http://kaiserfamilyfoundation.files.wordpress.com/2013/01/8378.pdf

Sommers, B. D., & Epstein, A. M. (2011). Why states are so miffed about Medicaid—economics, politics, and the "woodwork effect." *New England Journal of Medicine, 363*, 2085–2087. Retrieved from http://www.nejm.org/doi/pdf/10.1056/NEJMp1104948

Starr, P. (1982). *The social transformation of American medicine.* New York, NY: Basic Books.

State Health Access Data Assistance Center. (2013). *State-level trends in employer-sponsored health insurance.* Retrieved from http://www.rwjf.org/content/dam/farm/reports/reports/2013/rwjf405434

Vladeck, B. (2003). Where the action really is: Medicaid and the disabled. *Health Affairs, 22*(1), 252–258.

Zuckerman, S., McFeeters, J., Cunningham, P., & Nichols, L. (2004). Changes in Medicaid physician fees, 1998–2003: Implications for physician participation. *Health Affairs, W4*, 374–384. Retrieved from http://content.healthaffairs.org/content/early/2004/06/23/hlthaff.w4.374.full.pdf+html?sid=570a9424-22cb-4a02-98bb-5cdd10682f02

Index